On Your Own Terms

The Seniors' Guide to an Independent Life

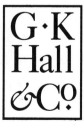

G·K Hall &Co

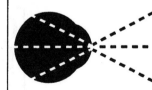

This Large Print Book carries the
Seal of Approval of N.A.V.H.

On Your Own Terms

The Seniors' Guide to an Independent Life

Linda D. Cirino

G.K. Hall & Co.
Thorndike, Maine

Published in 1996 by arrangement with William Morrow & Co., Inc.

This book is intended to offer choices for a broad range of readers and neither the writer nor the publisher pretends to be offering a solution to any individual's medical problems. Likewise, we do not mean to prescribe panaceas for avoiding illness. The information in this book is not intended to substitute for the advice and services of a trained health professional. All matters regarding your health require medical consultation and supervision. Your individual needs require consultation with a qualified professional on issues specific to your care to assure that your unique situation has been evaluated and so that the choices of care or treatment are appropriate for you, the reader. Mention of products in this book is not intended as endorsement or recommendations since we include a wide range of items that may not be suitable for every reader.

G.K. Hall Large Print Reference Collection.

The text of this Large Print edition is unabridged.
Other aspects of the book may vary from the original edition.

Set in 16 pt. News Plantin by Juanita Macdonald.

Printed in the United States on permanent paper.

Library of Congress Cataloging in Publication Data

Cirino, Linda D.
    On your own terms : the seniors' guide to an independent life / Linda D. Cirino.
    Large print ed.
        p.   cm.
    Includes index.
    ISBN 0-7838-1594-8 (lg. print : hc)
    1. Aged — United States — Life skills guides. 2. Aged — United States — Services for. I. Title.
[HQ1064.U5C47   1996]
646.7'9—dc20   95-39388

For my parents,
Sylvia Hyman Davis and Harold Davis,
my source of strength, high standards, and good examples

with love

Preface

It has taken me some time to realize that the apparent paradox that everyone needs a little help to live independently is actually a truism. In my own family we struggle against a penchant for stubbornness, stoicism, and silent suffering that makes asking for help difficult. With a book like this one, however, you can decide what you need and find out for yourself what suits your situation. My hope is that the ideas and resources collected here can provide you with options that will make your life less complicated and more comfortable and will enhance your ability to live on your own terms.

Acknowledgments

This book has been shaped by the intelligence and attention of a small group of professionals. A friend, Marion Komar, broached the topic to me after looking for such a book in vain. The idea was refined and packaged by Nancy Yost, an agent whose ongoing involvement with the project was a source of encouragement to me. Toni Sciarra edited the book, keeping the reader's needs in the forefront and with an unfailing instinct for achieving a clear, rational narrative. Editorial guidance from Deborah Jurkowitz at a crucial stage gave an organizational lift to the book and helped improve its accessibility. These professionals combined to help me produce a book we all hoped would fill a need for many readers.

Naturally the people who assisted me in assembling the resources that are the heart of the book — sending me material, answering questions, explaining how they work — were all important to presenting accurate information. Their names, organizations, products, and other information are found in the listings in the "Resources" sections.

While there is a certain amount of isolation inherent in writing, I am fortunate and grateful to have the companionship, advice, and support of my husband, Antonio Cirino.

Contents

PART TWO

PART THREE

PART FOUR

What Makes an Independent Life

Everyone's idea of independence is unique, but few would disagree about its importance. While what I need to live independently may be different from your needs, we both derive a sense of self-esteem by knowing we are in charge of our lives. An independent life is one in which you have control over what you do, and you decide how, when, and where to do it. People for whom such a life is important share certain traits:

- The *motivation* to take action
- Concern for *a healthy diet*
- A way of life that includes some *physical activity*
- Awareness of the elements of *a safe environment*
- An *alert mind*
- The foresight to consider *a planned future*

We have divided *On Your Own Terms* into parts that coincide with each of these distinguishing qualities.

PART ONE: "An Independent Spirit"

This abstract trait may be the most universally important for an independent life. All the gadgets, well-intentioned plans, and clever solutions are useless without the spark of gumption you need to adopt them. Nurture the part of you that wants to take initiatives, that has faith that we can affect our destiny, and that has a basic hope in a better future.

PART TWO: "Designing Your Diet"

Despite controversies among nutritionists and medical researchers we need a sane approach to selecting our food. Our goal is to stay healthy, strong, and competent.

PART THREE: "Staying Active"

The independent person remains active. We want to be able to get around, carry small packages, do daily chores, pursue a social life. Not everyone enjoys the same activities, but one way or another we must keep our joints and muscles functioning and be sure that our hearts and lungs are strong enough so that we can do what we want.

PART FOUR: "A Sense of Safety"

A safe home supports your independence. You need the freedom to navigate without fear, without barriers that put you at risk of accidents.

PART FIVE: "An Alert Mind"

We want to preserve our mental capacities to make rational decisions, and we want to keep our faculties at optimum levels.

PART SIX: "A Secure Future"

We need the confidence to control our destinies, to decide matters that affect us in the long run, as well as today and tomorrow. We want to know what financial and legal decisions we can make now to determine our future lifestyles, to assert our preferences for medical treatment, and to indicate how we want our worldly goods disbursed.

All these issues are significant and not easily or lightly resolved. You and I should reach out for any assistance in finding acceptable solutions to hard questions.

Fortunately we do not face such important decisions alone. Life is still the greatest adventure. Without a timetable, without a map, we each create our own unique experiences according to our individual choices. *On Your Own Terms* does not offer a blueprint to follow, but rather it empowers you by offering tools for designing the kind of future that suits you best. It is reassuring to realize that so many resources and so much information are available. You may need to try more than one product before finding just what you need, but I hope you keep experimenting. *On Your Own Terms* is a compendium of solutions, many of which may be just what you need to maintain your independence.

An Important Note About Resources

The items in the "Resources" sections are intended to be selective rather than encyclopedic. I indicate sources to facilitate your shopping from home, by phone or mail. Of course, you may find a local source — your hardware store or pharmacy — for many of the items mentioned.

Prices are included for comparison only, so that you can distinguish between items that cost $20 or $200. You will find the exact current price when you get in touch with the source. Remember, the prices in this book don't include postage, handling, or sales taxes.

I have tried to provide toll-free numbers to simplify contacting sources and manufacturers. I also have noted addresses in case you prefer to write a postcard or letter for further information or if the telephone number is no longer in service.

Many items are available through catalogs, an increasingly widespread method of marketing, and catalogs are listed wherever possible. You will find that catalogs are good places to browse for products and that catalog photos will often help you visualize an item. Often catalog companies rotate merchandise in response to the seasons or according to what seems to be selling at a given time. This may mean that a product mentioned in this book is no longer being offered in a particular catalog. If that is the case, inquire about another source or contact the manufacturer directly. Sometimes new or improved products may have superseded the ones that are no longer available. My experience is that catalog salespeople are helpful and will try their best to find what you need. Note that occasionally I mention a catalog as a resource in itself when the catalog company specializes in a particular area or item and has a variety of offerings from which to chose. For the complete address of each catalog, please see the Complete Listing of Catalogs.

The "Resources" sections include products, services, publications, and organizations and occasionally audiotapes, videotapes, and computer programs. (I have not reviewed tapes or computer software, but their selection is based on written descriptions or accompanying manuals.) To avoid too much duplication, if an organization is mentioned as a source for a publication, it may not be mentioned again, so it will be fruitful to read through all the resources in the sections that interest you. Most organizations respond to postcards requesting general information by sending membership brochures explaining their services and offering lists of their publications.

The books mentioned are in print, but interesting new books are continually being published, and your library may have them; older books are often good resources too.

Also keep in mind that the services and programs mentioned here may depend for funding on government or private sources; it is not uncommon for nonprofit groups to expand, cut back, or go out of business entirely according to changing priorities or social or political developments. One of the organizations in "Essential Resources," page 17, may be able to direct you by providing updated information. Please let me know if you discover such address or name changes or if you find other resources that are helpful; I am interested in your own solutions or products you find. Write to me c/o Hearst Books, William Morrow and Co., Inc., 1350 Avenue of the Americas, New York, NY 10019.

Notations in the "Resources" Sections

Many of the "Resources" sections refer you to another chapter in the book where you can find supplementary information or where a subject is discussed from a different point of view.

"FREE WITH SSE." When this appears in a resource entry, it means that you must include a self-addressed, stamped, business-size envelope with your request.

"BEST BUY." This is a subjective evaluation, indicating an especially useful, practical, or economical (sometimes even FREE) item.

Essential Resources

The following resources are so essential that I have included them here to avoid repeating them in every chapter and to make it easy for you to find help fast.

SERVICES

Federal Information Center Hot Line
The central directory assistance for all federal government services, programs, regulations, or referrals to agencies. The operator has the telephone number of the agency responsible for any subject you name.
(800) 688-9889.

Eldercare Locator
A service that provides a resource in your community that can help you with your specific problem or direct you to the proper contact. Through this service you can find local sources for housing guidance, legal assistance, home health care advice, or information on a wide variety of other services. A coordinated project of the Administration on Aging, the National Association of Area Agencies on Aging, and the National Association of State Units on Aging.
NAAAA, 1112 16th Street, NW, Suite 100, Washington, DC 20036, (800) 677-1116.

Combined Health Information Database (CHID)
A central reference source for health information and health education material. The database contains citations of printed resources compiled by various agencies of the federal government. Information is available on a wide variety of diseases and disorders.
The database can be accessed directly by computer by subscribing to CDP Online, 333 7th Avenue, New York, NY 10001, (800) 950-2035. Access is also available directly from the individual contributing agencies. For a list of these and more information, write CHID, National Institutes of Health, Box CHID, 9000 Rockville Pike, Bethesda, MD 20892.

National Health Information Center

Resources for health information, publications, or programs. Referrals from a database of organizations that provide health-related information. Includes federal clearinghouses and resource centers.

NHIC, P.O. Box 1133, Washington, DC 20013, (800) 336-4797.

PUBLICATIONS

The Center for Books on Aging

A mail-order source for more than 2,500 titles related to the field of aging. Books are listed by subject, such as home care, geriatric medicine, philosophy, and ethics.

FREE catalog. Center for Books on Aging, 1331 H Street, NW, Lower Level, Washington, DC 20005, (800) 221-4272.

"A Guide to Health and Consumer Toll-Free Hotlines," by Regan Bailey

More than a hundred toll-free numbers for information on health topics or consumer issues with a brief description of what each source has to offer.

$1. Hot Lines Guide, Essential Information, P.O. Box 19405, Washington, DC 20036.

"Who? What? Where? Resources for Women's Health and Aging," National Institute on Aging

A compilation of resources focusing on women's health concerns and information to improve the quality of their lives. Brief discussions of various topics are followed by the names of organizations and publications that would be particularly helpful for further information. Many publications are available directly from the NIA.

FREE. NIA Publication Information Office, P.O. Box 8057, Gaithersburg, MD 20898, (800) 222-2225.

ORGANIZATIONS

American Association of Retired Persons

A group whose scope and variety of interests may surprise you even if you already are a member. A look at the annual catalog, "AARP Publications and A/V Programs: The Complete Collection," gives an idea of the astonishing breadth of activities AARP is engaged in. Most publications are FREE if you send a postcard request. AARP sponsors programs that are carried out on a local level, such as FREE tax assistance, driver refresher training courses, and more. Members receive *Modern Maturity*, a monthly magazine, and access to AARP's pharmacy, financial, insurance, and travel services.

Documents that discuss various aspects of aging are available through an AARP database, AGELINE. AARP Online allows communication with the organization through computer information networks.

For more information about these or other AARP services, contact AARP, 601 E Street, NW, Washington, DC 20049, (800) 424-3410.

Next to being loved, the part of life most of us treasure is independence — having control over our futures, the freedom to make our own decisions.

— Beverly Chapman, *Orlando Sentinel*

Chapter 1

Embracing a Positive Outlook

"Forget negative thinkers; they drag you way down to their gloomy level. I intend to enjoy the rest of my life, even if I need something or someone to lean on. I'm afraid to get too close to naysayers; it may be catching."

A positive outlook is the key ingredient in living independently. It's like a powerful whirlwind that not only supports relationships with family and friends and buoys an inner sense of optimism but also generates the motivation for finding and implementing solutions to problems. What's more, it only strengthens with use.

Chances are if your outlook is positive, you'll agree with a number of the following statements:

- I don't care what they call me — senior citizen, older American, elderly — I don't label myself.
- My age is just a number.
- Many people are in worse shape than I am.
- I think my physical condition will improve.
- I look forward to each day.
- I can overcome a bad experience.
- I don't think my problems are unique.

Most older Americans find that getting older isn't as bad as they anticipated, according to a 1993 *Parade* magazine survey. In fact, negative views about aging were found among those between the ages of eighteen to twenty-four; older people themselves had fewer qualms about the future.

Research reveals that people with a positive attitude enjoy life more fully and recover better from illness. Your attitude reflects the habits and experiences of a lifetime, so it can take time and deliberation to transform negative thinking into a new, optimistic frame of mind. Here are some practical steps that can speed the process:

- Spend time with people who smile frequently.
- Say yes more often than no to invitations and suggestions of new activities.
- Make at least one positive comment each day.
- Plan for something you want to do in a week or so.
- Think about ways of improving or enhancing some daily activity: a special dessert, a flower or two in a vase, radio music for background.

Studies have shown that smiling — even just making the facial movements for a smile — can have beneficial results, physically and psychologically. Laughter causes blood pressure and heart rate to fall, improves the immune system, and reduces stress.

A belly laugh is healthy activity; some consider it a key to longevity. When you laugh heartily, the cardiovascular system is activated: your breathing rate increases and your heart pumps faster, sending more oxygen to the body's cells. According to a study from Stanford University, laughing one hundred or two hundred times a day provides the same health benefits as ten minutes of rowing. Laughing at yourself or smiling at a private thought when you are alone is a sign of a positive outlook.

Pets also contribute to a positive perspective, especially if you live alone, by providing a source of humor and a companion that needs your care and listens to your troubles. Many people find that the company of a bird, fish, cat, or dog lifts the spirit.

You might also look to popular role models or people you know who set positive examples to reinforce your own efforts. The grandmother in the cartoon series *For Better or for Worse* by Lynn Johnston tells her granddaughter, "All kinds of stuff happens when you get old, Elizabeth. People are like cars. Things wear out, things go wrong, things don't work . . . And see these spots on the backs of my hands . . . Rust!!" Millicent Fenwick, the diplomat and congresswoman and the inspiration for Garry Trudeau's Doonesbury character Lacey Davenport, told a reporter on her eightieth birthday, "You have to be tough; you have to keep in there with good humor. . . . Some are peppery and fight back, and then there are others who are wet smacks. My philosophy is to allow no self-pity and no brooding about the past."

A positive outlook implies having a stake in the future, a goal, a plan, or an objective that can give meaning to your life. The organizer of the New York City Marathon, Fred Lebow, found inspiration for battling serious illness by vowing to complete the more than twenty-six-mile-course himself. A small light in the distance can be enough to spark a positive approach.

Resources

Products

Talking Picture Frame Clock. Awaken to a beep or to the recorded voice of someone special. When open, one side holds a favorite photo, with a clock on the other side. $25. Sharper Image catalog, (800) 344-4444.

Publications

BEST BUY. Growing Wiser: The Older Person's Guide to Mental Wellness by Donald W. Kemper et al. A workbook that highlights the wisdom that comes with maturity with a view to enhancing self-respect. Raises issues in a practical format with exercises and encouragement for positive changes. Large print. $10. Healthwise, P.O. Box 1989, Boise, ID 83701, (208) 345-1161.

"Every day is a surprise package that I look forward to opening with anticipation. I try to live as if each day were my last."

A positive outlook makes you resilient enough to withstand life's inevitable challenges, including those related to getting older. The person who greets each birthday with more anticipation than anguish, more enthusiasm than embarrassment will take the decades lightly, as just a number, and relish the future. Of course, it's natural to experience days when you feel "blue," "sad," "low," or "out of sorts." Usually this is temporary and will pass in a day or two by itself.

Even though we use the word "depressed" for both, there's a big difference between a "bad mood" and clinical depression. Clinical depression, a disease that can be diagnosed and treated by a physician, lasts far longer than two weeks. If you suspect that you might be seriously depressed, consult a mental health practitioner.

There are things you can do to shake off a sad feeling, like giving in to your own best instincts. Even simple activities, such as satisfying the urge to buy a new hat or going to a movie, can often result in a brighter mood.

Ways to Combat a Sad Mood

Be active, stay busy. Keep to a regular schedule despite your mood.

Reach out to help others.

Exercise, even if you feel sluggish.

Reminisce. Recollecting events you have experienced, whether happy or sad ones, helps you recognize everything you have overcome, accomplished, and enjoyed during your lifetime. This can render the present more meaningful.

Your first moments awake can set the tone for the whole day. If you start the day with cheerful, positive thoughts, any physical problems you may have will seem more tolerable. Gentle exercises, meditation, or taking a few minutes to plan activities while you're still in bed can create a positive beginning for the day.

Resources

Suggestions for activities such as traveling, volunteering, and leisure pursuits that involve other people can be found in Chapter 18, "Continuing to Learn," and Chapter 19, "Creating Your Retirement."

Strategies for incorporating exercise into your life are mentioned in Part Three, "Staying Active."

Services

Legacies. A writing contest. Prizes are offered for short stories written by people sixty years of age and over on topics reflecting personal challenges, experiences, or role models. Write for contest rules. Legacies, 163 Amsterdam Avenue, No. 107, New York, NY 10023.

Publications

Opening Up: The Healing Power of Confiding in Others by James W. Pennebaker. An exploration of the health benefits of confiding life's events to others, through writing or orally. 1991. Avon.

SUPPORTIVE GROUPS

"My friends and family were sympathetic, supportive, but my group helped me the most. They had been through it before me or were going through it, as I was, and only they truly understood my problems. In the end the group knew more about how I felt than my family did."

The comfort of loved ones is indispensable in a crisis, yet support from a fellow sufferer, even a stranger, can be pivotal. Finding a support group of people who have had similar experiences to yours can help prevent isolation or despondency. There are more than five hundred thousand support groups focusing on nearly every type of life experience: illness, bereavement, emotional issues, addictions, and so on. Some are gatherings of people in the same age-groups; others cross age boundaries and bring together people with similar concerns. These groups provide their members with information, confidence, coping strategies, and strength from mutual sharing. You can form your own group if you can't find one near you.

Joining a support group can reduce stress and even improve the functioning of the body's immune system. While the motivation for joining generally springs from a desire to help yourself deal with a problem or change for the better, the ultimate satisfaction may be in realizing that you have something to offer that can help others. Inspiration and comfort can result from sharing insights and experiences. A support group can help you generate a positive outlook and provide suggestions for adjusting to new situations. Members can find relief just by expressing their thoughts in a reassuring atmosphere. The group is often a valuable source for locating equipment, alternative medications, innovative treatments, or homemade solutions others have devised to handle everyday problems.

Resources

Sources of medical information for health care consumers are noted in Chapter 21, "Planning Your Health Care."

Services

"Self-Help Clearinghouses in the United States and Canada." A list of phone contacts to find a support group near you. FREE with SSE. American Self-Help Clearinghouse, St. Clares-Riverside Medical Center, Denville, NJ 07834, (201) 625-7101.

Publications

"Ideas for Starting a Self-Help Group." FREE with SSE. American Self-Help Clearinghouse, St. Clares-Riverside Medical Center, Denville, NJ 07834, (201) 625-7101.

The Self-Help Sourcebook: A National Guide to Finding and Forming Mutual Aid Self-Help Groups. Contacts and descriptions for more than seven hundred and fifty national and model self-help groups and toll-free numbers. Updates are published every two years. $10. American Self-Help Clearinghouse, Attn: Sourcebook, St. Clares-

Riverside Medical Center, Denville, NJ 07834, (201) 625-7101.

Women and Divorce: Turning Your Life Around and Social and Emotional Issues for Mid-Life Women. Self-guiding workbooks with checklists and exercises for help in confronting transitional phases of life. $12 each. Information also is available about seminars on these subjects. The National Center for Women, Long Island University, Southampton, NY 11968, (800) 426-7386.

Directory of National Helplines: A Guide to Toll-Free Public Service Numbers. The directory has more than five hundred national help lines that provide information on social, economic, health, and environmental concerns. $7. Consumers Index, P.O. Box 1808, Ann Arbor, MI 48106, (800) 678-2435.

Growing Younger Handbook by Donald W. Kemper et al. A positive approach to reducing what the authors call "health" age by developing healthy habits. Suggests ideas to let you participate in maintaining your health. $10. Healthwise, P.O. Box 1989, Boise, ID 83701, (208) 345-1161.

Audiotapes

Self-Help Tapes. These tapes address a variety of supportive self-help goals, such as changing behavior patterns (particularly stress management), dealing with pain or other health issues, and developing "inner strength." Some require relaxation with eyes closed; others are suitable for use while driving or doing other activities. Most about $11. Source Cassettes, P.O. Box W, Stanford, CA 94309, (800) 52-TAPES (528-2737).

Organizations

National Self-Help Clearinghouse. Referral to and information about support groups nationwide. Also guidance for organizing a self-help group. NSC, Graduate School and University Center of the City University of New York, Room 620, 25 West 43rd Street, New York, NY 10036, (212) 642-2944.

Connecting by computer with others is a new way of finding people with interests you share and communicating with them without leaving your home. You may follow a subject that appeals to you: trading tips; exchanging experiences; doing research with others in distant places. This can be accomplished through the global computer network of networks, the Internet, often called the information superhighway. The network of computer users enables you to send messages, either to read later (electronic mail or E-mail) or for real-time conversation, and you can cruise a highway where you can stop and retrieve various collections of information (databases) or computer programs.

Connecting to the Internet is complicated, and as more refined and simplified hookups are devised, guidance is available from explanatory books written for the neophyte. Most people are finding access through one of a number of "gateway" services. These offer their own on-line networks, including shopping, travel information and reservations, and financial market information. These intermediaries facilitate connection to some aspects of the Internet, mainly the electronic mail exchange. Until more companies offer simplified access to this global network, computer users can gain experience in computer communication through the established services: Prodigy, CompuServe, America Online, and SeniorNet Online.

Resources

Guidance for locating computer technology that can enlarge or "speak" the text can be found in Chapter 16, "Enhancing Your Memory and Vision."

Services

Computer Learning Centers. Learn to use a computer at your own speed in classes for seniors. For the center nearest you, contact SeniorNet, 399 Arguello Boulevard, San Francisco, CA 94118, (800) 747-6848.

Prodigy. Shopping, travel, and news services. 445 Hamilton Avenue, White Plains, NY 10601, (800) PRODIGY (776-3449).

CompuServe. An enormous choice of reference databases and services, including news stories and airline reservations. 5000 Arlington Centre Boulevard, Columbus, OH 43220, (800) 848-8199.

America Online. A selection of services such as airline reservations, an electronic campus where courses are offered, and interactions among small business owners. 8619 Westwood Center Drive, Vienna, VA 22182, (800) 827-6364.

SeniorNet Online. Accessible through America Online. Mainly networking among seniors, help using your computer, articles of interest to seniors on health issues or retirement. Membership, $35. Additional monthly fee for access to computer network. SeniorNet, 399 Arguello Boulevard, San Francisco, CA 94118, (800) 747-6848.

Delphi. Access to many Internet networks and services. 1030 Massachusetts Avenue, Cambridge, MA 02138, (800) 695-4005.

Publications

Computers for Kids over Sixty by Mary Furlong and Greg P. Kearsley. Introduction to computer use and ideas for projects you can undertake using a computer. 1984. Available from SeniorNet, 399 Arguello Boulevard, San Francisco, CA 94118, (800) 747-6848.

The Internet Complete Reference by Harley Hahn and Rick Stout. A guidebook to finding your way through the networks of the Internet. 1994. Osborne McGraw-Hill.

The Whole Internet User's Guide and Catalog by Ed Krol. An instructional manual for connecting to the "superhighway." 1995. O'Reilly and Associates, Sebastopol, CA.

Chapter 2

Nourishing Relationships

Our lives are richer and sweeter and our outlooks more optimistic when our relationships are satisfying. Making plans and participating in activities with friends and relatives build intimacy and shared moments. Such person-to-person connections can alleviate depression, minimize physical complaints, and even have a salutary influence on the heart by reducing stress.

As we learn how to bridge generation gaps and come to terms with changes in our lives, we create new ways of interacting in our roles as child, parent, sibling, friend, and spouse.

YOUR GRANDCHILDREN

"My mom's name is Grammom."

Your grandchildren look to you as a major source of family values and traditions, a role that strengthens family ties. The 1990 census found 5 percent of all children in the United States living with their grandparents; that's 3.3 million children, not including an unknown number who are living with grandparents on an informal basis. Whether they participate intensively in their grandchildren's lives as substitute parents or full-time or part-time day caretakers or live at a distance, grandparents have an opportunity to develop a special relationship with mutual benefits. The communication gap is usually greatest between two neighboring generations, while the more distant ones often get along fine. For a grandchild, a grandparent is a more objective adult than a parent as well as a source of family history and traditions. While grandparents have special wisdom and unconditional love to offer their grandchildren, their grandchildren can help them connect with the contemporary issues and interests of a new generation.

If you are a grandparent, make a point of establishing a special place for yourself in your grandchild's life.

Ideas for Grandparents Who Live Near Their Grandchildren

- Offer to substitute for working parents at school affairs, athletic events, dental appointments, library story hours, or other regular occurrences.
- Sponsor and provide transportation to music, dance, or skating lessons.
- Watch a special TV program together every week.
- Begin an album of photos that you can look at together periodically. At the appropriate age, give the child the gift of a camera so that you both can add to the album.
- Share an interest of yours — stamp collecting, card games — and pursue it together.

Ideas for Grandparents Who Live at a Distance from Their Grandchildren

- Telephone at regular intervals, so that your call will be an anticipated occasion.
- Pick a holiday and spend it together every year.
- Find out the child's favorite TV program, watch it regularly, and discuss it on the phone or in letters.
- Send photos of things you do or see and comment on them. When the children come for a visit, show them the places you photographed.
- Record a story from a book and send the tape along with the book, or create your own drawings and story, to tape and send.
- Write often, and send stationery, stamps, and crayons. Enclose clippings or other personal items you think might be of interest.

Products

Write Connection Program. A letter-writing kit to encourage weekly correspondence between a child and an adult. Kit for children ages four to twelve includes letters, calendars, return mailer for child, stickers, and special crafts projects. A six-month kit, $15. The Write Connection Company, 22821 Lake Forest Boulevard, Building 100, Suite 433, Lake Forest, CA 92630, (800) 334-3143.

Educational Toys. A catalog of moderately priced toys selected to provide challenging, creative play for designated age-groups. Most are not motorized. GrandKids, 5042 Wilshire Boulevard, No. 556, Los Angeles, CA 90036, (800) 766-0020.

Family Journal. A structure for recording your family history through five generations. A format for your recollections and genealogy. $10. Miles Kimball catalog, (414) 231-4886.

Services

AARP Grandparent Information Center. Information on support groups and advice about custody, health insurance, or other services for grandchildren. Newsletter. GIC, 601 E Street, NW, Washington, DC 20049, (202) 434-2296. Until a toll-free number is activated, leave a message and your call will be returned.

Publications

Becoming a Better Grandparent and *Achieving Grandparent Potential.* Two courses designed to help grandparents gain satisfaction from their relationships with grandchildren. Issues and practical exercises are presented in a guide book for each course that can be used for self-guided study. $20 each. Sage Publications, P.O. Box 5084, Newbury Park, CA 91359, (805) 499-0721.

Grandparent Power by Arthur Kornhaber, M.D., with Sondra Forsythe. An analysis of the importance of the role of grandparents in their lives and the lives of their grandchildren. 1994. Crown.

From Generation to Generation by Phyllis Massing, Ph.D., and E. Rhoda Lewis. A how-to manual for creating an oral family history on audiotape or videotape. May be used as a guide for someone to interview you or for you to complete on your own. You may also discuss the topics suggested in writing if you prefer. Comes with audiotaped instructions. $25. LIFE STORIES/A Video Legacy, 16161 Ventura Boulevard, Suite 634, Encino, CA 91436, (800) 2-R-STORY (277-8679), or in Los Angeles call (818) 995-3315.

Recording Your Family History: A Guide to Preserving Oral History with Videotape and Audiotape by William Fletcher. Hundreds of questions from which you can create a family history, on your own or jointly with a relative. Actually designed for an interviewer, but the questions can be adapted for use on your own. 1989. Ten Speed Press.

Writing Your Life by Mary Borg. A guide to help you write your autobiography. Explains ways of stimulating your memory and gives instructions for "publishing" your book. $16. Cottonwood Press, 305 West Magnolia, Suite 398, Fort Collins, CO 80521, (800) 864-4297.

Organizations

Foundation for Grandparenting. Promotes an active role for grandparents in their families and communities. A weeklong summer camp for grandchildren and grandparents to enjoy together. Newsletter available. 53 Principe De Paz, Santa Fe, NM 87505.

Creative Grandparenting, Inc. A nonprofit group that encourages grandparents to interact with youngsters for mutual benefits. FREE introductory packet and sample newsletter. CGI, 609 Blackgates Road, Wilmington, DE 19803, (302) 479-5759.

National Federation of Grandmother Clubs of America. Organizes gatherings of grandmothers for charitable activities. For a club near you, contact the National Federation of Grandmother Clubs of America, 203 North Wabash Avenue, Chicago, IL 60601.

FRIENDS AND RELATIVES

Maintaining relationships — with old and new friends, siblings, cousins, children, etc. — is the prime antidote for loneliness and isolation.

Family quarrels often erupt with volcanic power and can leave lasting residues, reigniting or smoldering beneath the surface at family celebrations. These disputes sometimes linger well past the normal life span of an argument and cause a disproportionate amount of pain. Make the first move toward reconciliation, and you will be solidifying your meaningful past with your present and future. A family reunion is a valuable tradition that becomes richer the longer and larger it grows, transcending disputes.

Tips for Maintaining Long-Term Relationships

- Forget offenses after a month or two.
- Don't expect more than the other person can give.
- Don't stand on ceremony, waiting for a call, a letter, a thank-you note, a Christmas card, an invitation, etc.
- Don't undervalue or dismiss the importance of the relationship and the need to patch up differences swiftly when they surface.

Most relationships fall short of an ideal of mutual reciprocity where every phone call is soon returned and every letter promptly answered. To maintain your connection with friends and relatives, it's wise not to keep score at all, not to take offense easily, and never to forget that a door opens from both sides.

If you take the initiative for visiting and extending invitations, you can determine the style that's easiest for you. If meal preparations are daunting, have tea; if you tire in the afternoon, make a date for a morning walk; if you can't get out, suggest a card game or other activity.

If you live far from people you've known for a long time, you can begin to create a new circle of contacts through community programs, such as visiting companions. This program is usually available through a local office on aging and is designed to connect people who can benefit from spending time together. Pen pals also pair people with similar interests, and there are intergenerational programs that match Girl or Boy Scouts or other young people with older adults, providing mutual exchanges that stimulate and educate on both sides.

Products

Big Print Date Calendar Book. A large-format date book to accommodate large writing. Front and back pockets for notes, entire month on two facing pages, 9″ × 11″. $14. Lighthouse Consumer Products catalog, (800) 829-0500.

Big Print Address Book. Includes wide-tipped black pen for easy readability and heavyweight paper with half-inch-wide lines; spiral-bound, so it lies flat. $13. Sense-Sations catalog, (800) 876-5456.

Services

Intergenerational Programs. For contact with a community program near you where you can work with young people. Generations United, c/o CWLA, 440 1st Street, NW, Suite 310, Washington, DC 20001, (202) 638-2952.

YOUR AGING PARENTS

As we contemplate the prospect of longer lives for ourselves, our own parents may be entering old age. Your relationship with your parents changes in response to every new stage of life. Just when you begin to feel some effects of aging yourself, your parents may be looking to you for help.

Your goal for them, as for yourself, is to maximize their independence. When you, the child, become the nurturer, the situation requires diplomacy, delicacy, and restraint. You will be most supportive when your suggestions are in balance with your parents' readiness to accept them. As long as your parents are making their own decisions, they need your encouragement. The point at which parents can no longer manage on their own is time enough to take over the decision-making responsibilities.

Publications

Care Sharing Directory. A listing of professional geriatric care managers, caregiver support groups, and related health services. $20. For a single state listing, $2. Children of Aging Parents, Woodbourne Office Campus, Suite 302-A, 1609 Woodbourne Road, Levittown, PA 19057, (215) 945-6900.

Answers. A bimonthly magazine for adult children of aging parents. Articles on practical ways of dealing with problems and ways of facing emotional issues when you are helping an elderly parent. Sample copy FREE. *Answers* Magazine, 75 Seabreeze Drive, Richmond, CA 94804, (415) 924-4737.

Organizations

Children of Aging Parents. National clearinghouse for caregivers of the elderly provides information, referrals, resources, and emotional support. A monthly newsletter for members. CAPS, Woodbourne Office Campus, Suite 302-A, 1609 Woodbourne Road, Levittown, PA 19057, (215) 945-6900.

SEXUAL RELATIONSHIPS

"[S]exual passion, pleasure and playfulness are not just for the young and the beautiful. The empty nest may actually be a love nest."
— ANDREW GREELEY, novelist, priest

Sex can provide continuing pleasure and satisfaction throughout life. Partners can even explore ways of adapting to physical limitations within the intimacy and privacy of sex.

Some people easily find opportunities to satisfy their sexual needs, regardless of how events have affected their life's routine: loss of a spouse, moving to a new area, chronic illness. Sadly, others needlessly deny the sexual aspects of themselves, thinking that sexual activity is no longer possible for them.

The following are some oft-cited excuses for discontinuing sex:

- Loyalty to a dead spouse
- A belief against having more than one sex partner in life
- Objections to sex without marriage
- Negative body image caused by weight, mastectomy, hysterectomy, loss of muscle tone
- Apprehension about health problems: heart attack, stroke, pain, osteoporosis
- The effects of menopause on sexual response
- Problems having or maintaining erections
- The effects of medications on sexual interest
- Moodiness or fatigue

Experts say that age is no barrier to sexual enjoyment, and that a fifty-year-old has the same capacity as a twenty-year-old for achieving an orgasm. Some people find that sex actually improves with maturity. Negotiation, accommodation, and communication are part of a positive sexual experience, and all these skills ripen over the years. Studies show that most people who enjoyed sexual relations in their younger years would continue to do so throughout life. Women should consult a gynecologist, and men a urologist, concerning any problems that interfere with sexual relations.

Surveys on sexual activity among older people are far from scientific, but more than 80 percent of Americans between sixty and ninety-one years of age are found to be sexually active. Nature takes its course, it seems, without our advice. The medical results are positive too since sex raises the heart rate to about 130 beats per minute, the equal of sprinting up a flight of stairs in ten or fifteen seconds. So sex qualifies as good exercise.

Ways of Improving Sex

- Discuss special pleasure points and preferences with your partner.
- Consciously change something — the time of day, position, technique, location, or your attitude toward some sexual practices. Experiment with comfortable positions, and alternate active and passive roles with your partner.
- If you take medication, plan to have sex before or after you take it, depending on whether it soothes you or causes uncomfortable side effects.

- If a warm bath eases sore joints, schedule it before sex, or even share it with your partner.
- Keep active so that your joints retain their full range of motion.
- If you have limited energy, plan sex at your best time of day, and adjust your energy resources accordingly.
- To add variety, incorporate a vibrator or other means of stimulation.
- Remember that sex is a private, intimate experience, so you and your partner need not worry about how others might react to what you do.

Resources

Pointers for keeping limber and fit are noted in Part Three, "Staying Active."

Services

American Association of Sex Educators, Counselors and Therapists. Provides referrals to sex therapists in your area. AASECT, 435 North Michigan Avenue, Chicago, IL 60611, (312) 644-0828.

Sexual Function Health Council. Information and publications. C/o American Foundation for Urologic Disease, 300 West Pratt Street, Suite 401, Baltimore, MD 21201, (800) 242-2383.

Publications

150 Most-Asked Questions About Midlife Sex, Love & Intimacy by Ruth S. Jacobowitz. Discussion of issues couples face in sexual relations after age fifty, in particular the pros and cons of hormone therapy, overcoming the consequences of menopause, and erection problems. 1995. Hearst Books/William Morrow.

Sex over Forty. A monthly newsletter focusing on the sexual concerns of mature adults. Sample issue FREE. $72 per year. DKT International, P.O. Box 1600, Chapel Hill, NC 27515, (919) 929-2148.

How to Find Love, Sex and Intimacy After 50: A Woman's Guide by Dr. Matti Gershenfeld and Judith Newman. For single women over age fifty who are interested in beginning new relationships. Discusses concerns about finding single men, dating, having sex, and integrating a new partner into the family circle. 1991. Ballantine.

Love and Sex After 60 by Robert N. Butler, M.D., and Myrna I. Lewis, M.S.W. Looks at how to combat negative attitudes that may limit sexual enjoyment for people over age sixty. Examines changes that may occur and ways of adjusting to them so that you can continue the sexual aspect of life. 1993. Ballantine.

"Living and Loving: Information About Sex," Arthritis Foundation. Suggestions for improving sexual relationships for people with physical limitations or pain. FREE. AF, P.O. Box 19000, Atlanta, GA 30326, (800) 283-7800.

Growing Older Together: A Couple's Guide to Understanding and Coping with the Challenges of Later Life by Barbara Silverstone and Helen Kandel Hyman. A down-to-earth discussion of issues, including sex, that can change a couple's relationship along with some suggestions for confronting them. 1992. Pantheon.

Organizations

Sex Information and Education Council of the United States. Provides information and educational materials about sexuality. SIE-CUS, 130 West 42nd Street, Suite 2500, New York, NY 10036, (212) 819-9770.

Women and Sex

Women lose their mates at an astonishing rate compared with men, making it more likely that women will be without partners in their later years. For every hundred women over age eighty-five, there are only thirty-six men.

The belief that men should take the social initiatives can make finding a partner even more difficult for some women. Happily that is beginning to change. Single women who are leading active lives, involved in events and activities they enjoy, and who are generally happy and congenial are more likely to meet available men.

Women Alone — the Statistical Story

- About 85 percent of wives outlive their husbands. There are 11 million widows in the United States, compared with only 2.5 million widowers.
- Women over age forty-five are more likely than men to find themselves alone because of the death of a spouse or divorce. Between ages forty-five and fifty-four women are twice as likely as men to be widowed or divorced, and over age fifty-five three times more likely.
- About 70 percent of all persons forty-five and older living alone are women, and nearly 80 percent of those sixty-five and older living alone are women.
- In the over-sixty-five age group, for every hundred unmarried women there are twenty-seven unmarried men.
- About half of all women age sixty-five and older are widows.

Only about 20 percent of women experience uncomfortable symptoms from menopause, attributed to a sharp drop in the body's production of the hormone estrogen. Most notice only one or two, such as hot flashes, night sweats, insomnia, atrophy of vaginal tissue, reduction in vaginal lubrication, or mood swings.

Estrogen replacement has become a widely recommended treatment for relief of these discomforts. Hormone replacement therapy provides important additional health benefits: It cuts in half the risk of cardiovascular disease, the single leading cause of death for women over age fifty, and it prevents excessive bone mass loss that might otherwise lead to osteoporosis, a disease that causes brittle bones that are subject to fractures. You and your doctor must weigh the benefits and side effects of hormone replacement for your particular situation.

Women whose doctors counsel against the use of estrogen can use methods of lubricating the vagina and managing other menopausal symptoms that don't involve medication. More frequently than in the past women are joining support groups to share information and experiences with others. Hospitals have established "menopause clinics" that combine social, medical, and psychological services.

* By 1996 the results of a National Institutes of Health (NIH) study on the effects of hormone replacement therapy may add to the information available on the value of this treatment for women after menopause. Initial reports indicate that a combination of hormones may protect the heart without some undesirable side effects, such as an increased risk of uterine cancer.
* Another longer-term NIH study will follow the incidence of heart disease, osteoporosis, breast and uterine cancers in twenty-five thousand postmenopausal women taking various hormone therapies. This study will benefit the generation of women who reach menopause in the first decade of the next century.
* An inquiry into the natural history of menopause funded by the NIH will begin in 1995. It will attempt to chronicle the changes in ovarian function, how these affect the menstrual cycle, and why certain symptoms are experienced by some women and not others.
* Also funded by the NIH is the Women's Health Initiative to study medical problems experienced by postmenopausal women. The fifteen-year study involving 160,000 women ages fifty to seventy-nine will observe one group of women and test others for three therapies intended to prevent heart disease, osteoporosis, and breast and colon cancers.

Resources

Services

A List of Gynecologists in Your Area. Informational publications are also available. FREE with SSE. Resource Center, American College of Obstetricians and Gynecologists, 409 12th Street, SW, Washington, DC 20024.

Menopause Hot Line. Recorded messages on about three hundred topics relating to menopause. You may leave a message for answers to your specific questions. Publications available. National Menopause Foundation, 222 Southwest 36th Terrace, Gainesville, FL 32607, (800) MENO ASK (636-6275).

Publications

Menopause News. A bimonthly newsletter containing information and resources on hormone replacement therapy. $23 for subscription. 2074 Union Street, San Francisco, CA 94123, (800) 241-MENO (6366).

A Friend Indeed. A newsletter resource for menopause containing an exchange of information from contributors' personal experiences. Sample copy FREE. P.O. Box 1710, Champlain, NY 12919, (514) 843-5730.

Staying Healthy, Being Aware: Health Care After Forty. A handbook on women's health issues. Briefly discusses such topics as breast cancer, menopause, and other subjects from a woman's point of view. 1992. FREE. U.S. House of Representatives, Subcommittee on Housing and Consumer Interests, 717 House Office Building Annex, Washington, DC 20515.

"Estrogen Use," American College of Obstetricians and Gynecologists. Booklet explaining the role of estrogen and hormone replacement after menopause. FREE with SSE. ACOG, 409 12th Street, SW, Washington, DC 20024.

Taking Hormones and Women's Health: Choices, Risks and Benefits, National Women's Health Network. A view of estrogen replacement therapy from a feminist perspective. $5. NWHN, 1325 G Street, NW, Washington, DC 20005, (202) 347-1140.

"The Menopause Years," American College of Obstetricians and Gynecologists. Describes the process of menopause and related treatments. FREE with SSE. ACOG, 409 12th Street, SW, Washington, DC 20024.

The Silent Passage, Menopause by Gail Sheehy. An upbeat approach to the opportunities presented by the "change of life" as a positive beginning of a new stage of life. Includes a nontechnical description of how menopausal changes affect women and some treatments available. 1993. Pocket Books.

Hot Flash. A quarterly newsletter covering health and social issues of concern to midlife and older women. Sent to members. $25 for subscription. National Action Forum for Midlife and Older Women, P.O. Box 816, Stony Brook, NY 11790.

"The Healthy Heart Handbook for Women," National Heart,

Lung, and Blood Institute. Answers questions about women and cardiovascular disease, including self-help strategies and resources. FREE. NHLBI Information Center, P.O. Box 30105, Bethesda, MD 20824, (301) 251-1222.

"Silent Epidemic: The Truth About Women and Heart Disease," American Heart Association. Highlights the relation of estrogen to a woman's risk of heart disease, as well as other factors. FREE. AHA, 7272 Greenville Avenue, Dallas, TX 75231, (800) AHA-USA1 (242-8721).

Organizations

National Women's Health Network. Answers questions, provides publications, and lobbies for women's health issues. Members' newsletter. NWHN, 1325 G Street, NW, Washington, DC 20005, (202) 347-1140.

Men and Sex

In the past problems achieving or maintaining an erection were often considered psychological. Now more than 75 percent of impotence is thought to result from physical causes.

One third of men over age sixty, about twenty-five million American men, experience problems with erections. Adverse reactions to medication are responsible for as much as 25 percent of these instances. Other cases may result from such conditions as diabetes, high blood pressure, depression, and anxiety.

The good news is that 99 percent of impotence can be treated. More than 95 percent of men deny themselves and their partners sexual enjoyment rather than discuss the problem with a doctor. The main reasons for not seeking treatment for impotence are embarrassment and the belief that impotence is a normal consequence of aging and that little can be done for it.

Since the very word "impotence" projects blame on the person suffering from it, use of the alternative and more neutral term, "erectile dysfunction," is suggested by the National Institutes of Health.

A normal erection occurs when blood engorges the penis, causing stiffening until orgasm. If blood flow is insufficient for maintaining an erection, there are several possible solutions. An injection of medicine directly into the penis shortly before intercourse can relax arterial muscles to increase blood flow to the penis. Some oral medications may provide the same effect of relaxing the muscles to allow the blood vessels to accommodate more blood. Penile vacuum devices are cylinders that fit around the penis and create negative pressure by pumping most of the air out; this encourages blood to flow into the penis, causing an erection that is then maintained by placing a band at the base of the penis. Surgery has been used to improve blood circulation, and penile implants may provide a solution for some men.

Resources

Publications

Male Sexual Health: A Couple's Guide by Richard F. Spark, M.D. A review of available treatments for impotence and how to evaluate them for your own situation. 1991. Consumer Reports Books.

"A Patient's Guide for the Treatment of Impotence" by James B. Osbon. A comprehensive discussion of impotence and various treatments. Includes discussion of the company's product, a vacuum system. FREE. Osbon Medical Systems, P.O. Box 1478, Augusta, GA 30903, (800) 438-8592.

"Impotence: Patient and Professional Materials," National Kidney and Urologic Diseases Information Clearinghouse. A bibliography with abstracts of each publication mentioned. FREE. NKUDIC, 3 Information Way, Bethesda, MD 20892-3580, (301) 654-4415.

The Potent Male, Facts, Fiction, Future by Irwin Goldstein, M.D., and Larry Rothstein. A clear explanation of the body's functioning during erection and discussion of treatments for problems, including surgery and implants. 1990. Body Press/Price Stern Sloan.

"Impotence Answers: Where to Go, What to Ask," American Medical Systems. Discusses treatment alternatives and how to decide whether to seek help. FREE. Impotence Information Center, P.O. Box 9, Minneapolis, MN 55440, (800) 843-4315.

"Diagnosis and Treatment of Impotence" by H. Handelsman. Analysis of the safety, effectiveness, and uses of new technologies for diagnosis and treatment of impotence. FREE. Agency for Health Care Policy and Research, Publications Clearinghouse, P.O. Box 8547, Silver Spring, MD 20907, (800) 358-9295.

Organizations

Impotents Anonymous (IA); I-ANON, for partners. Provides a list of doctors near you who specialize in impotence. Informational brochures, help in locating support groups and local chapters. IA, 2020 Pennsylvania Avenue, NW, Suite 292, Washington, DC 20006, (800) 669-1603.

Impotence Information Center. Informational literature and names of urologists in your area. IIC, P.O. Box 9, Department A, Minneapolis, MN 55440, (800) 843-4315.

Chapter 3

Keeping in Touch

To maintain relationships and interact with your community, you must be able to share thoughts, feelings, comments, and experiences. All human contact is predicated on communication. Of course, everyone communicates instinctively by a gentle touch, a raised eyebrow, a written note, or a personal gift. Usually we think of communicating by having conversations, either in person or over the phone. One of the greatest challenges of later life is confronting a gradual loss of hearing acuity that can affect our enjoyment of many facets of life, but primarily interpersonal communications.

Many of us will identify with the poignant reaction of the great composer Ludwig van Beethoven to his progressive loss of hearing: "I could not bring myself to say to people: 'Speak up, shout, for I am deaf.' Alas! . . . If I appear in company I am overcome by a burning anxiety, a fear that I am running the risk of letting people notice my condition."

You will observe that Beethoven wasn't complaining about problems composing music; indeed, he continued to produce masterpieces for many years after he had begun to lose his hearing. It was in his social interactions that he suffered.

If, like Beethoven, you feel embarrassment at not sharing a conversation with friends, if you suffer humiliation or shame at not hearing well, if you isolate yourself from social situations because of hearing loss, you will jeopardize the positive outlook that is essential to your independence.

Actually age-related hearing loss is quite common, affecting one third of the population over age sixty-five, about fifteen million people. Beginning around age fifty, presbycusis — the irreversible and permanent loss of the nerve cells, or hair cells, that transmit sounds to the brain — causes noticeable hearing loss. The deterioration is evident in two aspects of hearing: loudness and tones. The volume of sounds you can hear is referred to as sensitivity and is measured in decibels (dB). Your ability to distinguish tones and thereby understand speech is called discrimination and is measured in hertz (Hz).

Normal conversation occurs in the 45- to 55-decibel range, and even sounds from 0 to 25 decibels are detectable by normal hearing.

Categories of Hearing Loss (in Decibels)

Slight, 0-25 dB: problems hearing a whisper or a conversation in a noisy surrounding.

Mild, 26-40 dB: problems hearing normal speech under adverse conditions. Distant speech or background noise may be hard to hear. (A watch ticks at 30 dB.)

Moderate, 41-55 dB: problems hearing loud speech. Speech may be heard at three to five feet but not understood well.

Severe, 56-80 dB: ability to hear only amplified speech. Very loud speech at close range is needed in order to follow a conversation, especially in a group setting. (A baby's cry is 60 dB.)

Profound, 81 dB or more: problems hearing amplified speech. Even talking loudly into the ear may not be understood. (Traffic sounds or noise in a factory are 90 dB; a lawn mower's engine is 100 dB; a rock band's music is 120 dB.)

If you lose hearing up to 25 dB, no hearing aid is necessary. For a loss of up to 40 dB a hearing aid may be helpful. For a loss of up to 55 dB a hearing aid is necessary. Lipreading is a useful adjunct to a hearing aid for loss up to 70 dB and becomes more significant for loss up to 90 dB.

Presbycusis is a combined hearing loss: One detects fewer soft sounds and fewer sounds in higher frequencies. Problems understanding speech begin when hearing loss is 3,000 Hz and above, and most people in their sixties are not able to hear over 1,000 Hz.

Examples of Tones (in Hertz)

Traffic noise	*250 Hz*
The letters m, d, b, n, ng, el, u	*300 Hz*
The letters z and v	*400 Hz*
A dog barking	*500 Hz*
The letters p, h, g, ch, sh	*1,500 Hz*
Telephone ringing, the letters k, t, f, s, th	*3,000 Hz*
Airplane roar	*4,000 Hz*
Flute music	*9,000 Hz*

WHO, ME? YOUR HEARING ACUITY

Part of the struggle of having a hearing loss is acknowledging it, first to yourself, then to people you meet.

In fact, it is often extremely difficult to detect that hearing loss is happening to you. Even though loss of vision also occurs gradually, a slight diminishment in hearing is not really noticeable. Usually the condition worsens until some event or a comment calls to your attention the fact that your hearing has already greatly declined.

Anyone over fifty-five should be alert to the following ten ways of noticing hearing loss.

Ten Signs of Possible Hearing Loss

1. You hear a ringing or other noises in your ear.
2. You feel as though you are talking loudly.
3. You often have to raise the volume on the radio or TV.
4. You complain that others aren't speaking clearly.
5. You can hear people speaking, but you can't understand their words.
6. You confuse similar-sounding words.
7. You find that you are watching people's lips or faces intently as they speak.
8. When someone remarks that he or she phoned or rang your doorbell, you realize that you were home and didn't hear it.

9. In a group conversation you don't always know who is talking and you lose the thread of a discussion.
10. You frequently ask others to repeat what they have said.

You also should be alert to these signs that you are failing to acknowledge a hearing deficit:

- A friend accuses you of not hearing something. (Hearing deficiencies are almost always noticed first by other people; you may be the last to know.)
- You pretend you understand even though you weren't able to follow a conversation.
- At an entertainment event you claim you weren't paying attention or were too tired to listen rather than admit you couldn't hear the play's dialogue or how the music sounded.
- People don't look at you when they speak to a group, sensing from your blank expression that you aren't following.
- You are told of an appointment you missed and realize you got the time, place, or date wrong.
- You think some people don't speak clearly.
- Social occasions take an unusual toll on you because conversation requires such concentration.

Hearing problems may begin with tinnitus, a persistent noise in the ears — ringing, buzzing, crackling — sometimes so distracting that it causes problems with the ability to concentrate. Thirty-six million Americans suffer the symptoms of tinnitus to various degrees of severity. Some people get relief from a tinnitus masker, which resembles a hearing aid and produces a sound like rushing water that covers the other sound created in the ear.

House alarms and devices that alert you to household sounds are detailed in Chapter 14, "Preparing for Emergencies."

Products

Products for People Who Are Hard-of-Hearing:
Accessolutions catalog, (800) 445-9968
Harris Communications catalog, (800) 825-6758
Hear-More catalog, (800) 881-HEAR (4327)
Hear You Are catalog, (800) 278-EARS (3277)
Potomac Technology catalog, (800) 433-2838

Services

Helpline. For information about communication disorders and a list of audiologists in your state. American Speech-Language-Hearing Association, 10801 Rockville Pike, Rockville, MD 20852, (800) 638-8255.

Dial-A-Hearing Screening Test. A completely private, self-scoring recorded test that sounds four tones to listen for in each ear. The toll-free number provides you with a local number to call. (800) 222-3277 (EARS).

Hearing Helpline. A toll-free hot line for questions about hearing loss and available remedies. FREE literature available. Better Hearing Institute, 5021-B Backlick Road, Annandale, VA 22003, (800) 327-9355 (EAR WELL).

National Information Center on Deafness. A centralized source of information on topics dealing with deafness and hearing loss. FREE list of brochures. NICD, Gallaudet University, 800 Florida Avenue, NE, Washington, DC 20002, (202) 651-5051.

Public Information Center. Answers inquiries about hearing aids and other issues affecting people with hearing problems. National Association of the Deaf, 814 Thayer Avenue, Silver Spring, MD 20910, (301) 587-1788.

Publications

"5 Minute Hearing Test . . . Especially for Seniors," American Academy of Otolaryngology — Head and Neck Surgery, Inc. A short questionnaire to help you evaluate whether you should have your hearing tested professionally. FREE. AAO, 1 Prince Street, Alexandria, VA 22314.

"Tinnitus" by Norman Lee Barr, Jr., M.D. A brief discussion of the causes and treatment of tinnitus. FREE. Better Hearing Institute, P.O. Box 1840, Washington, DC 20013, (800) EAR WELL (327-9355).

"Aging and Hearing Loss: Some Commonly Asked Questions" by William McFarland, Ph.D., and B. Patrick Cox, Ph.D. Explains several tests used to determine hearing loss. $1. National Information Center on Deafness, Gallaudet University, 800 Florida Avenue, NE, Washington, DC 20002, (202) 651-5051.

"Hearing and Older People," National Institute on Aging. A brief discussion of how to detect hearing loss, types of hearing loss, and current treatment choices. FREE. NIDCD Clearinghouse, 1 Communication Avenue, Bethesda, MD 20892, (800) 241-1044.

BEST BUY. "Have You Heard? Hearing Loss and Aging," American Association of Retired Persons. Ten-point hearing self-check. Describes some hearing impairments that accompany aging and provides information on coping with hearing loss and buying a hearing aid. FREE. AARP Publications, 601 E Street, NW, Washington, DC 20049.

"Hearing Loss: Personal and Social Considerations" by Helen Sloss Luey. A frank discussion of the changes in attitudes and communication styles hearing loss may require. SHHH Information Series No. 151. $2. Self Help for Hard of Hearing People, 7910 Woodmont Avenue, Suite 1200, Bethesda, MD 20814, (301) 657-2248.

"Managing Hearing Loss in Later Life" by Teena Wax, Ph.D., and Loraine Di Pietro, M.A. Discusses common reactions to hearing loss and practical ways of maximizing communication. $1. National Information Center on Deafness, Gallaudet University, 800 Florida Avenue, NE, Washington, DC 20002, (202) 651-5051.

"Communication Tips for Adults with Hearing Loss" by Harriet Kaplan, Ph.D. Practical advice about enhancing communication in a variety of settings. $1. National Information Center on Deafness,

Gallaudet University, 800 Florida Avenue, NE, Washington, DC 20002, (202) 651-5051.

Hearing Loss Handbook by David M. Vernick, M.D., and Constance Grzelka. A comprehensive discussion of hearing loss, including treatments, hearing aids, and assistive listening devices. 1993. Consumer Reports Books.

How to Survive Hearing Loss by Charlotte Himber. A firsthand account of a woman experiencing midlife hearing loss, including practical information on hearing aids and speechreading. 1989. Gallaudet University Press, Washington, DC 20002. Available from Harris Communications catalog, (800) 825-6758.

Missing Words? The Family Handbook on Adult Hearing Loss by Kay Thomsett and Eve Nickerson. A personal account of a woman's reactions to hearing loss, her experience with various aids to hearing, and how she conducts conversations by asking others to help her understand what they are saying. 1993. Gallaudet University Press, Washington, DC 20002. Available from Self Help for Hard of Hearing People, Inc., 7910 Woodmont Avenue, Suite 1200, Bethesda, MD 20814, (301) 657-2248.

What's That Pig Outdoors?: A Memoir of Deafness by Henry Kisor. One man's view of situations he faces daily because of hearing loss. The book provides insights into the concerns and sensibilities of people with hearing problems. 1990. Hill & Wang.

"Signaling and Assistive Listening Devices for Hearing-Impaired People" by Diane L. Castle, Ph.D. Describes various alternatives for people who can no longer depend on their hearing in everyday situations. FREE. Alexander Graham Bell Association for the Deaf, 3417 Volta Place, NW, Washington, DC 20007, (202) 337-5220.

Coping with Hearing Loss: A Guide for Adults and Their Families by Susan V. Rezen, Ph.D., and Carl Hausman. Practical information about purchasing a hearing aid and learning speechreading, including practice exercises. 1993. Barricade Books.

hearing health. A bimonthly publication about hearing loss and hearing issues. $14 year subscription. P.O. Box 2663, Corpus Christi, TX 78403.

Life After Deafness. A bimonthly magazine that serves as a support publication for late-deafened adults. Informational articles, humor, networking, hints, advice. $12 year subscription. 6773 Starboard Way, Sacramento, CA 95831.

Organizations

Self Help for Hard of Hearing People, Inc. A group that offers its members support, discounts, and publications and carries out lobby and educational activities on behalf of people with hearing problems. SHHH, 7910 Woodmont Avenue, Suite 1200, Bethesda, MD 20814, (301) 657-2248.

National Institute on Deafness and Other Communication Disorders Clearinghouse. A resource center for information about hearing, balance, smell, taste, voice, speech, language. Offers publications, a newsletter, and referrals to organizations with further information. NIDCD Clearinghouse, 1 Communication Avenue, Bethesda, MD 20892, (800) 241-1044.

Alexander Graham Bell Association for the Deaf. Provides members with guidance, newsletters and informational publications, self-help groups, and information on speechreading. 3417 Volta Place, NW, Washington, DC 20007, (202) 337-5220.

American Tinnitus Association. Will refer you to a support group in your area and will provide information. ATA, P.O. Box 5, Portland, OR 97207, (503) 248-9985.

STRATEGIES FOR IMPROVED COMMUNICATION

If you are diagnosed with a hearing deficit, you face the challenge of enlisting your friends, family, and others with whom you must communicate to help you understand them. This can be a stumbling block of self-defeating proportions for anyone who, like Beethoven, is reluctant to let others know about a hearing problem. People with positive outlooks, however, don't define themselves by their hearing ability. A sense of humor and strong motivation can help you learn to communicate in new ways.

Adjusting to hearing loss is more complicated than just increasing the TV volume or asking someone to speak more loudly. You will need to use a variety of methods to improve communication with others. Sometimes it involves asking for their help; at other times it will be up to you.

"I can't hear you with the water running." Everyone knows that a person washing dishes can't hear when someone speaks from another room. Everyone should also know that someone with hearing problems can have a conversation only with people in the same room. Those you live with must be told this so that they can try to comply; they must be reminded when they forget.

Furniture at home can be positioned so that people face each other. A circular arrangement gives a panoramic view of a whole group from each seat. Chairs with casters allow flexibility in moving closer to a speaker or away from a conflicting side conversation.

Sound-absorbing materials are preferable to sound-reflecting ones, which tend to multiply sounds and create echoes. Interior decoration choices should include upholstered furniture rather than acrylic, glass, or bare wood; drapes, curtains, and shades rather than unadorned windows; carpeting instead of bare floors. Acoustical tiles can be installed on the ceiling, and walls can be buffered with cork.

When hearing is unimpaired, the sound of one's own child calling from among dozens of children in a noisy playground is easy to isolate. This is due not only to parental instinct but also to our ability automatically to tune out sounds we don't want to focus on, like traffic noise or a person next to us who is talking. The same trick occurs with some conscious effort dozens of times a day when you can keep the radio going, listen for the doorbell, and react to the washing machine downstairs and to a footstep on the floor above. Since hearing declines slowly, you gradually lose this sound-selecting skill and must relearn it in order to focus on a conversation. As much background noise as possible should be eliminated so that you can concentrate on only one sound; turn off the air conditioning, a radio, the dishwasher. Choose a quiet restaurant, and try to sit in a corner, away from large walls of sound-reflecting mirrors or windows. This is particularly important when you use a hearing aid, which magnifies all ambient sounds.

Of course, to enhance speechreading, you must see to best advantage the face of the person who is speaking. Lighting should fall on the person's face, rather than from behind. Sitting in front of an unshaded window with bright light from behind creates a silhouette effect, putting the person's face in shadow. Exchange places in such a situation, draw the curtains, or turn on some room lights to counteract the silhouette effect.

Be sure to wear glasses, if you use them, whenever you need to hear well. You won't want to miss any details that might help you follow a conversation better, such as hand gestures or facial expressions.

Resources

Interior design and lighting suggestions are included in Chapter 12, "Adapting the Old Homestead."

Products that can provide closed-captioned programs on your television are listed in Chapter 18, "Continuing to Learn."

Speechreading

Speechreading, which incorporates lipreading but also includes observing facial expressions and hand gestures, is a skill that can greatly help communication when you have hearing problems. It isn't a substitute for using a hearing aid, rather it's one component of comprehension. You can learn speechreading, and with practice you can improve. Speak to yourself in the mirror first, to see how much lipreading you already know. First start by practicing with someone privately, then by watching TV, and finally with everyone.

Most people discover that without being conscious of it they have been relying on speechreading for some time in the course of their hearing's decline. On a clattering train, when loud music is playing from nearby speakers, or when a fire engine passes, it is natural to watch a person's lips as he forms his words, the expressions on his face, and his hand motions. These factors, plus verbal cues, are part of the way we understand conversation, even when we can hear well. Watch yourself speak in a mirror, and notice how many sounds look alike, such as the letters *p, b, m,* which are formed with the same mouth position. Seventy percent of English sounds are formed inside the mouth, reducing even more the value of lipreading alone. Speechreading must therefore include more than merely looking at a person's lips; you must decode a person's individual speech peculiarities to understand what is being said.

To use speechreading to best advantage, the speaker must be involved. A person with hearing problems needs to use clear and specific language when asking for assistance from other people. For example, "Please talk more slowly [loudly, clearly]. I can't hear you well"; "Please turn your face toward me. I can't understand what you are saying"; "Please spell that word. I don't hear what it is"; "Could you repeat that number? I couldn't hear it well."

Some large hospitals have facilities for teaching communication strategies, including speechreading. In some cases these clinics may offer hearing tests and other services more cheaply than elsewhere. Hearing therapy, either individual or group, can help you choose the methods of communicating — including speechreading and using a hearing aid — that suit you best.

Resources

Publications

"Introduction to Speechreading" by Mark Ross, Ph.D., and Karen Webb, M.S. An overview of speechreading. FREE with SSE. New York League for the Hard of Hearing, 71 West 23rd Street, New York, NY 10010, (212) 741-3143.

Videotapes

I See What You're Saying: A Practical Guide to Speechreading. One instructional tape and one practice tape provide strategies for understanding speech in various situations. Narrated by Gene Wilder. The 110-minute instructional tape and handbook, $85. The 65-minute practice tape, $50. Practice tape, instructional tape, and handbook, $120. New York League for the Hard of Hearing, 71 West 23rd Street, New York, NY 10010, (212) 741-3143.

Read My Lips. Self-paced instruction with everyday listening situations. Six 1-hour tapes, $195. Hear You Are catalog, (800) 278-EARS (3277).

Lipreading Made Easy by Audrey B. Greenwald, M.S. Practice material for lipreading. Eighteen captioned lessons. More than 2 hours long. $75. Alexander Graham Bell Association for the Deaf, 3417 Volta Place, NW, Washington, DC 20007, (202) 337-5220.

Learning Speechreading Videotape Series. Tapes cover all speech sounds and provide three practice sections. Four 30- to 50-minute tapes, $58 each. Hear You Are catalog, (800) 278-EARS (3277).

The first time you try a hearing aid you may discover a lost world of sound: the background noises that create your environment — birds singing, pots banging, people calling to one another, refrigerators humming.

Like other devices — glasses or contact lenses, a cane or a walker, a microwave oven — you have to learn how to use a hearing aid properly in order to reap its benefits. As many as 50 percent of those who have hearing aids don't use them because they never learned how they could most benefit from them, and nearly 75 percent of those who could improve their hearing by using aids don't have them because of a reluctance to let others know they have hearing problems.

A hearing aid doesn't correct hearing loss the way eyeglasses do for vision problems. The human ear perceives frequencies between 0 and 20,000 Hz, but a hearing aid range is between 200 and 6,000 Hz. The hearing aid is merely one strategy, and an imperfect one, to assist communication for people with hearing loss.

Since the mechanism of a hearing aid is relatively simple, it may seem that you merely insert the ear mold, hook up the receiver, put in the batteries, and turn it on to be in business. But you need to practice using it in a variety of situations in order to get used to it and learn how it can help when you need it. At first everything will seem much too loud, so you must gradually increase the volume as you adapt to hearing new sounds. As you become accustomed to using the hearing aid in various situations, you will notice progress. Though at times it may seem slow, your persistence will pay off if you stick with it.

The sound a hearing aid transmits is first received and amplified electronically, so it sounds like what you hear on a radio. It won't let you hear birds or other sounds *exactly* as you used to. In addition, a hearing aid makes *all* sounds louder. This is some help for people with sensitivity problems, but it can't help with sound discrimination. If many people are speaking at once, you have to learn, or relearn, how to focus on the person you want to hear.

The initial adjustment to a hearing aid involves becoming accustomed to sounds you haven't been used to hearing, particularly high tones, like the telephone. The adjustment process should begin in a quiet place. You can listen to how your own voice sounds, the sound of dishes being washed, the toilet flushing, and so on. Now talk to one visitor, then to more than one person at a time. Over a month or more, gradually begin to use the hearing aid full-time in a variety of situations.

Hearing aid technology has focused on making the device smaller, as a means of concealing it better. The smaller aids may respond to your vanity, but unfortunately they provide fewer features than larger ones. Behind-the-ear and in-the-ear hearing aids are the most popular; few people choose eyeglass aids or body aids anymore. In-the-canal aids are even smaller than in-the-ear and offer fewer features. The smaller size also requires smaller controls, which may be difficult for some people to manipulate. Most people discover that a hearing aid in each ear can provide a more natural background of sound.

You will need to compare aids according to their performance in four areas:

1. Gain: the amount of amplification. New models have automatic gain control, which reduces amplification in very noisy environments or when a loud noise like a fire alarm goes off, so that it isn't amplified and doesn't hurt your ear.
2. Frequency range: the ability of the aid to amplify sounds at the higher and lower tones. Tone controls allow you to adjust the frequency according to your needs at a given moment.
3. Maximum power output: the loudest volume setting.
4. Distortion: the accuracy of the sounds.

A T-switch, incorporated into the aid, will allow you to use the hearing aid with other amplifiers, such as the telephone and TV. You can simply flip the switch to avoid feedback from these devices.

Most hearing aids can amplify high-frequency sounds, such as *th, s,* and *f* and bird sounds and can filter out low-frequency background noise, such as a vacuum cleaner or an ocean's roar. So far, however, a hearing aid cannot block a restaurant's clatter so that you hear only the conversation at your table; in fact, the noise in the restaurant is also amplified.

This is a purchase that should *not* be made by mail order. Before you purchase a hearing aid, federal law requires that a doctor certify that your hearing may be improved with an aid, ruling out medical conditions that may need treatment. After a physician's examination and hearing tests by an audiologist, you should consult a hearing aid salesperson about which style and type are best for you.

The device must be fitted properly and should be accompanied by instructions and continuing support with advice about using the aid in various situations and responses to your questions and problems. A trial period, sometimes offered for a special fee, can help you be certain you haven't made a mistake. Although you will need time to get used to a hearing aid, the ear mold, and the unnatural sound, there are several shortcomings you shouldn't tolerate.

When to Return a Hearing Aid

When the aid doesn't help you hear better
When the aid hurts your ear, is too loose, or otherwise doesn't feel comfortable
When the sound is too loud
When the sound echoes or is metallic

The cost of a hearing aid is not reimbursed by Medicare or most private insurance plans, but it *is* deductible as a medical expense on your income tax. Hearing aids are available FREE for some American war veterans.

New Developments

* For people whose hearing loss is not remedied by a hearing aid, a cochlear implant may restore the ability to hear. This surgically implanted device transmits sounds by means of directly stimulating the auditory nerve, in the absence of hair cells that formerly triggered the nerve.
* Studies are being initiated to understand how newer technological advances in signal processing can be used to assist various components of hearing. This is particularly relevant to equipment designed to help people hear well in a noisy environment.

61

Products

High-Frequency Amplifier. A hunter designed this device to amplify animal sounds over other noises, without amplifying noise over 110 dB (like a gunshot). Weighs less than one ounce, worn behind the ear with a soft earpiece. $180. Walker's "Game Ear," Inc., P.O. Box 1069, Media, PA 19063, (800) 424-1069.

Super Ear Amplifier. A microphone receives sounds that are amplified with a pocket-size box to enable you to use stereo headphones to hear theater performances, TV, or classroom lectures. $26. Accessolutions catalog, (800) 445-9968.

Services

National Hearing Aid Bank. Used or reconditioned hearing aids are supplied to those who cannot afford to purchase them. Also offers grants or low-interest loans to purchase hearing devices or cochlear implants. HEAR NOW, 9745 East Hampden Avenue, Suite 300, Denver, CO 80231, (800) 648-4327.

Hearing Aid Helpline. Offers information on symptoms and treatments and a FREE literature kit. Answers questions about hearing loss and hearing devices and helps resolve problems with devices. Send for a list of your state's hearing instrument specialists, members of the International Hearing Society, an association of hearing aid professionals. IHS, 20361 Middlebelt Road, Livonia, MI 48152, (800) 521-5247.

Publications

"A Consumer's Guide for Purchasing a Hearing Aid" by Patricia Ann Clickener. A brochure providing a detailed list of what to expect during the fitting and choosing of a hearing aid. SHHH Information Series No. 102. $2. Self Help for Hard of Hearing People, 7910 Woodmont Avenue, Suite 1200, Bethesda, MD 20814, (301) 657-2248.

"How to Buy a Hearing Aid," National Association for Hearing and Speech Action. A question-and-answer guide to hearing problems and hearing aid selection. FREE. American Speech-Language-Hearing Association, 10801 Rockville Pike, Rockville, MD 20852, (800) 638-8255.

"How to Buy a Hearing Aid," *Consumer Reports* magazine. A step-by-step guide to determining what to look for when you are in the market for a hearing aid, including a description of features and advice on finding a reputable audiologist. $3. Consumers Union, Reprints Department, 101 Truman Avenue, Yonkers, NY 10703, (914) 378-2448.

"Hearing Aids," Department of Veterans Affairs. The results of the DVA's annual hearing aid testing program, which tests aids voluntarily submitted by manufacturers. FREE. DVA, Veterans Health Services and Research Administration, Washington, DC 20420.

"Hearing Aids: A Link to the World," Food and Drug Administration. Explains the functions and operation of hearing aids and what to consider when you purchase one. FREE. Center for Devices and Radiological Health, 1350 Piccard Drive, Rockville, MD 20850, (800) 638-2041.

"All about the New Generation of Hearing Aids" by Cynthia L. Compton, Lee Van Middlesworth, and Loraine Di Pietro. Describes various new types of hearing aids; how they work; advantages and disadvantages of each. $2. National Information Center on Deafness, Gallaudet University, 800 Florida Avenue, NE, Washington, DC 20002, (202) 651-5051.

"About Assistive Listening Devices," American Speech-Language-Hearing Association. A brief discussion of devices other than hearing aids that can help you hear better. FREE. ASLHA, 10801 Rockville Pike, Rockville, MD 20852, (800) 638-8255.

Organizations

Cochlear Implant Club International. A membership organization that provides information and support for people interested in cochlear implants. P.O. Box 464, Buffalo, NY 14223.

Hearing Dogs

A trained hearing dog can alert you to a ringing telephone, the doorbell, or other household and street sounds, such as timers, clock alarms, buzzers, and smoke alarms. Such a dog may provide the security and confidence that will allow you to remain in your own home. If you feel comfortable owning a dog, but don't think you need one with special training, you'll find that most dogs react instinctively to some of these noises.

Sources of dogs trained to assist people with a variety of needs are mentioned in Chapter 15, "Feeling Safe on the Road."

Publications

"Hearing Ear Dogs," National Information Center on Deafness. A list of Hearing Ear Dog training programs. $1. NICD, Gallaudet University, 800 Florida Avenue, NE, Washington, DC 20002, (202) 651-5051.

"Hearing Dog Programs," Self Help for Hard of Hearing People. $3. SHHH Publications, 7910 Woodmont Avenue, Suite 1200, Bethesda, MD 20814, (301) 657-2248.

"Directory of Animal Support Programs for People Who Have Disabilities." For visual and physical as well as hearing needs. FREE. Information Center for Individuals with Disabilities, Fort Point Place, 27-43 Wormwood Street, Boston, MA 02210, (617) 727-5540.

Organizations

Dogs for the Deaf, Inc. Provides trained dogs to deaf and hearing-impaired individuals. FREE. Dogs are rescued from the pound and trained to recognize sounds. 10175 Wheeler Road, Central Point, OR 97502, (503) 826-9220.

International Hearing Dog Inc. Dogs are placed FREE. Every state except Hawaii gives hearing dogs the same privileges as blind guide dogs. 5901 East 89th Avenue, Henderson, CO 80640, (303) 287-3277.

Delta Society. Promotes mutually beneficial contacts among people, animals, and nature. Provides information on taking care of pets, the health benefits of owning animals, and resources such as hearing ear dog programs. P.O. Box 1080, Renton, WA 98057, (800) 869-6898.

TELEPHONE CONVERSATION

The telephone is a social link as well as a safety link. Both incoming and outgoing aspects of the telephone must work for you — that is, you have to be able to hear both the ringing and the conversation.

In order to maintain your connections to friends and family, you can install an answering machine or service as a backup, in case you don't hear the phone ring. Some phone companies now offer voice mail services that incorporate an answering machine into your own phone. These can store messages for you while you are on the phone with someone else. Return call is a service that automatically redials the number of the last individual who called you, in case you don't get to the phone in time to answer. A fax, or facsimile machine, alleviates concerns about hearing messages correctly since the message is received in printed form.

A text telephone (TTY) eliminates the need to hear or speak by conveying messages you type on a keyboard and can see displayed on a screen. If you are telephoning another person with a TTY, both parties will be connected through normal telephone lines. A FREE relay service is provided by all telephone companies to allow TTY users to communicate with people using standard telephones. The Telecommunications Relay Service (TRS) provides a communications assistant who acts as an intermediary by conveying conversation from text to voice and voice to text, as needed.

Resources

Using the telephone to call for help, including personal emergency response systems, is discussed in Chapter 14, "Preparing for Emergencies."

Products

Phone Equipment and Components. Radio Shack, a nationwide chain of electronic supply stores, stocks a variety of reasonably priced amplifiers, big-button phones, automatic dialers, and other phone-related products.

Equipment and Supplies for Enhancing Communication by Telephone:

> Accessolutions catalog, (800) 445-9968
> Harris Communications catalog, (800) 825-6758
> Hear-More catalog, (800) 881-HEAR (4327)
> Hear You Are catalog, (800) 278-EARS (3277)
> Hello Direct catalog, (800) 444-3556
> Maxi-Aids catalog, (800) 522-6294

Potomac Technology catalog, (800) 433-2838

Text Telephones (TTYs)

AT&T Telecommunication Device. Via recorded message, informs callers without TTYs to use the relay service. Can print out a conversation and display messages on a screen. You can dial the phone directly from the keyboard. Basic device, $350. With answering machine, $450. With answering machine and printer, $600. Hello Direct catalog, (800) 444-3556.

Minicom IV Telecommunications Display Device. A basic model, easily portable. $240. Hitec Group International catalog, (800) 288-8303.

Superprint TDD. Saves and sends messages and prints out conversation. $480. Potomac Technology catalog, (800) 433-2838.

Portable Display Telephone Typewriter. Standard, $250. American Communication Corporation, 180 Roberts Street, East Hartford, CT 06108, (203) 528-9821.

Uniphone 1000. Combination text telephone and standard telephone with amplified handset. Enables hearing and hard-of-hearing usage with one unit. $230. Harris Communications catalog, (800) 825-6758.

Easy-to-Hear Phone Ringers

TelBell. Extravolume ringer sounds an old-fashioned ring rather than an electronic-sounding ring. Volume control. $20. Hello Direct catalog, (800) 444-3556.

Tel Warble. Volume control amplifies warble up to 90 decibels. $50. Hello Direct catalog, (800) 444-3556.

TelHorn. Horn or warble up to 105 decibels. $130. Hello Direct catalog, (800) 444-3556.

Adjustable Ringer. Ring volume, tone, and warble can be customized to the pitch that's best for you. $35. Potomac Technology catalog, (800) 433-2838.

Outdoor or Indoor Loud Bell. Hammer strikes two 4-inch gongs. $75. Hear You Are catalog, (800) 278-EARS (3277).

Super Phone-Ringer. Volume adjusts to 95 decibels, and tone is variable to suit individual requirements. $40. Harris Communications catalog, (800) 825-6758.

Auxiliary Mechanical Bell Ringer. To hear phone ring even where there is no extension, this plugs into phone jack. $12. Independent Living Aids catalog, (800) 537-2118.

No–Bell Ringer. Replaces ringer with music or other sounds. $100. Ann Morris Enterprises catalog, (516) 292-9232.

Flashing Light Signals for Telephone Ring

TelStrobe. A high-intensity flashing light to substitute for a ring. $90. Hello Direct catalog, (800) 444-3556.

Flashing Lamp Telephone Ring Alerter. Plug lamp and phone into alerter, and light will flash every time the phone rings. Also includes an on/off switch to operate the lamp. $33. Independent Living Aids catalog, (800) 537-2118.

Teleflash. A sensor you place near your phone's ringer signals you with a bright strobe light and a loud tone. Hello Direct catalog, (800) 444-3556.

Easy Dialing

Touchable Phone Buttons. Fits over push-button desk phones. Black with white numbers. $13. Visual Aids catalog. In eastern states call (212) 889-3141; in western states call (415) 221-3201.

Larger Push Buttons. For any standard phone. $8. Enrichments catalog, (800) 323-5547.

Stick-on Buttons. For push-button phones. Larger, easier-to-read numbers. FREE. AT&T Accessible Communications Products Center, 14250 Clayton Road, Ballwin, MO 63011, (800) 233-1222.

Large Number Overlay. For rotary phones. Doubles the size of numbers on rotary phones. FREE. AT&T Accessible Communications Products Center, 14250 Clayton Road, Ballwin, MO 63011, (800) 233-1222.

Big Button Phone. Three emergency numbers can be dialed automatically. Hearing aid-compatible. $50. Independent Living Aids catalog, (800) 537-2188.

Lighted Big Button Phone. Four emergency memory buttons, plus ten additional memory buttons; other features. $40. Bruce Medical Supply catalog, (800) 225-8446.

Operator Dialer. Only for push-button phones with three- by four-button arrangement. Press anywhere on the surface to reach an operator. FREE. AT&T Accessible Communications Products Center, 14250 Clayton Road, Ballwin, MO 63011, (800) 233-1222.

Databank Dialer. Pocket-size device dials with tones at the touch of a button after you key numbers and place it near the handset. Many features: stores 200 names, addresses, and phone numbers; clock and alarm. $50. Hello Direct catalog, (800) 444-3556.

Talking Phone. Hear the numbers as you dial to verify your accuracy. $34. Ann Morris Enterprises catalog, (516) 292-9232.

Voice Recognition Dialing. As you speak the name of the person whom you wish to call, the number is dialed automatically. For fifty voice-recall names, $330. Maxi-Aids catalog, (800) 522-6294.

Receivers

Phone Receiver Hand Grip. An open handle that can be mounted on the phone to provide an alternative to grasping receiver. Velcro or suction cups attachment. $6. Enrichments catalog, (800) 323-5547.

Speak Easy. Hands-free headset with volume control, a twenty-four-inch cord, and belt clip. $25. Independent Living Aids catalog, (800) 537-2118.

Handset Amplifier. Connects to both phone and handset, allows adjustment of volume more than three times that of a standard handset. $40. Hello Direct catalog, (800) 444-3556.

Amplified Handset. Hearing aid-compatible handset allows volume to be increased as much as 25 percent, up to 25 decibels, about three times normal levels. $50. Potomac Technology catalog, (800) 433-2838.

Telephone Amplifier. Adjustable volume. $8. Carol Wright Gifts catalog, (402) 474-4465.

Telephones and Jacks

Plug-In Phone Jack. Just plug unit into an outlet, and you can connect a second phone. $80. Hear-More catalog, (800) 881-HEAR (4327).

TeleTalker. Renders conversations both louder and clearer for someone with slight to severe hearing loss. Caller's voice is amplified up to thirty times without amplifying background noises. Separate volume and clarity controls. Large buttons. $300. Harris Communications catalog, (800) 825-6758.

Universal Phone. Large buttons, flashing light for incoming calls, volume control, three emergency number buttons. $80. Ann Morris Enterprises catalog, (516) 292-9232.

Cordless Telephone. Functions up to a thousand feet from base. $80. Independent Living Aids catalog, (800) 537-2118.

Clarity Phone. Makes speech sound louder and clearer by increasing the volume of only high-frequency sounds with adjustable tone equalizer. Hearing aid-compatible. Easy-to-hear low-frequency ring. $100. Accessolutions catalog, (800) 445-9968.

Tel-Ease Telephone. Ringer adjusts up to 90 dB and indicator light flashes when telephone rings. Handset volume can be amplified and is hearing aid-compatible. $100. LS&S Group catalog, (800) 468-4789, or in Illinois call (708) 498-9777.

Remote Control Speaker Phone. Answer and dial by pressing a single button. Includes volume control and backup battery. $500. Accessolutions catalog, (800) 445-9968.

Combination Answering Machine and Speakerphone. Digital recording eliminates need for tapes. $200. Hello Direct catalog, (800) 444-3556.

Speakerphone with Memory. Hearing aid-compatible phone that speed-dials ten numbers. Take calls over the speakerphone or with headset, purchased separately. $115. Hello Direct catalog, (800) 444-3556.

Services

"Facts About Telecommunications Relay Services," National Institute on Deafness and Other Communication Disorders. A list by state of telephone numbers for relay service. FREE. NIDCD Clearinghouse, 1 Communication Avenue, Bethesda, MD 20892, (800) 241-1044.

Directory Assistance for Text Telephone Users. An alternative to 411 to request your state's relay service number, text telephone numbers, or voice numbers. (800) 855-1155.

Tele-Consumer Hotline. Provides publications and assistance for telephone users, including a directory of services that relay messages between TTY users and hearing callers, as well as consumers' guides for telephone products. Fact sheets specifically designed for each state explain the telephone relay procedure and other special services and how to use them. Fact sheets available to help you choose a long-distance company and for sources that lend equipment or provide grants for special equipment. FREE with SSE. 1331 H Street,

NW, Suite 201, Washington, DC 20005.

AT&T Accessible Communications Products Center. Advice about solving communications problems with special telephones, ringers, handsets, signaling devices. Service and equipment available at discount prices. 14250 Clayton Road, Ballwin, MO 63011, (800) 233-1222.

Publications

Telephone Strategies: A Technical and Practical Guide for Hard-of-Hearing People by Diane L. Castle, Ph.D. Suggestions for understanding information given by phone and how to use phones when you have a hearing aid. $6.50. Self Help for Hard of Hearing People, 7910 Woodmont Avenue, Suite 1200, Bethesda, MD 20814, (301) 657-2248.

Official Guide to Buying, Connecting and Using Consumer Electronics Products, Electronic Industries Association. Information in laymen's terms to help you buy, install, and maintain such products as telephones, VCRs, and computers. $9. EIA Consumer Electronics Group/CE Book, 2500 Wilson Boulevard, Arlington, VA 22201, (703) 907-7626.

Organizations

Telecommunications for the Deaf, Inc. Provides information about purchasing and using text telephones (TTYs). Compiles a phone directory of TTY users and a list of state relay service numbers. 8719 Colesville Road, Suite 300, Silver Spring, MD 20910, (301) 589-3786.

Chapter 4

Looking Your Best

Everyone is influenced by first impressions, despite the wisdom of the adage that cautions us against judging the contents of a book by its cover. Making an effort to look one's best is a signal of self-esteem and a social greeting, a sign of receptivity to meeting and being among people.

Appearances may deceive, beauty be only skin-deep, but the faces we show the world reflect something from within. As a mirror of mood and self-worth, appearance is not a trivial matter.

CLOTHING

"Nothing fits!"

Changes in body shape that are due to a gradual loss of muscle tissue may occur after age sixty. This accounts for a loss of weight after age fifty-five that is not necessarily accompanied by a slimmer shape. Body fat deposits also change as fat accumulates in deeper sites, while subcutaneous fat thins. Breasts change their shape, the waist thickens, the abdomen or stomach protrudes, and buttocks flatten. Changes in posture and loss of height from compression of vertebrae or loss of bone mass also affect the way clothes hang on your body.

The fashion industry's focus on the youth market creates problems for the mature body, particularly for women. Not only do clothes fit differently, but certain styles seem inappropriate for a mature lifestyle. Many people have the disheartening experience of trying on everything in their sizes and thinking that nothing fits or looks appropriate. This explains why some people wind up wearing clothes that look unfashionable — worn out, out of style, and "old."

Problems Selecting Clothes

- Colors may be perceived differently because of the clouding of the lens of the eye as cataracts develop. You may be buying sharper, brighter, or uncoordinated colors because it is harder for you to distinguish accurately among them.
- Stores and departments where you used to shop don't stock clothes that fit you well.
- Clothes are difficult to put on because of rows of buttons, long zippers up the back, etc.
- Current fashions are too "young"-looking.
- Clothes that fit well are too "old"-looking.

Women's clothing sizes are based on measurements taken during World War II of women in the military, nearly all of whom were under fifty years old. In 1992 the Institute for Standards Research conducted a nationwide sizing study to create the first database of body measurements of women age fifty-five and older for apparel sizing. This should result in the introduction of a new size category designed for seniors based on the proportional changes that were documented in measurements of shoulder, back length, bust, waist, abdomen, and upper arm. Interviews with the seven thousand women who were measured confirmed that they were dissatisfied with the fit of clothing and sewing patterns. Most of the differences from the earlier measurements were due to postural changes, spinal curvature, and relocation of muscle and fat. Until those new fashions are available, however, there are some steps you can take to look your best and feel good about it.

Gray hair and pale skin can be enlivened by wearing clothing in bright colors and avoiding earth tones, like gray, camel, brown, and off-white.

Available handy devices can help with various aspects of getting dressed: buttoning, zipping, pulling up pants, socks, or stockings, and putting on shoes. A dressing hook (a wand with a hook at one end) can be inserted in the loops in the waistbands of skirts or pants to pull them up. When a button hook is inserted through a buttonhole, it can be looped around to drag the button back through. This is not difficult when the button is on the front of a garment.

Shirt cuff buttons can be bypassed completely by attaching the button permanently to the *outside* of the buttonhole and using a Velcro attachment to close the cuff. As an alternative, elastic thread looped around the button will allow expansion so you can get your hand through the cuff without having to undo the button.

A zipper pull is a wand that hooks on to the zipper tab and raises or lowers the zipper as you pull. Some zippers, particularly back zippers, may need an extra loop or ring added to the tab.

A shoehorn helps your foot slide into a shoe. You may brace the shoe against a wall to provide some resistance as you push your foot in. The shoehorn or a bootjack also can be used to help push your shoe off without bending. Tying and untying shoelaces can be avoided with a lace clip, fashioned like a western tie holder, that locks the laces in place and loosens them when it is pulled up. Elastic shoelaces expand easily to release your foot without being untied, and some shoes have Velcro closings or can be adapted by gluing on Velcro closings.

Sweatpants or jogging suits, usually generously cut, with elastic waists and cuffs, are comfortable to wear and easy to get in and out of. Today's casual lifestyle is reflected in the widespread acceptance far from athletic fields of these sporty outfits, many of which are quite elegant.

Clothes shopping can be exhausting, particularly when it involves the repeated trying on of garments. Most people find that friends are the best shopping helpers. Let your friend know what you need most, be it an objective and truthful eye, help with dressing, or simple reassurance.

Mail-order catalogs offer underwear, shoes, and clothing for a large range of occasions and requirements. Catalog shopping allows you to evaluate clothes in the privacy of your home, at your own pace. Most mail-order clothing establishments try to help you select the sizes and colors you need when you order by phone. Usually they have liberal returns or exchange policies. Of course, it's wise to clarify the company's policy before you place an order. If you are able to sew your own clothing or can make alterations in a ready-made garment, you can also buy by mail the equipment and supplies for this.

Resources

Ideas for minimizing changes in body shape through physical activity can be found in Chapter 9, "Achieving the Four Elements of Mobility," and Chapter 10, "On the Move."

Products

Dressing Aids

Implements to Help with Dressing:
>AdaptAbility catalog, (800) 243-9232
>AfterTherapy catalog, (800) 235-7054
>Easy Street catalog, (800) 959-EASY (3279)
>Enrichments catalog, (800) 323-5547
>Maxi-Aids catalog, (800) 522-6294
>TASH ADL catalog, (416) 686-4129

Bracelet Helper. Holds one end of a bracelet while you attach the clasp. $5. Carol Wright catalog, (402) 474-4465.

Stocking Pull-On. Elastic straps attach to top of the stocking, and a plastic insert allows your foot to slide through to the toe. Then you pull the stocking up, using the straps. Carol Wright catalog, (402) 474-4465.

Button Aid and Zipper Pull Set. Choose either 1/2- or 7/8-inch-diameter handles. $4. Enrichments catalog, (800) 323-5547.

Zipper Pull. For inconvenient zippers, especially back zippers. Includes ten rings to attach to zipper tabs. $10. Bruce Medical Supply catalog, (800) 225-8446.

Button Helper. $4. Carol Wright catalog, (402) 474-4465.

Shoe Horns. Stainless steel version comes in 18-, 24-, or 30-inch lengths, about $8. 16-inch plastic, $2. Enrichments catalog, (800) 323-5547.

Clothing

T-shirt. Two Velcro-fastening side seams. Short-sleeved, choice of colors. $20. Very Special Clothing catalog, (800) 283-3094.

Clothes for Men and Women Who Use Wheelchairs or People with Continence Problems. All wash-and-wear, easy closings, such as snaps, wraparound styles, or Velcro closings. Pantsuits, pajamas, slips, underwear, stockings, socks, slippers, and shoes available. Fashion Ease catalog, (800) 221-8929.

Women's Underwear and Casual Clothes:
National Wholesale Company catalog, (704) 249-0211
Sears Home HealthCare catalog, (800) 326-1750

Clothing for Wheelchair Users. Avenues catalog, (800) 848-2837.

Women's Stockings. Includes a large choice of support styles, shoes, underwear. Support Plus catalog, (800) 229-2910.

Women's Suits, Pants, Tops, Skirts. In sizes from small and petite to tall, large, and half sizes. Blair Mail Order catalog, (800) 458-6057.

Men's and Women's Suits and Dresses. All with Velcro closings, elasticized waists. JC Penney's Easy Dressing Fashions catalog, (800) 222-6161.

Women's Natural-Fiber (Mainly Cotton) Underwear and Casual Clothes. Back to Basics Soft-Wear catalog, (919) 682-8611.

Sewing Items

My Double Dress Form. Waist adjusts for size and for high or low waist. Petite, small, or medium, $120. Full figure, $130. Atlanta Thread and Supply catalog, (800) 847-1001.

Mr. Ardis Male Tailoring Form. Adjustable chest, waist, hips, and neck. $120. Atlanta Thread and Supply catalog, (800) 847-1001.

Hook and Loop Tape. Twenty-five-yard reels each, hook or loop, choice of color. ⅝ inch, $10. Atlanta Thread and Supply catalog, (800) 847-1001.

Needle Threader. For both hand and machine needles. 25 cents. Atlanta Thread and Supply catalog, (800) 847-1001.

Witch Automatic Threader. You position the needle and thread and press a button to operate; a blade is placed to cut the thread. $2. Easier Ways catalog, (410) 659-0232.

Work Holder. A flexible post clamps to the table and holds a frame for sewing or embroidering or a knitting or crochet needle as you work. $60. Cleo of New York catalog, (800) 321-0595.

Publications

Dressing with Pride by Evelyn S. Kennedy. Step-by-step instructions for adapting clothes for your needs. Also shopping and dressing tips. $15. Promote Real Independence for the Disabled and Elderly (PRIDE), Box 1293, 391 Long Hill Road, Groton, CT 06340, (203) 445-1448.

SKIN

The skin's appearance is affected over time by exposure to the sun, the loss of fat under the skin's surface, and a slowing in the renewal of skin cells. These result in the loss of skin tone, dry skin, "liver spots," and bruises that seem to arise "from nowhere."

Skin cells in a person over age sixty are renewed over a sixty-day period, a process that takes only thirty days in a young adult. This translates into the slower creation of new cells and the longer retention of older ones, making the skin less elastic and drier. Thinner skin provides less protection for fragile blood vessels, resulting in easier bruising. Large bruises can appear even when you don't remember bumping into anything. A decline in the network of capillaries — the smallest of the body's blood vessels that supply the skin — reduces blood flow to the skin. This causes a translucent or pallid appearance, a more rapid reaction to cold temperatures, and slowness in warming up.

You can find new ways of maintaining your appearance, using magnifying mirrors to see better or products that reduce the effort you need to expend to shave, apply makeup, or accomplish other grooming tasks.

Although an electric razor does not provide the close shave you may be used to getting with a regular razor and shaving cream, consider experimenting with one if you have been getting a "nick" every day. New battery-powered razors are designed for use with shaving cream, so you can keep the familiar feeling as you make the transition. A shaving cream or gel may be easier to dispense from a tube than from a canister. To simplify the process further, squeeze a supply into the sink and scoop it up. You can hold the razor steady and move your face, rather than the other way around, if it seems easier.

Women may need to experiment with new cosmetics; blush, a brighter lipstick, and some color around the eyes may help the paleness that comes from reduced blood flow to the skin. A porcelain base under makeup will neutralize a ruddy look or sallowness. Subtle applications of blue mascara and blue pencil around the eyes enhance the white of the eye and reduce the appearance of redness under or around the eye. If you can't decide whether you have overdone your makeup, inadvertently creating a "clown" face, check with a trusted friend or a cosmetics adviser in a department store.

You may develop a skin sensitivity to ingredients in some cosmetics or skin care products, because of either changes in the product's formulation or alterations in your skin's chemistry. Experiment with products made without fragrance or preservatives, like the Basis brand. Protect your hands from soaps, sun, and wind by wearing gloves and using hand creams, preferably one containing sunscreen.

Resources

Products

Magnifying Mirror. Two-sided chrome mirror. One side magnifies two and one-half times, swivels to a regular mirror. Angle adjusts, arm extends from six to twenty-eight inches, and base attaches firmly with suction. Folds flat. $13. Visual Aids catalog, (212) 889-3141.

Lighted Triple Mirror. Fluorescent lights illuminate central mirror and two swiveling side mirrors. Includes outlet for other appliances. $35. LS&S Group catalog, (800) 468-4789.

Variable Magnification Mirror. Adjust magnification from 1× to 5× or any point in between by rotating the mirror's frame. Attaches to tabletop with suction cups. Position with eight-inch-long flexible arm. $35. Comfort House catalog, (800) 359-7701.

Personal Care Magnified Lighted Mirror. Magnifies three times. $70. Self Care catalog, (800) 345-3371.

Five Power Magnification Compact Mirror. Measures 2¼-inch diameter, with regular mirror too. $12. Visual Aids catalog, (212) 889-3141.

Magnifying Make-Up Glasses. Lenses flip down to allow viewing through one lens while you make up other eye. $10. Bruce Medical Supply catalog, (800) 225-8446.

Adjustable Tilt Mirror. Stainless steel frame with piano hinges allowing easy positioning for seated or standing use. Available in various sizes. 16 by 30 inches high, $105. Adaptations catalog, (800) 688-1758.

Wrinkles

Preventing wrinkles would be easy if we never used our facial muscles, but when we crinkle our eyes in a squint, crease our cheeks in a smile, or raise our eyebrows in question, we eventually acquire wrinkles. Smokers in particular get fine lines around the mouth; frowners get frown lines. Smoking more than triples the average person's likelihood of developing premature facial wrinkles. Exposure to the sun *plus* smoking increases the risk twelvefold.

While it's hard to find anyone who welcomes a wrinkle, people react differently when wrinkles appear. Some people regard wrinkles as well earned and are philosophical about them, others feel a diminished sense of self-worth, and still others would do anything to recover their youthful, smooth-skinned looks. This last group is the target of manufacturers of products claiming to eliminate wrinkles, make the user look younger, and reverse the aging process. The main focus in such campaigns is on smoothing the skin by restoring collagen, the substance in cells that supports the skin.

Some wrinkle treatments are only of temporary value, and some are completely worthless. For temporary improvement of wrinkles, options include:

Autologous fat transplants. In this process collagen from your own body is injected to fill deep wrinkles or scars. Depending on the rate at which your body reabsorbs the collagen, the results last from six weeks to three years, longer for younger people.

Collagen injections. Collagen derived from cowhide is an effective means of puffing out a wrinkle temporarily. Individuals respond to the treatment differently: The collagen may take several weeks to smooth the wrinkle, and it may be reabsorbed and lose its value at different rates.

Retin-A. This cream, gel, or liquid is available only by

prescription and is approved by the FDA only for treatment of acne, but it has also been found to remove fine, recent wrinkles. Sometimes it causes unpleasant skin reactions during the first weeks of use, and its long-term safety is not known.

Electric stimulation machine. Mild electric current is applied to the skin to smooth wrinkles temporarily or to encourage the skin's regeneration. Improvement from electric stimulation of the skin has not been scientifically proved. NOTE: The FDA has found electric stimulation of facial *muscles* to make them contract UNSAFE and ineffective for facial toning.

Moisturizer. Deep wrinkles may become less noticeable when a moisturizer is used regularly, as the skin becomes smoother, more pliable, and less dry.

Be alert to these items that are worthless for wrinkle repair and may not be safe to use:

Creams that contain collagen or elastin. These cannot penetrate to cells beneath the surface of the skin where collagen and elastin have been depleted.

Liquid silicone injections. This widely used method of eliminating wrinkles has not been approved for use on humans.

Amino acids and liposomes. These substances have not been found to have any long-term benefit to the skin as ingredients in lotions or creams.

Resources

Products

Cosmetics:
Beautiful Times catalog, (800) 223-1216
Home Health Products catalog, (800) 284-9123

Natural Soaps and Cosmetics. Walnut Acres catalog, (800) 433-3998.
Automatic Liquid Dispenser. When you place your hand under the sensor, liquid soap, shampoo, or lotions can be dispensed automatically. Mounts on wall or sits on countertop for use in shower or kitchen. $45. Home Trends catalog, (716) 254-6520.

Publications

Cosmetics Buying Guide by Andrew J. Scheman, M.D., and David L. Severson. Lists ingredients by brand name, indicates which substances may cause allergic reactions, and evaluates products' claims. 1993. Consumer Reports Books.

Skin Spots

The sun takes a cumulative toll on the skin. Damage to the skin occurs because of exposure to the sun's ultraviolet A (UVA) and ultraviolet B (UVB) rays. UVA rays penetrate deeply, though slowly, into the skin. UVB rays are more quickly damaging. Parts of the body that have been exposed to the sun develop brown spots as the result of changes in the skin's pigmentation.

Types of Skin Discolorations

- Freckles.
- Beauty marks or moles: darker freckles. Most light-skinned adults have fifteen to twenty moles.
- Liver spots or lentigines: flat, colored spots, darker than a freckle, lighter than a mole. Usually appear on the face or back of the hand.
- Dysplastic spots: moles with irregular borders and various shades of color. These are more likely to become malignant than single-color moles with even borders.

NOTE: Any changes in the color or shape of spots or any spots that itch or bleed should be seen by a physician and possibly a dermatologist.

Avoiding exposure to the sun is the only way to avoid getting more spots. To do this, apply sunscreen daily, even when it's cloudy. Check the sun protection factor (SPF) value on the package. With SPF 15, for example, you can expose yourself to the sun fifteen times longer than without sunscreen before getting a sunburn. Use at least one ounce of sunscreen to cover your face, hands, neck, ears, and body. Ultraviolet rays can penetrate thin clothing, several feet underwater, and can reflect off sand, snow, water, and concrete, so sunscreen should be used regardless of weather or season. Apply it half an hour before exposure to the sun so that it can be absorbed by the skin and will be less likely to be washed away by perspiration. If possible, avoid exposing your skin to the sun, even with sunscreen, between 10:00 A.M. and 3:00 P.M.; schedule your outdoor activities with this in mind.

Some people are allergic to PABA, the ingredient in sunscreen that protects against UVB, and experience puffiness and red, rashy, or itchy skin reactions. Sunscreens that contain substances, such as benzophenones and anthranilates, are less likely to provoke allergic reactions. For people whose skin reacts adversely to benzophenone, two products without it or PABA are Clinique's City Block SPF 13 and Hawaiian Tropics Baby Faces Natural Sunblock. These contain a derivative of zinc oxide that rarely causes allergic reactions. Look for sunscreens with "broad-spectrum" protection. These include protection from both UVA and UVB rays.

Ask your physician or pharmacist if any medication you are taking is a photosensitive drug that may make your skin subject to extreme sunburn with only mild exposure to the sun.

Wear clothing with a tight weave to limit the penetration of the sun's rays, as well as a hat or visor, gloves, and lip balm containing sunscreen.

Resources

Products

Sunwatch. A watch-size monitor that measures the amount of UVB rays you are exposed to and indicates how much longer you can remain in the sun without damaging your skin. Comes with wristband, clip, and battery. $40. Real Goods catalog, (800) 762-7325.

SPF 32 Sunscreen. UVA rays blocked with transparent zinc oxide, PABA-free, fragrance-free, alcohol-free, waterproof. Two 3-ounce tubes, $18. Self Care catalog, (800) 345-3371.

Sun Protection Lotion. Made with plant extracts and oils and without PABA. SPF 8, 15, or 30. $6 to $8 for 4 ounces. Beautiful Times catalog, (800) 223-1216.

SPF 30+ Clothing. Blocks more than 97 percent of the sun's

UV rays. Polo shirts, $60. Sweatshirts, $50. Long pants, $60. Wide-brim hat, $40. Lightweight. Sun Precautions catalog, (800) 882-7860.

Desert Rhat Hat. Protects from sun and wind, breathable top and side mesh for ventilation, long visor, detachable neck portion. $38. Self Care catalog, (800) 345-3371.

Hat. Flexible hat with 3¼-inch-wide brim, floats. $40. Self Care catalog, (800) 345-3371.

Solar Shields Sun Glasses. Wraparound top and side. Can be worn over your own glasses or by themselves. $20. Self Care catalog, (800) 345-3371.

Services

National Cancer Institute Hot Line. Provides current information on the disease and research, offers publications. (800) 4-CANCER (422-6237).

Organizations

Skin Cancer Foundation. FREE brochures and self-examination instruction. SCF, 245 5th Avenue, Suite 2402, New York, NY 10016, (212) 725-5176 or (800) SKIN-490 (754-6490), an answering service.

Dry Skin

After age sixty-five everyone has dry skin. For women this change usually occurs following menopause and the decline of estrogen. Skin becomes dry as the result of a decrease in the production of oil glands in the body. Dry skin is unattractive, but more significant, it can cause itchiness, cracks, and bleeding, sometimes leading to infection in severe cases.

Conditions That Tend to Worsen Dry Skin

- Exposure to the sun or wind.
- Overheated rooms.
- Low humidity. Air conditioners and radiator heat tend to dehumidify rooms.
- Overzealous or frequent washing with harsh soaps, overly hot water, or too-vigorous rubbing.

Moisturizers work by preventing the loss of water from the skin, rather than by adding anything to the skin itself. The best moisturizer for dry skin is petroleum jelly, or Vaseline. It penetrates the outer layer of the skin and keeps it soft.

Suggestions for Alleviating Dry Skin

Increase the humidity in your home by using a humidifier, keeping the heat moderate, growing houseplants, putting trays of water on the radiators.

Apply lotions or creams to moist or damp skin.

Wash your face no more than twice a day, lathering with your hands rather than a washcloth.

Moisturizers with the following ingredients are the most effective against dry skin: urea, alpha-hydroxy acids, lactic acid, glycolic acid. Some brand-name products that are worth trying: Crème-Mousse Hydratante, Nivea, Lubriderm, Curél. The first choice should be a cream, followed, in order of descending preference, by an ointment or a lotion. Gels often contain alcohol, which may add to the dryness.

Mineral oil is an effective makeup remover that can be washed off in turn with a nonsoap face cleanser like Cetaphil, Phresh 3.5, or Foaming Face Wash. Soaps that are less harsh on the skin include Dove, Superfatted Basis, Purpose, Oilatum, and Neutrogena.

Resources

To reduce drying due to sun exposure, consult the products mentioned for skin spots, pages 81–82.

Products

Natural Skin Creams. Beautiful Times catalog, (800) 223-1216.

Body Brush. Boar bristles stimulate cell renewal, slough off old skin. Long handle. $14. Fuller Brush catalog, (800) 522-0499.

Publications

"Preventing Dry Skin and Other Skin Problems." A brief overview of skin problems and ways of avoiding dry skin. FREE with SSE. Elder-Health, University of Maryland, School of Pharmacy, 20 North Pine Street, Baltimore, MD 21201.

HAIR

Hair begins to change color and thickness at widely varied ages and to widely varying degrees. Many men enjoy a "distinguished" graying at the temples, and women may find a silver streak dramatic.

If you plan to cover the gray, the most natural look comes from coloring only the gray one shade lighter than your natural hair. This will avoid a too-harsh look against paler skin tone. Since hair is never only one shade, blending shades will result in the most natural appearance, and leaving some streaks of gray can add credibility. There are several types of hair color, do-it-yourself or professionally applied, wash in and wash out, semipermanent, and permanent — at least until new growth occurs. Of the forty million American men with gray hair, only 8 percent color it. A darker hair color may help camouflage thinning hair by making it appear fuller.

Twenty million American women and thirty million American men experience hair loss, mainly because of heredity and not related directly to age. Women's hair usually thins over the entire head, while men experience bald spots on the crown and receding hairlines. Thinning hair can be disguised by keeping the hair cut shorter or having a permanent to keep the hair curly and covering the bare scalp.

Only one product, Rogaine, a prescription drug, has been proved to restore hair. After a minimum of four months of twice-daily application of Rogaine to the scalp, new hair can grow by stimulating the blood flow to existing hair follicles. Once use is discontinued, however, the new hair falls out and is not replaced. This is the only product approved by the FDA for regrowing hair; all other creams or lotions do not work. However, the success of Rogaine is greater for people who are just beginning to lose their hair than for those with long-term thinning or baldness.

Products

Quick-Dry Hair Towel. Towel is more absorbent than regular towels. $20. Self Care catalog, (800) 345-3371.

No-Rinse Shampoo. Massage shampoo into hair, and towel-dry. For times when you can't easily use water on your hair. 12 ounces. Three for $20. Avenues catalog, (800) 848-2837.

Dispenser for Shampoo, Conditioner, Liquid Soap, Body Oil. Installs in shower so that you can avoid bending to reach various containers. Each section holds 14 ounces. Four sections, $30. Two sections, $23. Seventh Generation catalog, (800) 456-1177.

Hair Brushes. Variety of shapes, all with natural boar bristles and wood handles. $25. Fuller Brush catalog, (800) 522-0499.

Hands Free Hair Dryer. Dryer sits in a base and can be angled and adjusted in height. $35. Lighthouse Consumer Products catalog, (800) 829-0500.

Designing Your Diet

Chapter 5

Hearty Appetite

"My eating habits are no better than a teenager's. The only complete meal I eat is when I eat out with friends. The rest of the time I just snack at one thing or another. I never cook anymore; I just reheat things."

"Foods just don't taste the same anymore."

The ideal of "three squares" a day may not describe a complicated nutritional plan, but it does remind us that eating three substantial meals each day is vital for a healthy and vigorous way of life. To maintain our energy and to complete our chores and activities, we need nourishment from a variety of foods. Sometimes this may mean renewing a lackluster appetite or learning to deal with sore teeth or new dentures that make it difficult to chew. It's important to find ways of keeping up our interest in meals.

WHAT'S ON YOUR MENU?

Are you among the 30 percent of people over age sixty-five who skip at least one meal a day? There are many reasons for missing a meal: lack of energy, lack of funds, lack of interest, lack of teeth, lack of food in the pantry. If you don't eat enough, you might experience weakness and debilitation and dehydration and then be at higher risk of illness or reduced ability to bounce back from a cold or the flu. Some people turn to food for consolation when they feel blue, while others can't eat at all during personal crises. Loss of appetite may also be due to an illness or may be a side effect from a medication. If you suspect this, consult your doctor.

Appetite Checklist

If any one of the following statements describes you, even some of the time, you should be on guard against unnecessarily putting your independence in jeopardy.

- You have cut back on food as an economy measure.
- You have lost interest in food.
- Teeth or denture problems prevent you from enjoying your meals.
- Your pantry is sparsely supplied because you can't get out or because shopping is too physically demanding.
- Your moods affect your attitude toward food. You are too depressed to think about food.
- You find cooking too boring or preparations too difficult.
- Food looks and tastes less appetizing than in the past because of changes in your vision or sense of taste.
- You hate to eat alone.
- You lack the energy or knowledge to prepare meals.

While you needn't be alarmed if you experience a blunted appetite now and then, be careful that a skipped meal or two doesn't become the routine.

We depend on the interrelated senses of smell and taste to make food appetizing, but the sense of smell begins to decline at age forty-five, accelerating after age sixty-five. Since a seventy-five-year-old has half the number of taste buds of a twenty-year-old, flavors take longer to register in the mouth, making food less appealing. Smoking also dampens a person's ability to distinguish flavors.

Herbs and spices, particularly fresh ones, enhance both the smell and the taste of foods and can stimulate the appetite. Look carefully at the ingredients of premixed spice combinations, especially if some spices are difficult for you to digest or if you need to limit sodium.

- Arrange to meet friends at mealtimes, either at restaurants or in alternating homes, as a weekly event.
- Invite a friend or relative who is alone for a meal.
- To alleviate the cooking burden, renew the old idea of potluck suppers or lunches.
- Have your main meal at lunchtime if you are more likely to feel energetic then.
- Challenge several friends to an afternoon of Scrabble or a card game, preceded by lunch.

In addition to herbs, flavors that can awaken your palate include lemon juice, maple syrup, bacon-flavored bits, and butter flavoring.

Eating can be a sociable activity, from which the pleasure comes as much from the occasion as from the food itself. Company at the table can often revive a dull appetite.

A healthy diet can be compromised by relying too much on convenience foods or fast foods. While it may seem too much trouble to prepare fresh foods for only one or two, supermarket produce sections include vegetables washed and cut up for cooking, ready-to-eat salads, and single-serving portions. Foods that can't be conveniently purchased or made in small portions, like lasagna or roasts, can be divided with a friend. For economy, consider sharing with a friend a five-pound bag of onions or potatoes.

If your repertory in the kitchen is limited to preparing a fried egg or frozen pizza, you need to take some steps to ensure that you get a more nutritious diet. Prepared convenience foods are loaded with sodium and may not conform in other ways to your dietary requirements. If you've never learned to find your way around a kitchen, it's not too late to experiment. Ask a friend to teach you how to make the foods you like, buy an elementary cookbook and follow the instructions, or join an adult cooking class for beginners. Propose an exchange with a friend who can cook. In exchange for some lessons in the kitchen, you will teach something you know how to do well. Cooking can also be a great socializing opportunity: pancakes for grandchildren; barbecued chicken for friends; cookies for tea. Experiment on yourself, and take responsibility for this important aspect of your life.

If you lack the energy or appetite to finish a normal-size meal, adopt the six-snacks-a-day system: Eat smaller meals more frequently; eat your salad and dessert between regular meals. If cooking tires you, prepare your meal ahead of time, and set it aside so that you feel rested at mealtime.

In order to be able to eat a variety of nutritious foods — fresh apples, hard rolls, crunchy celery — you need strong teeth and jawbones. Problems with your teeth can not only affect appearance and speech but can also interfere with a proper diet.

Only thirty years ago nearly 60 percent of people over age sixty-five had lost all their teeth. Now less than 40 percent of sixty-five-year-olds have none of their own teeth left — a remarkable improvement. Gum disease, a result of plaque buildup that leads to infection in the gum and ultimately to bone loss and tooth loss, is the major factor in tooth loss for people over sixty-five.

If dental problems affect your choice of foods, you risk losing your usual sources of vitamins, particularly if you eat fewer fresh fruits or vegetables. Favoring soft foods because you have difficulty chewing crunchy or crisp foods may result in problems with constipation. One study discovered that people who switched to soft, processed foods because of difficulty chewing tended to have higher blood pressure levels.

If you have difficulty grasping the toothbrush handle or find flossing hard on your arms or fingers, consider more frequent visits to a dentist or hygienist to help keep your teeth clean. Build up your toothbrush handle with foam padding or a foam hair curler to make it easier to hold, or substitute an electric toothbrush. To be sure you can see where to floss, add to the wattage of your bathroom lighting.

In addition to good home dental care, you can eat in ways that are beneficial to your teeth:

- Choose foods with a natural cleansing action for the teeth (all low fat and low calorie): celery, carrots, lettuce, radishes, cantaloupe, oranges, raw cauliflower, pears, raw peppers, plums.
- Choose foods that fight cavities by counteracting the acids in the mouth that wear down tooth enamel, all usually high-fat, high-calorie, high-sodium: cheese, peanut butter, nuts, seeds,

olives, dill pickles. They should be consumed in limited quantities.
- Avoid foods that provide food for bacteria, especially during nighttime hours: sweets, fruits, or starchy foods.

Even if you no longer have your own teeth, you still need regular dental care. Since Medicare does not cover dental expenses, you may be inclined to view the expense of a dentist as optional. This is a false economy that can lead to serious and expensive consequences in the long run.

If you do lose your teeth, you will need dentures in order to chew your food, form your words clearly, and maintain your normal facial appearance. Dentures, however, are a poor substitute for original teeth. Even the best-fitting ones have a tendency to slip and slide, either because your gums change shape or because the underlying bone loses density and provides less support. Ill-fitting dentures resulting from changes in your mouth can irritate the gums and create problems with chewing and speaking, so regular visits to your dentist are still important. Dentists in some communities have outfitted mobile dental offices that enable you to receive professional dental care in your home. Your local dental society may help you locate a dentist who makes home visits in your area.

Dentures require a period of adjustment for cheek and tongue muscles to help keep them in place. Denture teeth also feel different from natural teeth. Gradually you will progress from chewing only soft foods to returning to your normal diet. To protect your dentures should they fall during cleaning, place a cushioning towel in the sink, or fill the basin halfway with water.

Smart Dental Care Economies

- Effort expended on regular flossing, brushing, and denture care may save expenditures for dental treatment.
- Visit a dentist once, rather than twice, a year.
- Prior to treatment, negotiate monthly payments with your dentist.
- Use dental school clinic services.
- Contact your state dental association to locate free or low-cost clinics or special services for people over sixty-five.

Problems with bad breath are usually due to odor from foods you have eaten. If you still have a sour taste in your mouth after brushing and flossing, try a mouthwash for temporary relief. Plaque and bacteria increase when saliva is insufficient to cleanse the mouth and, besides bad breath, can lead to tooth decay and gum disease. "Dry mouth" was once thought to be a consequence of aging, possibly caused by a decline in saliva production, but this has been disproved. Dry mouth can result from some medications, particularly those for hypertension, or from disease and is not a normal condition of aging. If dry mouth is a problem for you, consult your dentist and your doctor.

For the sixty-one million Americans who suffer heartburn or acid indigestion, an old-fashioned after-dinner stroll may avert the discomfort. The burning sensation in the chest occurs when the sphincter muscle between the esophagus and the stomach relaxes, allowing stomach acid to leak up into the esophagus. Simplistic though it sounds, the force of gravity when you stand up helps the acid return to the stomach.

Some people find relief from heartburn by limiting the citrus fruits, mint, or tomatoes in their diet. Chocolate contains a muscle relaxant that may affect the operation of the sphincter muscle. Fried or fatty foods, alcohol, and coffee have also been known to cause heartburn.

SURVIVAL PANTRY

If a blizzard, a busy life, or illness keeps you from getting to the grocery, you can relax if you have a Survival Pantry. The one outlined below enables you to stockpile enough food to keep yourself nourished for nearly a week. A Survival Pantry can be a source of security: You know that there is food for several meals on hand and in a safe place.

The pantry should contain some foods you always use, some that you may need for a special diet, and some that provide concentrated nourishment. Although most of the foods are chosen for their long shelf lives, every six months the food from the Survival Pantry should be rotated into your regular pantry and replaced with fresh items (note that most food products these days have expiration dates stamped on the packages). Should a real emergency, such as a power

outage, occur, most of the items in the pantry are edible as is —
that is, without heating or cooking.

The Survival Pantry traditionally created by the Boy Scouts and
Girl Scouts includes a five-day supply of food and at least five quarts
of water for each family member. For your purposes, consider small
packages of the pantry items, even if it is less economical, and
two gallons of fluids for each person, which include water for re-
constituting instant milk or adding to soups. The following items
will provide a basic Survival Pantry:

Instant nonfat dry milk. Instant milk can be a lifesaver even on
an ordinary day when you find your milk has soured and there's
none for your morning coffee or cereal.

Small cans or paper cartons of milk and juice. In the juice department
of the supermarket you will find small cartons of 1 and 2 percent
milk wrapped in cellophane and dated for a fairly long shelf life.
A selection of juices is also packaged in easy-to-store single-serving
cartons.

Water in small plastic (refillable) bottles. These are more convenient
than the heavy gallon jugs since you open only what you need.

Five cans of soup. Choose lentil, bean, split pea, vegetable, or beef.
These varieties are good sources of protein and are substantial
enough to constitute a main course.

Three cans of broth or tomato soup. These can be used alone or in
place of water as cooking liquid for rice or pasta.

*An assortment of canned pasta dinners, canned stews, tuna fish, and
salmon.* These are filling and would be substantial main course
meals.

A pound of rice and a pound of pastina. These starches can be
cooked in tomato soup or topped with spoonfuls from a jar of
tomato sauce.

Dried mixes for pancakes, muffins, gelatin, and custard. These items
provide carbohydrates and are satisfying foods.

*Lunch box sizes of dried fruits, canned fruits, canned vegetables, and
beans.* In the absence of fresh produce, these are good sources of
vitamins and minerals.

Processed cheese spread, peanut butter, and crackers. Sources of protein, these items can be stored at length on the shelf.

Instant oatmeal or dry cereal. When you don't feel good, these

95

breakfast foods are easy to digest, comforting to eat, and preferable to skipping a meal.

These suggestions provide more nutritional value than snack food and can keep up your energy level until you can restock your regular food items at the supermarket. When you don't feel like cooking, you can also use some of the more substantial main dishes in the Survival Pantry — for example, canned fish, vegetables, and soups. Your own Survival Pantry will be tailored to your needs, of course, but the idea is to be in control of your food supply even when you can't get out to shop.

Resources

Suggestions for developing a positive attitude are enumerated in Chapter 1, "Embracing a Positive Outlook."

Thoughts to consider for maintaining social contacts are offered in Chapter 2, "Nourishing Relationships."

Products

Kitchen Whiz. Calculates amounts to increase or decrease a recipe; converts measurements, such as teaspoons to tablespoons or pounds to ounces and from American to metric and more. $30. King Arthur Flour catalog, (800) 827-6836.

Microwave Hot Plate. Keeps food warm at the table after you heat it in the microwave for three minutes. Outer rim doesn't get hot. $25. Improvements catalog, (800) 642-2112.

Covered Cake Pan. Cook, store, and transport a cake in one 13″ × 9″ × 3¼″ pan with its own lid. Lid can be used as a baking sheet too. $10. Signatures catalog, (909) 943-2021.

Disposable Toothbrush with Toothpaste. When you are away from home and need to brush your teeth, use this individually wrapped toothbrush, which dispenses a gel toothpaste when you push on the handle. Fifty for $18. Self Care catalog, (800) 345-3371.

Automatic Toothbrush. Four brushes clean inner and outer surfaces, top and bottom teeth, and chewing surfaces simultaneously at three hundred strokes a minute. Rechargeable battery. $80. Oralgiene USA, 10920 Wilshire Boulevard, Suite 330, Los Angeles, CA 90024, (800) 933-ORAL (6725).

UltraSonex Toothbrush. Removes up to 97 percent of plaque with "ultrasonic" action. Includes recharging base. $100. Bruce Medical Supply catalog, (800) 225-8446.

Aqua Floss. Liquid flosser that pulses 950 times a minute. High or low pressure. $45. Self Care catalog, (800) 345-3371.

Braun/Oral-B Dental Hygiene Set. Toothbrush and oral irrigator. $160. Self Care catalog, (800) 345-3371.

Sword Floss. Floss is already stretched across a gap, so it's ready to use. Disposable. Thirty-two pieces, $1.60. AARP Pharmacy Service catalog, (800) 456-2277.

Portable Flosser. Battery-operated pulsating water appliance. $40. Self Care catalog, (800) 345-3371.

Emergency Preparedness Kit. Includes enough food for one person for three days, water, a flashlight, a body heat retaining blanket and more. Five-year shelf life. $40. Safety Zone catalog, (800) 999-3030.

Survival Kit. Three days of food, six packets of water, Mylar emergency blanket, for one person. $18. Real Goods catalog, (800) 762-7325.

Services

Nutrition Program for the Elderly. A federally funded program that provides one nutritious meal each day for anyone age sixty or older, regardless of income. Special diets may be available. Transportation may be provided to a neighborhood center where meals are served. Meals will be delivered to your home if you fall ill and cannot get to the center. If you are homebound and no one is available to cook for you, you may receive Meals on Wheels. FREE. Office on Aging, in the county listings of your telephone book or Eldercare Locator Service, (800) 677-1116.

Home Dental Services. To locate dentists equipped to make home visits in your area, contact your local dental society or the American Dental Association, 211 East Chicago Avenue, Chicago, IL 60611, (312) 440-2593.

Dental Clinics. To find clinics in your area, contact the American Dental Association, 211 East Chicago Avenue, Chicago, IL 60611, (312) 440-2593.

Geriatric Dentist. To locate a dentist with a special interest in treating older patients, contact your local dental society or the American Society for Geriatric Dentistry, 211 East Chicago Avenue, Suite 1616, Chicago, IL 60611, (312) 440-2660.

Publications

"Cooking Solo: Menus and Recipes for One or Two That Follow the Dietary Guidelines to Lower Cancer Risk," American Institute for Cancer Research. Suggestions for shopping and cooking to maintain a healthful diet when you eat alone. FREE. AICR, 1759 R Street, NW, Washington, DC 20009, (800) 843-8114.

Dad's Own Cookbook by Bob Sloan. Information on shopping, kitchen equipment, and cleanups; suggestions for including children in the cooking experience. Recipes. 1993. Workman Publishing.

"Heartburn." A fact sheet that briefly explains causes and treatments of heartburn. FREE. National Digestive Diseases Information Clearinghouse, 2 Information Way, Bethesda, MD 20892-3570, (301) 654-3810.

Chapter 6

Choosing Foods for a Healthy Heart

"I've seen food fads come and go over the years. I can remember the rice diet and the wheat germ craze. I always felt that if I ate a variety of foods, in the course of a week I would have enough vitamins and minerals."

"There is so much cross talk about which foods will make you sick, which ones prevent diseases, I can't remember it all, so I just ignore it all."

No subject is more fraught with controversy and confusion than food. The head-spinning claims and inevitable counterclaims made for one nutrient or another are impossible to ignore: foods that we cannot and should not live without; foods that will extend our lives; foods that are dangerous to our health. As for what's true and what's not, only time will tell. In the meantime, we must eat.

In the last few decades the government and other scientific bodies have agreed that if Americans limit the amount of fat in their diet, they will reduce their risk of heart disease. This is positive news that may protect us from the number one killer since 1910, responsible for half of all deaths in this country since 1949. To reflect the accumulation of research, the Department of Agriculture devised a

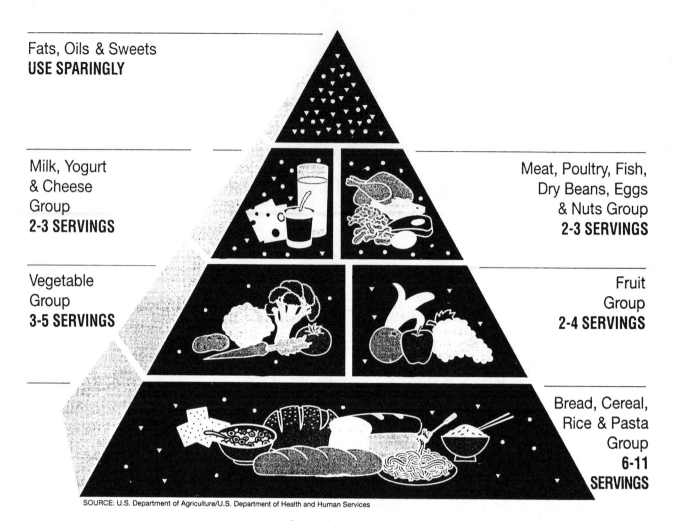

Food guide pyramid

graphic representation of new dietary guidelines — the Food Pyramid — depicting which foods to emphasize and which to eat little of.

The encouraging news is that between 1968 and 1991 the death rate from coronary heart disease dropped 53 percent, attributed to the public's understanding of the need to reduce smoking, eat low-fat foods, and get more exercise, as well as the availability of modern medical techniques, such as the coronary bypass, angioplasty, and new drugs. Risk of heart disease drops dramatically by 50 to 70 percent for anyone, regardless of age, who quits smoking; after five years his or her heart mortality rate will be equal to that of the lifelong nonsmoker. Estrogen replacement can protect postmeno-pausal women from heart disease, the leading killer of women over age fifty. These medical advances and lifestyle changes may be re-sponsible for the decline in the death rate from heart attack by more than 32 percent between 1981 and 1991. Still, according to the American Heart Association, in 1991, 923,422 Americans died from diseases of the heart and blood vessels, accounting for 42.7 percent of all deaths. Among women cardiovascular disease was the leading cause of death (45.3 percent).

In 1988 *The Surgeon General's Report on Nutrition and Health* called attention to a link found between saturated fat in the diet and high levels of blood cholesterol, a type of fat. Blood supply to the heart is restricted when plaque builds up on artery walls; this is found to occur mainly in people with high blood cholesterol.

Fat, then, is at the tip of the Food Pyramid and is the item to limit the most. A high measurement of cholesterol in the blood results from eating more fat and cholesterol than the body utilizes.

A Cholesterol Glossary

Blood cholesterol or serum cholesterol: cholesterol in the blood

Dietary cholesterol: cholesterol found in foods of animal origin

Total cholesterol: a measurement of two cholesterol-carrying proteins in the blood — LDL and HDL

Low-density lipoprotein (also known as LDL cholesterol or "bad" cholesterol): the protein that carries cholesterol in the blood and deposits it on arterial walls, forming a plaque

High-density lipoprotein (also known as HDL cholesterol or "good" cholesterol): a beneficial protein that carries cholesterol away from the blood for elimination from the body

---

Saturated fat — mainly those fats that are solid at room temperature — is the biggest contributor to blood cholesterol and should not constitute more than 10 percent of daily calories. Consuming poly-unsaturated fats and monounsaturated fats may be preferable for controlling blood cholesterol levels, yet these fats add calories, which may lead to overweight, another factor that raises the risk of heart disease as well as other serious diseases. That's why the government recommends limiting *all* fats, as a group, to no more than one third of our daily calories.

A Fat Glossary

Saturated fat: solid fat like butter and lard. Leads to higher levels of total cholesterol and LDL cholesterol.

Polyunsaturated fat: liquid oil like sunflower oil. Has been found to lower total blood cholesterol levels.

Monounsaturated fat: oil like canola or olive oil. Has been found to lower LDL cholesterol levels without lowering HDL cholesterol levels.

From a blood sample a laboratory can determine the number of milligrams (mg) of cholesterol in each deciliter (dl) of blood, the total amount of HDL and LDL.

Cholesterol Test Results

A total cholesterol level of 200 mg/dl or less is considered "Desirable."

A total cholesterol level of between 200 and 240 mg/dl is considered "Borderline-High" and should be controlled with diet and exercise.

A total cholesterol level of 240 mg/dl or more is considered "High" and may require medication if proper diet and exercise fail to effect a significant improvement.

Source: The National Cholesterol Education Program of the National Heart, Lung, and Blood Institute, which recommends this interpretation of the test results.

The results of a cholesterol test may vary depending on the foods you ate the day before or even the time of day the blood sample was taken. In winter results were found to be as much as 5 percent higher than in summer.

If, like more than 50 percent of Americans over the age of twenty, your total cholesterol level is found to be more than 200 mg/dl, analyzing your HDL and LDL levels will indicate if you're at risk for developing heart disease. A high level of HDL cholesterol (at least 35 mg/dl) is considered desirable. In contrast, *low* levels of

LDL cholesterol (less than 130 mg/dl) are considered favorable for reducing the risk of heart disease. Individuals with a total blood cholesterol level over 240 mg/dl are more than twice as likely to develop heart disease than those with total blood cholesterol levels of 200 mg/dl.

Blood cholesterol levels tend to increase until age sixty for men and age seventy for women, after which they remain stable. A 1994 study, however, found no increased health risk from high blood cholesterol levels for people in their seventies and eighties. This result implies that people over age seventy may be less concerned if they have high cholesterol levels and are otherwise healthy. It is not yet known whether a high blood cholesterol level in older age groups can respond to dietary changes or medication or even whether those treatments are necessary. New studies will address the question of whether reducing cholesterol levels and blood pressure in people over age sixty prevents heart disease.

If an individual's total blood cholesterol level is lowered by 1 percent, the risk of heart disease would be reduced by 1.5 to 2 percent. The government's goal is to reduce the national incidence of coronary heart disease by 20 percent or more by advocating a diet that could lower by 10 percent the average total blood cholesterol level, currently 205 mg/dl. Government experts tell us that by eating foods low in fat and cholesterol, in addition to maintaining normal weight, refraining from smoking, and getting sufficient exercise, we can reduce the risk of coronary artery disease, stroke, diabetes, cancer, and atherosclerosis, five of the ten main causes of death in America. (The other five: motor vehicle and other accidents, lung diseases, pneumonia and influenza, suicide, and liver disease.)

Following the Food Pyramid guidelines may provide other health benefits as well — for example, alleviating constipation, helping with weight control. Since the dietary guidelines are intended to provide recommendations for the general public, you may decide to reduce certain elements of your diet even further. The recommendations suggest you include a variety of foods in your diet, some in moderation, but radical change is not necessary for general health. Of course, allergies or sensitivities to certain foods or specific medical conditions may dictate certain restrictions for you.

Naturally the Food Pyramid should be only a starting point in our efforts to eat healthy meals and avoid heart disease. The truth is, we eat pretty much the same foods day in and day out, gravitating in the supermarket to the items we have consumed many times before. To change your eating patterns, you'll need to develop new habits and find new foods. If you want to make changes and stick with them, revolutionize your diet one food at a time. Get used to a new item slowly to give its taste a chance to become familiar before you make other changes. The dietary guidelines are targets for a week of meals, not necessarily a rigid formula for each day or each meal.

GUIDELINES FOR A LOW-FAT DIET

Like a palace revolution, the "balanced" diet — equal parts from four basic food groups — has been overthrown and replaced by one based on the pyramid shape. The new diet encourages us to choose most of our food from complex carbohydrates and fruits and vegetables, a smaller amount from meat and dairy products, and as little as possible from oils, fats, and sweets. We have to learn how to adjust our palates and habits to conform to this diet.

The guidelines represented by the Food Pyramid encourage a diet with less fat and less cholesterol resting on a substantial foundation of six to eleven servings each day of complex carbohydrates — pasta, whole grains, breads, cereals, rice, and potatoes. Eating complex carbohydrates helps satisfy the appetite so that we are less likely to eat foods found higher up on the pyramid. Sixty percent of the calories we consume daily should come from this group of foods.

By themselves, carbohydrates aren't high in calories, but we tend to flavor them with high-calorie and high-fat sauces and spreads. Potatoes, rice, and bulgur are cholesterol-free, as are spaghetti and other pastas made without eggs. Fresh egg noodles can be made using liquid egg substitute or only egg whites.

Plain breads and rolls contain little saturated fat, but your consumption of breads made with cheese or butter, such as croissants, doughnuts, muffins, biscuits, and buttery rolls, should be restricted. Look for chewier, crustier types, such as bagels, rolls, and English muffins, and whole wheat, rye, pumpernickel, oat, French, and sourdough breads. Rather than add a little butter or margarine, both of which carry eleven to twelve grams of fat in each tablespoon, use jam, jelly, or honey, which have no fat.

Benefits of Complex Carbohydrates

- They may help reduce blood cholesterol levels.
- The more complex carbohydrates in your diet, the less fat you are likely to include.
- As a source of dietary fiber carbohydrates may alleviate constipation and other digestive problems.
- Carbohydrates are a source of energy, as measured in calories.
- Most foods high in complex carbohydrates and fiber are low in fat.
- Rice and grains are cholesterol-free, as is pasta made without eggs.

NOTE: One serving of complex carbohydrates consists of: one slice of bread; half a bagel, roll, or English muffin; half a cup of cooked cereal, rice, or pasta.

Our daily menu should include five to nine servings of fruits and vegetables, forming the second stratum of the Food Pyramid. Fruits and vegetables (except for avocado) derive less than one third of their calories from fat.

Benefits of Fruits and Vegetables

- They contain dietary fiber that can alleviate constipation and improve digestion.
- Raw, they act as a natural cleanser of teeth, and they massage gums.
- Except for avocado, they contain no fat.
- They are low in sodium.
- They contain most of the vitamins and minerals our bodies need.

NOTE: One serving of fruits and vegetables consists of: one cup of raw salad greens; half a cup of cooked greens; half a cup of cooked dried beans or peas; one medium-size apple or other fresh fruit; half a cup of berries or cut-up fruit; three-quarter cup fruit juice (not a drink with water as the main ingredient).

In general, fresh fruits and vegetables are more nutritious than canned, which often contain unnecessary sugar or salt added during processing. If you use canned products, look for labels indicating "No added salt" or "No sugar." Frozen vegetables, without sauces, can be a time-saver and are useful when certain fresh vegetables are not in season. Processing diminishes the nutritional benefits of these foods, however. Let's compare, for example, the iron content of one cup of spinach:

Raw spinach	6.4 milligrams iron
Canned spinach	4.9 milligrams iron
Frozen spinach	2.9 milligrams iron

The rest of the Food Pyramid, as it narrows toward the tip, describes foods that should be a limited part of your diet since they contain fats, cholesterol, and sweets. Limit dairy products — milk, yogurt, cheese, ice cream — to two to three servings a day. One serving of a dairy product would be one cup of milk or yogurt or one and one-half ounces of cheese. Although they are reliable sources of calcium, dairy foods contain fat, particularly saturated fat, and cholesterol, which may contribute to clogged arteries.

Since nearly half the calories in whole milk come from fat, nonfat or low-fat dairy foods are better choices that still provide calcium. (For more about calcium, please see Chapter 7, "Following a Special Diet.") Naturally, choosing low-fat dairy foods necessitates excluding butter, cream, and ice cream, all of which contain an even larger percentage of saturated fat than whole milk.

Note that even in 2 percent milk more than 30 percent of the calories are from fat, so it can't be considered low-fat. Protein-fortified skim milk available in many supermarkets has 352 milligrams calcium and 10 grams of protein, instead of the 300 milligrams calcium and 8 grams of protein in regular skim milk. The result has a taste and appearance that are hard to distinguish from whole milk and is suitable for use in coffee, where ordinary skim milk may seem insufficient.

Instant nonfat dry milk (not to be confused with *powdered* milk) is easy to store and cheaper than regular milk. This is one of the items we suggest you include in your Survival Pantry (see page 95). When reconstituted and refrigerated, instant milk may be used in place of skim milk. The taste of the milk can be improved by

A Comparison of Selected Milks (8-ounce servings)			
	Calories	**Fat**	**Cholesterol**
Whole milk	150	8 grams (72 calories or 49% of total calories)	35 milligrams
2% milk	120	5 grams (45 calories or 35% of total calories)	20 milligrams
1% milk	100	2 grams (18 calories or 18% of total calories)	10 milligrams
Skim milk	85	Less than 1 gram (less than 9 calories or 0.04% of total calories)	5 milligrams

adding more dry milk than is called for in the instructions on the box (try about one cup more for each quart). The fat content won't be affected, of course, since this type of milk is fat-free, but the flavor will be enhanced.

Sherbet, sorbet, and frozen yogurt are good lower-fat desserts to use in place of ice cream. Read the labels of these products in case ingredients such as pecans or chocolate chips have increased the fat content.

Cheese, unless it is low-fat or part-skim, has almost as high a percentage of saturated fat as ice cream. In response to the public's heightened awareness of the need to limit cholesterol and saturated fats, cheese producers are reducing the fat in their cheeses or are using fat substitutes. New food labels will help you select cheese that contains no more than two grams of fat per ounce. Some cheeses made with low-fat or skim milk are: dry-curd cottage cheese, farmer cheese, part-skim mozzarella or ricotta, dry grated cheese like Parmesan or sapsago.

Beware of cream substitutes like nondairy coffee creamers, sour cream substitutes, and whipped toppings. These may contain coconut, palm, or palm kernel oil, which are high in saturated fat.

Sharing the third level of the Food Pyramid with dairy products are other major sources of saturated fat and cholesterol: meat, poultry, fish, eggs, and nuts. (Because this group is defined to include protein-rich foods, beans are included here, even though they *don't* contain saturated fat or cholesterol. Beans are legumes, of course, and could be grouped with complex carbohydrates.) A healthy diet would include only two to three servings a day of these foods. One protein-rich serving: two ounces of meat, poultry, fish, beans, or nuts; one egg yolk; two tablespoons of peanut butter; half a cup of cooked beans.

Eating less meat and poultry is a sure way to reduce the saturated fat in your diet. Organ meats, such as liver, and delicatessen meats, such as salami, sausages, and bacon, are particularly high in fat and cholesterol. The leanest choices are veal (9 grams of fat per 3-ounce cutlet) and skinless poultry (3 grams of fat per 3-ounce chicken breast). A well-trimmed round of beef (8 grams of fat per 3-ounce portion), pork (8 grams of fat per loin chop), or lamb (6 grams of fat per loin chop) might be good second choices. Fish (1 gram of fat per 3-ounce flounder fillet) is another low-fat option.

Fat Content of Chicken

Dark-meat chicken contains the same amount of fat as beef. One cup of dark-meat chicken without skin and visible fat contains 14 grams of fat, which is about three quarters of the total daily fat requirement, according to the pyramid. One third of the fat in chicken is saturated fat.

Some meat products should be eaten rarely because they are very high in fat. Deli meats (11 grams of fat in two slices of salami), bacon (9 grams of fat in three slices), hot dogs (13 grams of fat in one frankfurter), and sausage (5 grams of fat in one link) are some examples.

While blood cholesterol levels are primarily affected by the saturated fat in our diet, nutritionists recommend that we also limit food with high amounts of cholesterol, which is found in all animal products. Meat, poultry, fish, and eggs are the most cholesterol-rich sources.

Experts suggest restricting cholesterol to 300 milligrams a day — approximately the amount of cholesterol found in a single egg yolk (272 milligrams)! Liver (410 milligrams of cholesterol per 3-ounce serving) and other organ meats (164 milligrams of cholesterol per 3-ounce serving of heart) are high in cholesterol. Even chicken has 100 grams of cholesterol in a 4-ounce serving, the same amount as lean beef.

Liquid egg substitutes enable you to enjoy cholesterol-free egg dishes, like omelets, as well as cakes or other recipes requiring eggs. Rather than use two whole eggs in an omelet, try a whole egg and the white of one or two other eggs for increased volume. (If you decide to use only the whites of eggs, the yolks can be used as a hair conditioner: Comb the yolks through your hair after a shampoo, and then rinse.) Many brands of egg substitutes, some containing no fat or cholesterol, are available in supermarkets, in the refrigerator and freezer sections.

Beans are a good source of protein, calcium, soluble fiber, and other nutrients while contributing little fat and no cholesterol to your diet. They also generate a full feeling that helps you limit the amount of other foods you eat. Since most Americans eat more meat than beans, if we shifted our dietary patterns by adding a serving or two of beans a week, our overall consumption of meat and other fat-laden products might decline.

Most beans, either canned or prepared from dried beans, contain only a gram of fat per cup. These include many varieties, such as black, Great Northern, lima, pea or navy, pinto, red kidney, white, chickpeas, and the related legumes, split peas and lentils. Of course, beans cooked with additional fatty flavorings or meats will have additional fat.

Since humans lack the enzyme needed to digest two components of beans, gas builds up in the intestines. Because of this, people have different degrees of unpleasant side effects, mainly flatulence. Sometimes this problem can be ameliorated by adding small quantities of beans at a time to the diet, a tablespoonful or so in soups or salads, for example. Also, try boiling dried beans for five minutes and leaving them in the water for a few hours. Then discard the water, and cook them in fresh cold water. Beano, a product that contains the missing digestive enzyme, can be added to your first mouthful of beans to eliminate the negative effect.

While nuts have no cholesterol, they do contain fat, especially if they are roasted in oil. In some nuts the fat is mainly monounsaturated, so although nuts are high in calories, they may be a better choice than food high in saturated fat.

Fat Content of an Ounce of Selected Nuts		
	Total Fat (Grams)	Monounsaturated Fat (Grams)
Almond	15	9.6
Brazil nuts	19	6.5
Cashews	13	7.7
Filberts	18	13.9
Macadamia nuts	22	17.1
Peanuts	14	6.9
Pecans	19	12.0
Pistachios	14	9.3

The peak of the pyramid, representing what should be the tiniest segment of our diet, includes fats, oils, and sugar. Fats also contribute more calories by weight to our diet than other food: Each gram of fat contains nine calories, while each gram of carbohydrate or protein contains only four calories. Limiting fats and increasing other more healthful categories of foods therefore permit you to eat more food to consume the same number of calories.

Saturated fats are solid at room temperature. Lard (the fat found around meat and poultry) and butter are two examples. Monounsaturated fat is found in olive and canola oils. Polyunsaturated oils used frequently in commercial salad dressings are derived from safflower, corn, soybean, cottonseed, sesame seed, and sunflower seed. These oils are preferable to saturated fats.

Three tropical oils — coconut oil, palm kernel oil, and palm oil — are the highest of all oils in saturated fats. Use of these oils is slowly being eliminated by the food industry, but they may still be found in certain products that require deep-fat frying, as well as in cookies, crackers, whipped toppings, coffee creamers, cake mixes, and frozen dinners. The label must list any of these oils if they are an ingredient in a product. In some cases they may be listed as an alternative ingredient — for example, "vegetable oil *or coconut oil.*"

While margarine is preferable to butter because it contains no animal fat, it is not a preventive for heart disease. It contains no cholesterol, but it is made of fats, mainly polyunsaturated fats, and is not healthy if consumed in unlimited quantities. Margarines that list liquid oil as the first ingredient, followed by partially hydrogenated vegetable oils, are the lowest in saturated fat. During the hydrogenation process, in which margarine becomes solid at room temperature, a substance called transfatty acid that is thought to increase blood cholesterol levels is formed. It is preferable therefore to use margarine in liquid or semihard form, if possible. Diet margarine should list liquid oil as the second ingredient, after water; because of its water content, it can be used only as a spread, not for cooking. A butter-flavored powder can be sprinkled on hot foods at the table if you want to eliminate fat and cholesterol without losing the taste.

In place of butter, many people have been substituting oils, such as olive and canola, which are higher in monounsaturated fat. The annual use of butter declined between 1985 and 1990 from 4.9 pounds per person to 4.4 pounds per person. Olive oil use rose from 0.59 pound per person to 0.8 pound per person per year. While olive oil contains less saturated fat than butter and no cholesterol, it still contains 14 grams of fat per teaspoon. Using olive oil doesn't lower cholesterol, although as a source of monounsaturated fat it may increase levels of HDL.

Sugar shares the uppermost triangle of the Food Pyramid with fats and oils. Mainly a cause of tooth decay and a contributing factor in weight gain, sugar has few nutritional virtues other than the sweetness it imparts to foods.

Substituting a bunch of grapes for a piece of cake or candy is a totally incongruous suggestion to someone who adores sweets. If you can't resist sweets, try to select cakes and cookies that contain lesser amounts of fat. A fat substitute made from milk protein or egg whites and skim milk (Simplesse) is used in some low-fat foods, like cheese, ice cream, and other dairy products.

When you consider sweets in light of the pyramid's recommendation that no more than 30 percent of calories should come from fat, you can revise your choices rather than eliminate them altogether. If you also need to restrict your sugar consumption to control diabetes, weight, or tooth decay, you can use one of the three sugar substitutes currently available: saccharin (marketed as Sweet'n Low or Sugar Twin); aspartame (called Equal); and acesulfame potassium (available as Sunette).

Fat Content of Selected Sweets

	Grams of Fat	Calories
1 tablespoon maple syrup	0	122
2 tablespoons molasses	0	85
½ cup gelatin dessert	0	70
1 tablespoon honey	0	65
1 ounce jelly beans	Trace	105
1 tablespoon jam	Trace	55
1 slice raisin bread	1	65
1 ounce chocolate fudge	3	115
1 slice pound cake	5	120
1 brownie	6	95
1 wedge devil's food cake	8	235
4 chocolate chip cookies	9	180
1 serving chocolate pudding	11	205
1 doughnut	13	230
1 slice fruit pie	18	405
1 slice cheesecake	18	280
1 wedge carrot cake	21	385

LOW-FAT COOKING

Success in reducing the fat in your diet depends not only on selecting low-fat foods but on preparing foods in a low-fat manner and using unsaturated fats whenever possible. Try some of the following cooking methods and tips for reducing fat.

Stir-fry. Stir-fry onions or chopped ingredients quickly in a non-stick pan with no added fat or with a *quick* spritz of vegetable oil spray (spraying for seven seconds provides the equivalent of the fat in one pat of butter). Transfer some olive oil to a spray bottle, rather then buy aerosol cans of vegetable oil.

Grill, poach, steam, broil, roast, or bake. These are the preferred low-fat methods for cooking meat, poultry, or vegetables, either at home or when ordering in a restaurant. Before grilling, broiling, or roasting, place meats on a rack so that the fat drips into the pan below.

Roasting. Searing meat at a high temperature to brown it before roasting only seals in the fat. A leaner method is to roast it on a rack at 350 degrees and baste it, using such fat-free liquids as wine, tomato or lemon juice, or, if it seems unavoidable, a poly- or monounsaturated oil.

Microwave or steam. No added fat is needed when you microwave or steam, and both methods retain the nutrients in foods. If you braise, of course, you can skim off the fat after the food has cooled.

Fat-free gravy. Blend one tablespoon of cornstarch with a cup of broth. Heat another cup of broth in a saucepan, and stir in the cornstarch mixture, simmering until it thickens. For a buttery taste, use butter-flavored powder after the sauce is cooked.

Salad dressings. Four tablespoons of commercial salad dressing contain the same amount of fat as a piece of apple pie. In a restaurant, ask for dressing on the side, and be stingy with it. At home, thin prepared salad dressing with lemon juice or, for mayonnaise-type dressing, an equal amount of plain nonfat yogurt. Try to develop a taste for only oil and vinegar or for lemon juice with lots of herbs rather than bottled salad dressing.

Eggs. In baking, substitute two egg whites in most recipes calling for one egg yolk, or use one whole egg plus two egg whites for every two eggs. Liquid egg substitutes are suitable for making French toast, pancakes, and omelets.

Recipe Substitutions

Replace	With
1 tablespoon butter	1 tablespoon margarine or ¾ tablespoon vegetable oil★
1 cup shortening	⅔ cup vegetable oil
1 whole egg	2 egg whites
1 cup sour cream	1 cup plain yogurt
1 ounce baking chocolate	3 tablespoons cocoa plus 1 tablespoon margarine

★If the butter is to be creamed with sugar, use margarine; use vegetable oil when the recipe calls for melted butter or for frying or sautéing.

To help us select a low-fat diet as described by the Food Pyramid, federal laws require more explicit nutrition information on virtually all food packages.

Nutrition Facts

Serving Size ½ cup (114g)
Servings Per Container 4

Amount Per Serving

Calories 90	Calories from Fat 30

	% Daily Value*
Total Fat 3g	5%
Saturated Fat 0g	0%
Cholesterol 0mg	0%
Sodium 300mg	13%
Total Carbohydrate 13g	4%
Dietary Fiber 3g	12%
Sugars 3g	
Protein 3g	

Vitamin A	80%	•	Vitamin C	60%
Calcium	4%	•	Iron	4%

• Percent Daily Values are based on a 2,000 calorie diet. Your daily values may be higher or lower depending on your calorie needs:

Calories		2,000	2,500
Total Fat	Less than	65g	80g
Sat Fat	Less than	20g	25g
Cholesterol	Less than	300mg	300mg
Sodium	Less than	2,400mg	2,400mg
Total Carbohydrate		300g	375g
Fiber		25g	30g

Calories per gram:
Fat 9 • Carbohydrate 4 • Protein 4

Nutrition information guide

The label is intended to provide guidance to fat content, particularly saturated fat, and whether a food is a good source of carbohydrates. This should help you decide which foods to choose to increase carbohydrates and reduce fats in your diet. The most important information, "Calories from Fat," will help you select foods that get less than a third of their calories from fat.

The following table shows the amount of total fat and saturated fat in grams allowed under the guidelines. The table helps you estimate the amount of fat allowed for the number of calories you consume.

Daily Fat Allowances According to Calories Consumed		
Calories per Day	Total Allowable Fat (Grams)	Allowable Saturated Fat (Grams)
1,200	40	13
1,500	50	17
1,800	60	20
2,100	70	23
2,400	80	27

This does not mean that you *must* include the specified amount of fat in your diet in order to be healthy. On the contrary, the guidelines recommend a realistic amount that most Americans can adopt without needing to make radical changes in their diets. To function properly, your body needs only about one tablespoon of vegetable oil a day, equivalent to 14 grams of fat, 2.1 grams of saturated fat.

The label is designed to simplify comparisons between different products and help you figure out how much of your daily dietary needs a product provides. Nutrients are listed by grams and percentages of daily value — the percentage of a nutrient the food provides in one serving for a diet of two thousand calories a day. As a reminder, the label includes the grams of nutrients for both a two-thousand- and twenty-five-hundred-calorie diet.

Claims for foods, like "low-salt" or "low-fat," are now based on uniform criteria. Since vegetable products by definition have no cholesterol, no such claims about them can be made; "light" foods must have a third fewer calories or 50 percent less fat than comparable products.

Serving sizes on the new labels have been standardized, so that manufacturers can't claim fewer calories by using smaller servings. Health claims are also regulated, so that if the label indicates a product will help lower your risk of heart disease because it contains soluble fiber, you can depend on it.

While the labels contain a lot of information, you can focus on the nutrients that are important to your own diet and quickly determine which foods are healthy for you.

Resources

Mail-Order Foods

Organic Foods. A wide variety of fresh, dried, and canned foods. Cookies, soups, beans, granola, spices, vegetables. Also frozen turkeys and beef. Walnut Acres catalog, (800) 433-3998.

Vegetarian Foods. Harvest Direct, P.O. Box 4514, Decatur, IL 62525, (800) 835-2867.

Fat-Free Foods. Snacks, candies, sauces, and other foods made without added fat. The ingredients and nutritional specifications of all items are listed in the catalog. Fatwise catalog, (800) 733-8822.

Complex Carbohydrates

Sourdough Bread. A variety of shapes to order by mail. Sunberry Baking catalog, (800) 833-4090.

High Nutrition Mixes. Naturally fortified bread, pancake, cookie, and cake mixes. Recipe variations. Catalog lists exact ingredients, calories, sodium content, and nutritional analyses. Wheatless and salt-free mixes for breads available, as well as low-sodium bread mixes and soup mixes. HeartyMix catalog, (908) 382-3010.

Baking Mixes for People with Food Allergies. These mixes contain no milk, eggs, or salt; some contain no wheat flour. Pastas, breads, and other products for special dietary needs are available. Kingsmill Foods catalog, (800) 633-3438.

Flours, Pancake and Muffin Mixes. Also a source for nonfat dried milk, gluten-free flours, and other special ingredients. Great Valley Mills catalog, (800) 688-6455.

Bread Baking Ingredients and Equipment. Bread mixes, flours, pans, and so forth for home baking. King Arthur Flour catalog, (800) 827-6836.

Fruits

Oranges and Grapefruits. Monthly shipments of Florida citrus fruits from November through June. Half bushel (about twelve fruits), $25 per month. Hale Indian River Groves catalog, Indian River Plaza, P.O. Box 217, Wabasso, FL 32970.

Citrus Fruits. Oranges, grapefruits, and tangerines sent November through May. Quarter bushel, about eight oranges, five grapefruits, $22. Leo & Paul, Inc., 635-I Gator Drive, Lantana, FL 33462, (800) 443-7635.

Chemical-Free Fruit. Oranges and grapefruits grown without pesticides or chemicals. Half bushel mixed, $22. Environmental Fruit Company, 2780 East Oakland Park Boulevard, Fort Lauderdale, FL 33306, (800) 564-8993.

Tomatoes. Eight vine-ripened tomatoes. $18. Leo & Paul, Inc., 635-I Gator Drive, Lantana, FL 33462, (800) 443-7635.

Vegetables

Tomatoes and Onions. April to June, eight each, $26. Leo & Paul, Inc., 635-I Gator Drive, Lantana, FL 33462, (800) 443-7635.

Cheese

Sonoma Jack Brand Lite Cheeses. These cheeses have one third less fat, cholesterol, and calories and one half the salt of the regular line of cheeses. Garlic, hot pepper, pesto, and traditional jack flavors. An assortment of nine-ounce wedges, $20. Sonoma Cheese Factory catalog, (800) 535-2855.

Cabot Brand Cheddar Cheese. Three versions, each with fewer calories, less fat, less cholesterol than the regular line of cheddar. From two to five grams of fat per ounce, eight-ounce bar, about $8. Cabot Creamery catalog, (802) 563-2650.

Beans

Bean Soup Mixes. Different varieties, with flavorings and recipes included. Also chili. Enough for eight servings, $4. Buckeye Beans and Herbs catalog, (800) 449-2121.

Beano. Enzyme for digesting beans. FREE sample. AkPharma, Inc., P.O. Box 111, Pleasantville, NJ 08232, (800) 257-8650.

Low-Fat or Low-Calorie Foods

Smithers Low-Cal, Fat-Free Broths. Chicken, vegetable, or beef, six ounces per packet. Low-sodium varieties available. Forty packets, $20. Two hundred packets, $52. Bruce Medical Supply catalog, (800) 225-8446.

Egg Whites

Just Whites. Powdered dried egg whites. Each eight-ounce container is equivalent to the whites from 4 dozen eggs. Instructions included. Two eight-ounce cans, $10. Fatwise catalog, (800) 773-8822.

Products

Measures, Tools, and Tables

Egg Separator. Balance this straining device over a bowl, break the egg onto it, and the white will fall into the bowl while the yolk remains on top. $2. Lighthouse Consumer Products catalog, (800) 829-0500.

Tactile All-Purpose Food Scale. One raised dot marks each ounce up to eighteen ounces and three dots every four ounces. Also measures grams. $20. Lighthouse Consumer Products catalog, (800) 829-0500.

Electronic Food Scale. Either ounces or grams with digital display. Cuisinart. $70. A Cook's Wares catalog, (412) 846-9490.

Talking Kitchen Scale. Electronic voice announces measurements up to eleven pounds in half-ounce increments. Removable bowl. $137. Lighthouse Consumer Products catalog, (800) 829-0500.

Slimmer Skimmer. A fat-removing ladle. Fat enters the ladle through perforations on one side and is poured out the lip on the other side. Stainless steel. $9. A Cook's Wares catalog, (412) 846-9490.

Fat Separator Cup. Pour soup or gravy into cup; wait until fat rises to the surface; then pour nonfat liquid via spout that drains directly from the bottom. Four-cup capacity, $14; 1½-cup capacity, $8. Wooden Spoon catalog, (800) 431-2207.

Fat Finder Calculator. The percentage of calories from fat appears in a window of this vinyl calculator when the inner circle is aligned with the total number of calories and the outer circle is aligned with the number of grams of fat in a food. Small print. $4. Collage Video Specialties catalog, (800) 433-6769.

"Nutritional Analysis of Cheeses and Other Dairy Products,"

American Institute for Cancer Research. A slide chart that lists the protein, fat, sodium, calcium, and calorie content of a variety of cheeses, milks, and milk products. FREE. AICR, 1759 R Street, NW, Washington, DC 20009, (800) 843-8114.

Health Counts: A Fat and Calorie Guide, Kaiser Permanente. Calories, fat, and percentage of fat listed for twenty-five hundred foods. Includes weight loss tips and ideas for low-fat eating. 1991. John Wiley.

Fat and Cholesterol Counter, American Heart Association. A pocket-size reference. Includes sodium content of foods. Easy-to-read print. 1991. Times Books/Random House.

"The Eating Smart Fat Guide," Center for Science in the Public Interest. A sliding gauge that indicates the number of grams of saturated fat, total fat, and total calories for more than 250 foods, including brand-name frozen and fast foods. The size of a business envelope, with small print. $4. CSPI, 1875 Connecticut Avenue, NW, Suite 300, Washington, DC 20009, (800) 237-4874.

"Fat-O-Stat," American Heart Association. A diet quiz to reveal fat you may not realize you eat and a dozen ways to lower the fat in your diet. AHA, 7272 Greenville Avenue, Dallas, TX 75231, (800) AHA-USA1 (242-8721).

BEST BUY. *Nutritive Value of Foods*, U.S. Department of Agriculture. A listing of more than seven hundred foods with a comprehensive breakdown into component nutrients, including cholesterol, calories, saturated, monounsaturated, and polyunsaturated fats. Includes vitamin and mineral contents. Home and Garden Bulletin No. 72. $3.75. Superintendent of Documents, U.S. Government Printing Office, Washington, DC 20402.

"Food Plans That Lower Cancer Risk," American Institute for Cancer Research. A slide chart that details how much of different foods to include in different diets and for different age-groups. FREE. AICR, 1759 R Street, NW, Washington, DC 20009, (800) 843-8114.

"Guide to Beverages," American Institute for Cancer Research. A slide guide that indicates calories, sodium, and vitamins A and C content of about two hundred drinks, including brand-name sodas and alcoholic drinks. FREE. AICR, 1759 R Street, NW, Washington, DC 20009, (800) 843-8114.

Grocery Shopping Guide by Nelda Mercer, M.S., R.D., Melvyn Rubenfire, M.D., and Lori Mosca, M.Ph., M.D. A consumer's manual for selecting foods lower in total fat, saturated fat, and cholesterol. Indicates which foods, by brand names and product names, conform to recommended nutritional guidelines. Foods that are high in sodium and good sources of fiber are noted, as well as foods that contain egg yolks. The print is large enough to read easily. You can make your shopping decisions at home without having to worry about reading and studying labels in the supermarket. $20. MedSport, University of Michigan Medical Center, P.O. Box 363, Ann Arbor, MI 48106, (313) 998-7400.

The Low-Fat Supermarket by Judith Scharman Smith, M.S., R.D., and Scott D. Smith, M.D. A listing of more than four thousand products found in a supermarket that contain less than 30 percent of their calories from fat. Indicates calories, sodium, cholesterol, and amount of fat in products by brand name. Also suggests cooking tips and fast-food options for low-fat nutrition. $11. 1993. Starburst Publishers, P.O. Box 4123, Lancaster, PA 17604, (800) 441-1456, orders only.

Services

The Meat and Poultry Hot Line. Recorded messages on various nutrition-related topics, not only meat and poultry. Safety hints on handling, preparation, storing, and cooking of meat, poultry, and eggs; advice on labeling, nutrition, and other issues, including special information about planning for an earthquake. A dietitian or nutritionist will answer specific questions. Publications are available. U.S. Department of Agriculture, (800) 535-4555, in Washington, DC, (202) 720-3333.

HEARTLINE. Information on foods to choose to prevent cardiovascular diseases and stroke. American Heart Association, (800) AHA USA1 (242-8721).

National Health Information Center. Database of resources for information, publications, or programs about health issues. NHIC, P.O. Box 1133, Washington, DC 20013, (800) 336-4797.

HCF Foundation Hot Line. The initials HCF stand for "high carbohydrate fiber," and the hot line deals with questions relating to the role of diet in health, particularly cholesterol and high blood pressure. Brochures and newsletter. (800) 727 4HCF (4423).

The Nutrition Hot Line. Registered dietitians answer within two days questions about food, nutrition, dietary requirements, not necessarily related to cancer. FREE publications. Shopping list pads and a vitamin reminder notepad are also available FREE. American Institute for Cancer Research, 1759 R Street, NW, Washington, DC 20009, (800) 843-8114.

American Cancer Society Hot Line. Information about preventing cancer with dietary changes. (800) ACS 2345 (227-2345).

Food Allergy Center Hot Line. Information on food allergies and treatments. (800) YES RELIEF (937-7354).

University of Alabama at Birmingham Food Hot Line. Dietitians or dietetic technicians will answer food and nutrition questions within a day. (800) 231 DIET (3438).

Alliance for Food and Fiber Hot Line. The produce growers' trade association offers recorded messages and an opportunity to record questions, which will be answered within a day. (800) 266-0200.

Consumer Nutrition Hot Line. The American Dietetic Association, a professional organization of dietitians and nutritionists. Registered dietitians answer questions and make referrals to dietitians near you. Publications. Nutrition reading list. National Center for Nutrition and Dietetics, 216 West Jackson Boulevard, Chicago, IL 60606, (800) 366-1655.

The Food and Nutrition Information Center. Answers questions about specific foods, nutrition, the Food Pyramid, or food labels and will supply brief reading lists on a variety of topics. National Agricultural Library, 10301 Baltimore Boulevard, Room 304, Beltsville, MD 20705.

Publications

"The Food Guide Pyramid," Human Nutrition Information Service. Explains the various elements of the nutrition guidelines, serving sizes, choices for a healthy diet. Home and Garden Bulletin No. 252. $1. Consumer Information Center, Dept. 159-Y, Pueblo, CO 81009.

"Check Your Smoking I.Q.: An Important Quiz for Older Smokers," National Heart, Lung, and Blood Institute. A true-false quiz with answers that relate the benefits of quitting smoking to your health. FREE. NHLBI Information Center, P.O. Box 30105, Bethesda, MD 20824, (301) 251-1222.

"Eat Right to Lower Your High Blood Cholesterol." A pamphlet containing a simplified discussion of cholesterol. A detachable shopping list can be taken to the supermarket as a reminder of which foods to choose. FREE. National Cholesterol Education Program, NHLBI Information Center, P.O. Box 30105, Bethesda, MD 20824, (301) 251-1222.

"New Lean Toward Health," National Center for Nutrition and Dietetics. This brochure offers suggestions for reducing dietary fat and explains how to calculate the grams of fat you should include in your daily meals. FREE. NCND, 216 West Jackson Boulevard, Suite 800, Chicago, IL 60606, (800) 366-1655.

"The Facts About Fat," American Institute for Cancer Research. Brief discussion of fat and your diet. Includes a chart that shows the amount of fat you can consume depending on the calories in your diet. FREE. AICR, 1759 R Street, NW, Washington, DC 20009, (800) 843-8114.

Dr. Dean Ornish's Program for Reversing Heart Disease. A discussion of how to remove plaque from arteries and prevent it from forming through a combined program of meditation, exercise, and diet. Includes a two-hundred-page cookbook with mainly vegetarian recipes, with nutritional analyses of calories, total fat, saturated fat, and cholesterol. 1990. Random House.

American Heart Association, Low-Fat, Low-Cholesterol Cookbook, edited by Scott Grundy, M.D., Ph.D. Each recipe is analyzed for protein, carbohydrate, fat (saturated, polyunsaturated, and monounsaturated), sodium, calories, and cholesterol. The book includes the American Heart Association/National Heart, Lung, and Blood Institute diets and diets for different calorie needs. 1989. Times Books.

High Fit — Low Fat by Lizzie Burt and Nelda Mercer. This book includes menus and an analysis of each recipe per serving for calories, protein, fat, and carbohydrates. $14. MedSport, University of Michigan Medical Center, P.O. Box 363, Ann Arbor, MI 48106, (313) 998-7400.

"Step by Step: Eating to Lower Your High Blood Cholesterol." Easy-to-understand presentation of the cholesterol issue. Appendices list the cholesterol and fat contents of a variety of common foods. Some tips on how to lower blood cholesterol levels through changes in diet. The back cover includes a reminder chart with lists of foods to favor, others to eat seldom. FREE. National Cholesterol Education Program, NHLBI Information Center, P.O. Box 30105, Bethesda, MD 20824, (301) 251-1222.

Heartline. A newsletter for heart patients. Other publications. The Cleveland Clinic Foundation, 9500 Euclid Avenue, Cleveland, OH 44106.

"So You Have High Blood Cholesterol . . ." This pamphlet describes the significance of the results of blood cholesterol tests. 1992. FREE. National Cholesterol Education Program, National Heart, Lung, and Blood Institute, P.O. Box 30105, Bethesda, MD 20824, (301) 251-1222.

"Nutrition and Your Health: Dietary Guidelines for Americans," U.S. Department of Agriculture. Explains why you should follow this eating plan. 4th Edition due 1996. FREE. Food and Nutrition Information Center, National Agricultural Library, 10301 Baltimore Boulevard, Room 304, Beltsville, MD 20705.

"Be Your Best: Nutrition After Fifty," American Institute for Cancer Research. This brochure presents an overview of nutritional needs, food sources, and recipes. FREE. AICR, 1759 R Street, NW, Washington, DC 20009, (800) 843-8114.

Organizations

American Allergy Association. Information and self-help techniques for people with food and chemical allergies. AAA, P.O. Box 7273, Menlo Park, CA 94026, (415) 322-1663.

National Cholesterol Education Program. Information about cholesterol. National Heart, Lung, and Blood Institute, P.O. Box 30105, Bethesda, MD 20824, (301) 251-1222.

American Heart Association. Local branches provide information, referrals, publications, and support groups. AHA, 7272 Greenville Avenue, Dallas, TX 75231, (800) AHA-USA1 (242-8721).

Center for Science in the Public Interest. Publications on nutrition and diet. CSPI, 1875 Connecticut Avenue, NW, Suite 300, Washington, DC 20009, (800) 237-4874.

Chapter 7

Following a Special Diet

"At first my hand automatically reached for the salt-shaker, and everything tasted funny to me without it. Now I don't even think about it."

"I don't treat myself as a sick person. Limiting my diet isn't so radical. I just do the best I can."

In addition to concerns about fat, many of us have medical conditions that require us to shape our diets according to particular nutritional needs. Your doctor may recommend that you increase, avoid, or limit certain foods as part of a treatment program, such as including more calcium to forestall brittle bones, restricting salt in an effort to normalize high blood pressure, adding more soluble fiber to improve digestion, or consuming fewer calories to control weight.

LOWERING YOUR USE OF SODIUM

The role of salt, or, more accurately, sodium, in the diet of a person with high blood pressure is often misunderstood. Sodium by itself doesn't *cause* high blood pressure, also called hypertension, but sometimes, for some people, limiting salt can help lower blood pressure. Consuming less sodium may reduce the pressure the cells of the body exert against blood vessels, easing the flow of blood and lessening the effort needed by the heart to circulate blood. High blood pressure is particularly dangerous since it doesn't announce its presence with warning symptoms before heart disease or a stroke occurs. Hence its awful nickname, the silent killer.

One third of all cases of heart disease and one half of all cases of stroke can be eliminated through effective blood pressure management. For every five- or six-point reduction in blood pressure, your risk of heart disease declines 20 to 25 percent and your risk of stroke declines 30 to 40 percent.

Weight control may be an effective way to lower blood pressure for overweight people; cells heavy with fat deposits exert pressure on the walls of blood vessels, causing blood to move less freely about the body.

Alternatives to Foods High in Sodium	
Replace	**With**
1 tablespoon margarine — 132mg	1 tablespoon vegetable oil — 0
1 tablespoon blue cheese salad dressing — 164 mg	1 tablespoon oil and vinegar — a trace
1 tablespoon bottled mustard — 195 mg	Homemade mustard (1 teaspoon dry mustard plus 1 tablespoon vinegar) — a trace
4 medium green olives — 312 mg	3 small pitted black olives — 68 mg
1 cup canned green beans — 326 mg	1 cup fresh green beans — 5 mg
½ cup canned mushrooms — 400 mg	1 cup fresh mushrooms — 3 mg
¼ pound salted peanuts — 418 mg	¼ pound unsalted roasted peanuts — 5 mg
3 ounces corned beef — 802 mg or 1 beef hot dog — 639 mg	3 ounces lean beef — 55 mg
1 medium dill pickle — 928 mg	1 small gherkin — 107 mg
1 packet bouillon — 1,019 mg	1 packet dehydrated onion soup — 635 mg
1 teaspoon salt — 2,196 mg	1 teaspoon soy sauce — 439 mg

Attempts to treat high blood pressure with stress management, relaxation training, meditation, biofeedback, self-hypnosis, or such supplements as calcium, magnesium, potassium, and fish oil may work in isolated cases for short periods but have not been proved medically sound. Medication is sometimes necessary to control high blood pressure.

Reducing your use of table salt is a significant way of restricting sodium in your diet. While the human body needs a mere 200 milligrams of sodium a day to function, the average American consumes as much as 6,000 mg of sodium each day, or 1 *tablespoon* of salt. A quarter of a teaspoon of salt contains 500 mg of sodium.

The National Academy of Sciences recommends that people with normal blood pressure consume between 1,100 and 3,000 mg of sodium per day ½ to 1½ *teaspoons* of salt). A sodium-restricted diet may range from 500 to 3,000 mg a day. Since 75 percent of the sodium in American diets is derived from processed foods (plus 15 percent from using the saltshaker and 10 percent found naturally in foods), you should note the sodium content on nutrition labels of canned and frozen foods. A product that is "sodium-free" has less than 5 mg of sodium in each serving, while "low-sodium" foods have 140 mg or less sodium per serving. You may be shocked by the high amount of sodium in some foods.

Other foods high in sodium:

1 tablespoon ketchup — 156 mg
3 ounces canned sardines — 425 mg
2 slices braunschweiger — 652 mg
8 ounces cottage cheese — 920 mg
3 ounces ham — 1,000 mg
1 cup canned chicken noodle soup — 1,107 mg
¼ pound cheeseburger — 1,200 mg
7 ounces tuna, oil- or water-packed — 1,500 mg
1 cup canned sauerkraut — 1,560 mg
¼ pound pretzels — 1,680 mg
3 ounces smoked salmon — 1,700 mg

Also high in sodium: all shellfish (except oysters), anchovies, canned soups, canned gravies, canned sauces, frozen TV dinners, delicatessen meats, sausages, hot dogs.

Some foods low in sodium: fresh vegetables (except artichokes), vegetable oils, fresh fruits, jams and jellies, spices and herbs, cooked breakfast cereals, shredded wheat, pasta and egg noodles, popcorn, rice, dried beans, peas, lentils, poultry, uncured meats.

As with any changes in your eating patterns, you may accustom yourself to new tastes more easily if you reduce your use of salt gradually over a month or two. As you do so, you can flavor foods by increasing your use of other seasonings. The following ingredients will lend flavor to foods even in small amounts: lemon juice, oregano, paprika, garlic, minced onion, basil, and dill.

Adding no-sodium bouillon to your cooking water can flavor vegetables and rice. In baking, one and a half teaspoons of low-sodium baking powder can substitute for one teaspoon of regular baking powder, which contains sodium bicarbonate and sodium aluminum sulfate. Potassium bicarbonate, available at drugstores, can replace baking soda, which contains sodium bicarbonate. Low-sodium milk powder, available at drugstores, is an alternative to regular milk.

Resources

Products

Salt Sensor. Gives an instant readout of the percentage of salt when the point of this thermometer-style gadget is inserted into a food. Battery-operated. $25. Sears Home HealthCare catalog, (800) 326-1750.

Services

Mrs. Dash Sodium Information Hot Line. Dietitians answer questions about sodium, high blood pressure, and nutrition. The hot line can provide the sodium contents of ten thousand foods. Brochures available. (800) 622-DASH (3274).

High Blood Pressure Information Line. Recorded messages with suggestions from the National Heart, Lung, and Blood Institute about prevention and treatment of high blood pressure. (800) 575-WELL (9355).

Publications

Recipes for the Heart: A Nutrition Guide for People with High Blood Pressure by Lucy M. Williams. Although the emphasis in this book is on sodium reduction, a nutritional analysis of each recipe includes fat, calories, potassium, calcium, and carbohydrates as well as sodium.

The recipes are simple and require few ingredients and few steps; most are complete on a single page. The book has lists of the sodium contents of various foods and fast foods. This spiral-bound book lies flat and is typeset in a medium type size. $14. 1990. Sandridge Publishing, 15348 Sandridge Road, Bowling Green, OH 43402.

Craig Claiborne's Gourmet Diet by Craig Claiborne with Pierre Franey. Recipes for people who are watching the salt, fat, sugar, and cholesterol in their diets. The "Trompe le Palais" chapter includes some excellent suggestions for how to "fool the palate" when you don't cook with salt. Each recipe includes an analysis of calories, sodium, fat, and cholesterol per serving. A twelve-page appendix gives the nutritional analysis of dozens of foods. 1980. Times Books.

"Facts About How to Prevent High Blood Pressure," National High Blood Pressure Education Program. A simplified explanation of the effects of high blood pressure and dietary and lifestyle changes that can help prevent it. FREE. National Heart, Lung, and Blood Institute Information Center, P.O. Box 30105, Bethesda, MD 20824, (800) 575-WELL (9355).

"How You Can Help Your Doctor Treat Your High Blood Pressure," American Heart Association. A pamphlet that briefly explains the medical aspects of high blood pressure including a list of medications frequently prescribed and their side effects. List of food choices according to sodium content. AHA, 7272 Greenville Avenue, Dallas, TX 75231, (800) AHA-USA1 (242-8721).

"High Blood Pressure: Treat It for Life," National Heart, Lung, and Blood Institute. A discussion of high blood pressure and how to treat it with diet, exercise, and medication. FREE. NHLBI Information Center, P.O. Box 30105, Bethesda, MD 20824, (301) 251-1222.

"High Blood Pressure and What You Can Do About It" by Marvin Moser, M.D. A detailed discussion of high blood pressure and common treatments. FREE. 1994. High Blood Pressure Information Center, P.O. Box 30105, Bethesda, MD 20824.

"Health Alert: Sodium," National Council on the Aging. Suggestions for cutting back on sodium in your diet and a quiz to check your use of salt. FREE. NCOA, 409 3rd Street, SW, Suite 200, Washington, DC 20024, (202) 479-1200.

Organizations

National Heart, Lung, and Blood Institute Information Center. Information on cholesterol, heart disease, and high blood pressure. NHLBI, P.O. Box 30105, Bethesda, MD 20824, (301) 251-1222.

American Heart Association. Information about cardiovascular disease and stroke. AHA, 7272 Greenville Avenue, Dallas, TX 75231, (800) AHA-USA1 (242-8721).

National Stroke Association. Information about stroke prevention, facts about stroke, support groups, and answers to your questions. Publications available. NSA, 8480 East Orchard Road, Suite 1000, Englewood, CO 80111, (800) STROKES (787-6537).

CONTROLLING YOUR WEIGHT

Weight control isn't an issue of personal choice, a matter of ego or pride, or a fashion or fad of the moment. It's one risk factor that you can control. Thirty-four million American adults are officially obese, more than 30 percent above normal or desirable weight. One way to determine your ideal weight is to calculate as follows: For women, begin with 100 pounds for your first five feet in height and add 5 pounds for each additional inch; for men, begin with 106 pounds for your first five feet in height and add 6 pounds for each additional inch.

It's easy to be frustrated by proclamations and diet books that oversimplify a very complex subject. A lifetime of eating habits, your personality, lifestyle, and other health issues can make controlling weight difficult — difficult, perhaps, but not impossible. The basic principle of weight control is to balance the number of calories burned with the amount of calories in the food you eat. Following the recommendations of the Food Pyramid may help reduce the number of calories you consume per day by reducing your fat intake. Embarking on an exercise program has been found to be an essential component of any effort to lose weight.

To control your weight by limiting the total number of calories in your daily meals, you have to decide on how many calories you should consume each day.

Daily Calorie Needs for Men and Women

	Over Age 50	Over Age 75	Minimum
Men	2,400	2,050	1,650
Women	1,800	1,600	1,200

To *maintain your weight,* calculate a daily diet of 15 calories per pound of body weight. To *lose weight,* calculate a diet of 10 calories per pound of body weight. To *gain weight,* calculate a diet of 20 calories per pound of body weight. Then *subtract 10 percent* for each decade you are over age fifty.

SOURCES: The Food and Nutrition Board of the National Research Council and the *1990 Merck Manual of Geriatrics.*

Seven Simple Weight Control Strategies

1. *The 5 percent solution.* Think of the weight you need to lose in 5 percent blocks. For each block, allow a generous and achievable time period (expecting to lose not more than 1 pound each week) within which to accomplish it. Wait a few months before beginning to lose another 5 percent block. Example: You weigh 150 and want to lose a total of 30 pounds. First lose 8 pounds in two months, stay at 142 pounds for two months, and lose 7 pounds in the next two months.

2. *The balance beam.* Develop a balance of intensity between your diet and your exercise programs. When sticking to your diet seems particularly onerous or when you can't seem to lose another pound, add one extra exercise session. Alternatively, keep your exercise routine unchanged and make a substitution in your diet to cut back on some calories. This reinforces your control over your weight.

3. *The understudy.* Deprivation, especially with food, is never easy as a long-term proposition. Substitution can be a simpler method; let the understudies have center stage. Replace a cup of ice cream (270 calories) with a cup of ice milk (185 calories). Instead of a slice of carrot cake (385 calories), try a slice of pound cake (120 calories). By gradually incorporating these substitute foods

into your diet, you won't feel that you have suddenly banished treats from your life.

4. *Larger portions.* If smaller servings don't satisfy your eye or your stomach, try larger servings of a food with fewer calories. For example, you may prefer a normal-size portion of ice milk rather than a tiny bit of ice cream, or you might enjoy a salad generously flavored with low-calorie dressing rather than use only a touch of a higher-calorie one.

5. *More is better.* Eating more frequent meals, or small meals plus snacks, fills you up and counters feelings of deprivation.

6. *Weighing in.* Weighing yourself regularly can be uplifting and serve as reinforcement. However, decide whether you are the type who will become obsessed by the scale or whether you can use it to serve a positive purpose. Think about keeping within *a range* of five pounds so that you give yourself some leeway. Don't become a slave to the numbers. Remember, if you are exercising, you may be losing fat and gaining muscle with no change in your weight. Worrying about every half pound gained or celebrating every half pound lost is not productive in the long run.

7. *Fight the fat, forget the weight.* The variables of metabolism and body makeup can render the scale's message irrelevant. If you would rather monitor your size than your weight, find out your percentage of body fat and work to reduce it. A health club can calculate your body fat percentage by using a caliper to measure a fold of skin, or you can do it yourself at home. Alternatively, try on an item of clothing and monitor the way it fits as you progress.

As some people age, they notice slight or gradual weight changes, as well as redistributions of the amount of fat and muscle on their bodies. You should consult a doctor if you experience a sudden loss of weight.

Resources

Physical activity as an adjunct to managing your diet to control your weight is examined in Chapter 10, "On the Move."

131

Products

Doctor's Office-Style Scale. Sliding weights balance a bar. $200. Sears Home HealthCare catalog, (800) 326-1750.

Sitting Scale. Weigh yourself sitting down and read the result after you get up. $85. Sears Home HealthCare catalog, (800) 326-1750.

Scale with Waist Level Dial. $115. Sears Home HealthCare catalog, (800) 326-1750.

Electronic Bigfoot. Scale with two-inch-high digital display. $85. Sears Home HealthCare catalog, (800) 326-1750.

Weight Talker III. Voice synthesizer scale speaks your weight, up to 288 pounds, and indicates weight loss or gain. $75. Lighthouse Consumer Products catalog, (800) 829-0500.

Calipers. A do-it-yourself device for monitoring body fat. The package includes a Body Fat Interpretation Chart that gives percentages for men and women by age-group. $20. Accu-Measure, Inc., P.O. Box 4040, Parker, CO 80134, (800) 866-2727.

Skinfold Caliper. To check your body fat by measuring your "pinch." Instruction manual included. $11. Lowfat Lifeline, P.O. Box 1889, Port Townsend, WA 98368, (360) 379-9724.

Body Fat Tester. Place tester on upper arm and digital display shows percent body fat. Progress charts included. $100. Safety Zone catalog, (800) 999-3030.

Services

Weight-Control Information Network. Provides information about the prevention and treatment of obesity, weight management, and diet programs. WIN, 1 WIN Way, Bethesda, MD 20892, (301) 951-1120.

Publications

"Understanding Adult Obesity," National Institute of Diabetes and Digestive and Kidney Diseases. A fact sheet that discusses various ways of evaluating your weight, including a chart for determining your body mass index. Also discusses some causes and risks of overweight. FREE. Weight-Control Information Network, 1 WIN Way,

Bethesda, MD 20892, (301) 951-1120.

"Why Can't I Lose Weight?," American Dietetic Association. This pamphlet provides some weight control suggestions. FREE. ADA, 216 West Jackson Boulevard, Chicago, IL 60606, (800) 745-0775.

The Duke University Medical Center Book of Diet and Fitness by Michael Hamilton, M.D., M.PH., et al. A famous weight loss program in book form, including meal plans and recipes. 1990. Fawcett Columbine.

Take Control of Your Weight by Steven Jonas, M.D. Guidance in designing a weight loss program according to your individual goals, your metabolism, and your eating habits and needs. 1993. Consumer Reports Books.

"Get Fit, Trim Down: Losing Weight and Following the Dietary Guidelines to Lower Cancer Risk," American Institute for Cancer Research. Suggestions for ways to lose weight by eating a healthy diet. FREE. AICR, 1759 R Street, NW, Washington, DC 20009, (800) 843-8114.

"The Facts About Weight Loss Products and Programs," Food and Drug Administration. What to look for and what to avoid in selecting a program for weight control. Also, where to lodge complaints about misleading weight loss claims and where to obtain more information. FREE. FDA, Consumer Affairs, 5600 Fishers Lane, HFC-110, Rockville, MD 20857, (301) 443-3170.

"A Guide to Losing Weight," American Heart Association. Suggestions to help you assemble menus that can assist you in achieving a healthy weight and still eat healthy foods. FREE. AHA, 7272 Greenville Avenue, Dallas, TX 75231, (800) AHA-USA1 (242-8721).

ADDING DIETARY FIBER FOR DIGESTION

The complex carbohydrates that constitute the base of the Food Pyramid include starches, discussed earlier, which are digested by the body, and dietary fiber, the indigestible complex carbohydrates in plant cell walls. Dietary fiber, whether soluble (like that in fruits, vegetables, and oat bran) or insoluble (like that in wheat bran and whole grains), has several important health benefits.

Benefits of Dietary Fiber

- Alleviates constipation and discomfort from hemorrhoids by making the stool softer and heavier and helping it pass through the colon more easily and swiftly.
- Contributes to weight control by making you feel full and by reducing calories, since foods high in dietary fiber are low in fats.
- Protects against diabetes by helping control the level of sugar in the blood.
- Protects against heart disease by helping lower blood cholesterol levels.
- Protects against colon cancer in ways not yet fully understood.

The average American's daily diet includes about 12 grams of dietary fiber, about one third of the amount considered essential. The recommended amount is 20 to 35 grams a day, or at least 11.5 grams for each thousand calories. Consuming more than 50 grams of dietary fiber, however, may cause important vitamins and minerals to pass through your system without being absorbed by your body.

Most people must give their intestinal tracts time to adjust to an increase in dietary fiber. Diarrhea, bloating, cramps, and flatulence are evidence of the laxative effect of dietary fiber. Each person must proceed cautiously and in accordance with his or her own body's reactions. When you add dietary fiber to your diet, do so slowly, one food at a time in small quantities, over a period of weeks or months. Be sure to drink plenty of water — at least two glasses at mealtimes — when you are eating fiber-rich foods. Even a small amount of additional fiber may have a noticeable effect on constipation, hemorrhoids, and other digestive complaints.

The National Research Council recommends adding dietary fiber from food sources in preference to consuming concentrated fiber, as found in remedies sold in drugstores.

Selected Fiber-Rich Foods

	Grams of dietary fiber
3 dried figs	9.5
½ cup cooked kidney beans	9.0
½ cup cooked pinto beans	8.9
⅓ cup oat bran	7.8
½ cup cooked lima beans	6.6
½ cup canned chickpeas	6.5
5 dried dates	3.6
1 medium orange	3.1
1 medium potato with skin	3.0
1 tablespoon wheat bran	1.5

NOTE: There is no dietary fiber in meat and dairy products. Fruits and vegetables contain fiber, but their juices do not. Foods don't have to be raw and crunchy to contain fiber.

Add a handful of beans to your soups or salads as a first step in increasing your fiber intake. Use a real potato rather than the instant variety, or substitute raw spinach for some of the lettuce in your salad.

Your digestive system may respond to variations in your diet as well as to your level of physical activity or changes in your daily schedule. The idea of a bowel movement a day is considered outdated as a measure of health; constipation is now defined as five to seven days without a bowel movement.

Possible Causes of and Ways to Relieve Constipation

Possible Cause	Resources
Certain medications	Check with your doctor to see if you can take an alternative medication.
Overuse of laxatives	Prevent loss of muscle tone in the intestines by not depending on laxatives.
Lack of exercise	Exercise can stimulate intestinal activity.
Insufficient fluid intake	Increasing fluid consumption can soften stools.
Slowed intestinal activity	Speed intestinal activity with more dietary fiber, exercise, and fluids.
Insufficient dietary fiber	Be sure you are eating enough to stimulate digestion.

Options for physical activity are explored in Part Three, "Staying Active."

Services

National Digestive Diseases Information Clearinghouse. Information, referrals, and publications on subjects such as constipation, heartburn, ulcers. NDDIC, 2 Information Way, Bethesda, MD 20892-3570, (301) 654-3810.

National Kidney and Urologic Diseases Information Clearinghouse. Information regarding digestive problems. NKUDIC, 3 Information Way, Bethesda, MD 20892-3580, (301) 654-4415.

Publications

"Rough It Up," Center for Science in the Public Interest. A slide chart that lists the fiber and fat content of about 270 foods; includes brand names and fast foods. $4. CSPI, 1875 Connecticut Avenue, NW, Suite 300, Washington, DC 20009, (800) 237-4874.

"Fiber Facts," American Dietetic Association. A pamphlet that discusses fiber in the diet, suggests daily servings of fiber, and lists the amounts of fiber in various foods. FREE. ADA, 216 West Jackson Boulevard, Chicago, IL 60606, (800) 745-0775.

"Health Alert: Fiber," National Council on the Aging. Guidance to selecting foods that are good sources of fiber. FREE. NCOA, 409 3rd Street, SW, Suite 200, Washington, DC 20024, (202) 479-1200.

The Complete Book of Better Digestion: A Gut-Level Guide to Gastric Relief by Michael Oppenheim, M.D. An upbeat, nontechnical discussion of digestive problems and their treatments. 1990. Rodale Press.

"Constipation." A fact sheet that briefly describes the causes and treatment of constipation. FREE. National Digestive Diseases Information Clearinghouse, 2 Information Way, Bethesda MD 20892-3570, (301) 654-3810.

Organizations

American Dietetic Association. FREE publications, nutrition information. Referrals to registered dietitians in your area. ADA, 216 West Jackson Boulevard, Chicago, IL 60606, (800) 366-1655.

LOW-CARBOHYDRATE DIETS
TO CONTROL DIABETES

Diabetes is a disease that results in too-high levels of blood sugar, either from an insufficient supply of the hormone insulin, which functions to reduce levels of glucose in body tissues (Type I Diabetes), or from an inefficient breakdown and utilization of carbohydrates by the body (Type II Diabetes, also called adult-onset diabetes). The eleven million Americans with Type II Diabetes usually are not required to take insulin but are treated with weight control, diet, and exercise.

Unfortunately it has been estimated that nearly half of the Type II cases, occurring mainly in people over age fifty, are undiagnosed and untreated. The consequences of untreated diabetes are serious; diabetes is the seventh most frequent cause of death in the United

---

American Diabetes Association Quiz

Add the numbers in parentheses for statements that apply to you.

1. I have been experiencing one or more of the following symptoms on a regular basis: excessive thirst (3), frequent urination (3), extreme fatigue (1), unexplained weight loss (3), blurry vision from time to time (2).
2. I am more than thirty years old (1).
3. My weight is equal to or above that listed in a height/weight chart (2).
4. I am a woman who has had more than one baby weighing over nine pounds at birth (2).
5. I am of Native American descent (1).
6. I am of Hispanic or African-American descent (1).
7. I have a parent with diabetes (1).
8. I have a brother or sister with diabetes (2).

If your total is less than 5, you are at low risk for diabetes, but you should remain alert to the danger signs. If you score more than 5 points, you may have, or be at high risk for, diabetes, and the ADA recommends that you see your doctor immediately.

States, the principal cause of blindness and kidney disease, and the second major cause of amputations (after traumatic injury). People who have diabetes are at twice the risk of others for stroke and heart attack.

The American Diabetes Association has devised a self-screening quiz that helps you evaluate your risk of diabetes. It's worth a few minutes of your time to discover if you're among those who are unaware they have diabetes.

People with adult-onset diabetes have to follow a carefully monitored diet that limits the amount of carbohydrates — sugars and starches — as well as protein, fat, and calories, according to a doctor's or nutritionist's instruction.

Resources

Products

Sugarless Foods

Fifty 50 Products. Cookies sweetened with fructose. Half the company's profits are contributed to diabetes research. For further information, Fifty 50 Foods, P.O. Box 89, Mendham, NJ 07945, (201) 543-6115.

Low-Sugar, Low-Fat Foods. Cookies, candies, cake mixes, and other items either unsweetened or with the type of sweetener used listed. Nutritional analysis of each product is given in the catalog. Diabetic Food Emporium, Ltd., 51 Cleveland Street, Hackensack, NJ 07601, (800) 285-3210.

Clearbrook Farms Sugar-Free Preserves. Fruits sweetened with fruit juice concentrates. No artificial flavors, colors, sweeteners, or preservatives. Each 7.25-ounce jar, $5. A Cook's Wares catalog, (412) 846-9562.

Fruit Butters, Spreads, and Sauces. The sauces and butters have seven calories per teaspoon. Each 10-ounce jar, $5. Also fudge sweet toppings. Sweetened with concentrated fruit juices, these toppings are said to taste like chocolate, but contain only sixteen calories per teaspoon and no sugar. Each 10-ounce jar, $6. Wax Orchards catalog, (800) 634-6132.

Sugar-Free Chocolate. Variety of chocolate products sweetened with fruit juice or other sweeteners. For example, 12 ounces assorted,

$17. 10 ounces fudge, $12. Delty Sugar Free Chocolate catalog, (800) 962-3355.

Services

Sugarfree Center Hot Line. Answers questions about sugar in the diet and offers publications. P.O. Box 21735, Roanoke, VA 24018, (800) 972-2323.

NutraSweet Consumer Center. Information on fat substitutes and sugar substitutes and recipes. NutraSweet Company, P.O. Box 830, Deerfield, IL 60015, (800) 321-7254.

National Diabetes Information Clearinghouse. This arm of the National Institutes of Health provides referrals to other organizations and information to the public about diabetes and its complications. Among the useful publications available: "The Diabetes Dictionary"; "Cookbooks for People with Diabetes," an annotated list of cookbooks; and "Diet and Exercise in Noninsulin-Dependent Diabetes Mellitus." "Diabetes in Adults" or "Noninsulin-Dependent Diabetes" provide a good explanation of the medical basis of adult-onset diabetes. FREE. NDIC, 1 Information Way, Bethesda, MD 20892-3560, (301) 654-3327.

Television Programs

"Living with Diabetes," CNBC/American Medical Television. A cable program that features interviews with celebrities who have diabetes. News about research, and tips on diet and health. Sundays, 2:00 P.M. ET.

Publications

Diabetes Self-Management. A bimonthly magazine that follows the latest news and technology of interest to people with diabetes. $12 year subscription. P.O. Box 52887, Boulder, CO 80321.

"Diabetes and Food: A Guide for People with Non-Insulin-Dependent Diabetes Mellitus," American Dietetic Association. This pamphlet offers guidance for meal planning and food choices. FREE. ADA, 216 West Jackson Boulevard, Chicago, IL 60606, (800) 745-0775.

Books About Diabetes and Nutrition. One source for books about food topics and diabetes issues. FREE catalog. Chronimed Publishing,

P.O. Box 59032, Minneapolis, MN 55459, (800) 848-2793.

Organizations

American Diabetes Association. Publications, including cookbooks, aids for planning meals, support groups, local chapters. ADA, 1660 Duke Street, P.O. Box 25757, Alexandria, VA 22314, (800) 232-3472.

STRENGTHENING BONES WITH CALCIUM

We encourage children to drink plenty of milk as a source of calcium while their bones are growing, but now it is understood that the need for calcium continues throughout adulthood. Gradual loss of bone density begins as early as age thirty, when fewer and fewer lost bone cells are replaced. The stronger your bones are when the process of bone cell replacement slows, the stronger they will be in your seventies and eighties. After age fifty you can try to limit the loss by exercising and increasing calcium in your diet. After age sixty the loss tapers off until bone mass stabilizes at age eighty. By seventy, women will have lost more than 20 percent of the bone they had at thirty; men will lose about 10 percent.

Osteoporosis describes a condition of weakened or brittle bones already beyond the reach of dietary changes. It means that bone loss has progressed to a degree that the bones are susceptible to fracture in situations that normally wouldn't result in a fracture.

Low-density vertebrae may painfully collapse and be crushed together. Osteoporosis may announce its presence with the gradual formation of a widow's hump and eventually may lead to a bent-over posture. Early indications of weakened bones may manifest themselves in chronic back problems, broken ribs, tooth loss, or changes in the jawbone that may be noticeable on dental X rays. Slipping on a patch of ice, falling at home, or tripping on a step may result in a fracture. Frequently such falls result in hip fractures, commonly in the tip of the femur or thighbone which ends in the ball upon which the hip rotates. Each year about 1.3 million fractures occurring in people age forty-five and older are attributable to osteoporosis.

A study reveals that six months after a hip fracture only 25 percent of patients are fully recovered, 50 percent need assistance with their daily activities, and 25 percent require nursing home care. Yet few people know they have weakened bones before they actually suffer fractures caused by osteoporosis.

Women are more frequently victims of osteoporosis than men; their bones are less dense by nature, and estrogen, one of the hormones that regulate the level of calcium in the blood, gradually diminishes after menopause. Estrogen is also important for the body's production of vitamin D, which helps metabolize calcium.

If calcium in the blood is lost through the urine and not enough is added through the diet, it will be resorbed from the bones to maintain stable levels in the blood. Women who are prescribed estrogen at menopause may avoid the precipitous bone loss that can occur during the five to seven years after menopause. Overweight women may be less subject to severe bone loss because some estrogen is produced by fatty cells, even after menopause.

Statistics indicate that osteoporosis is pervasive among people around age fifty. One third of all postmenopausal women, some fifteen to twenty million women, will develop osteoporosis, and one out of every two women over fifty will experience a fracture attributable to osteoporosis.

In 1994 an expert panel of the National Institutes of Health advised an increase in the recommended dietary allowance of calcium for adults from the current 800 milligrams per day to 1,000 mg per day for women over age fifty who take estrogen, all women age twenty-five to age forty-nine, and men age twenty-five to age sixty-four. The recommended amount of calcium for women age fifty who don't take estrogen and men age sixty-five and over is 1,500 mg per day.

Simultaneously increasing calcium and decreasing fat in the diet are a real challenge, since so many foods high in calcium are also high in fat. Some choices from the table below of low-fat or nonfat sources may allow you to get sufficient calcium without adding fat.

Three or four servings of high-calcium foods may be enough to equal your daily quota. If you dislike most dairy products, try them in new ways that fool your palate. Sneak foods with extra calcium into your menus: shakes made with powdered nonfat milk; soups with collard greens; chunks of tofu or cheese added to salads, soups, and omelets; nonfat milk added to soups and other items when possible; a slice or two of cheese in sandwiches; or pancakes made

Low-Fat and Nonfat Sources of Calcium

	Milligrams of Calcium	Grams of fat
1 cup Hi-Calcium 2% milk	700	5
1 cup nonfat yogurt	452	Trace
1 cup low-fat yogurt	415	4
1 cup cooked frozen collard greens	357	1
6 ounces Yoplait breakfast low-fat yogurt	348	Trace
½ cup part-skim ricotta	340	9
6 ounces calcium-fortified orange juice	300	1
8 ounces skim, 1%, 2% milk	300	Trace, 3, 5
½ cup ice milk	140	3
½ cup 2% low-fat cottage cheese	80	4
1 tablespoon instant nonfat milk	52	0

with skim or 1 percent milk rather than water. If you make soup stock, the addition of two teaspoons of vinegar will draw calcium from meat bones.

Calcium is more efficiently utilized by the body when it is ingested in small amounts, so spread the servings throughout the day, and include some at each meal, plus a snack or two. It is particularly important to have a large late-night calcium-rich snack since bone loss takes place at a higher rate when the body is at rest.

Some people have unpleasant gastric reactions after eating dairy products. About half of people over age fifty experience some reaction to dairy products: gas or cramps, diarrhea, or feeling full or bloated. By age seventy nearly 70 percent will have problems digesting the lactose (a sugar in dairy products) because of a deficiency in lactase, a digestive enzyme. Yet even those who are lactose-intolerant may be able to consume small amounts of dairy products, perhaps an eight-ounce glass of milk per meal or a serving of yogurt.

If you suspect you have problems digesting milk products, reduce the amount you consume by a little each day until you reach a level your system can tolerate without discomfort. Some people find goat's milk more easily digested than cow's milk. Dairy companies are marketing milk with lactase added during processing to break down the lactose and make it easier to digest. Lactase enzyme tablets also can be added to milk to help you digest lactose.

Calcium is an important component of bone formation, but it doesn't add to bone mass on its own. Some factors facilitate the body's utilization of calcium, and others work against it. Vitamins C and D, estrogen, and exercise have been found to combine with calcium to enhance bone formation. On the other hand, other factors seem to inhibit bone formation. For example, frequent use of laxatives discourages absorption of calcium by speeding up the passage of food through the intestines, as does excessive fiber, sodium, animal protein, fat, or phosphorus in the diet. Steroids and some medications and certain medical conditions may impede the utilization of calcium in the body. Smoking is another factor identified in reducing calcium absorption. Researchers are uncertain about the role of alcohol and caffeine in calcium absorption.

The body absorbs calcium more easily from certain sources. For example, calcium is more easily absorbed from skim than regular milk, and even though cooked frozen spinach has 277 milligrams of calcium, it is not in a readily accessible form. Some sources of calcium that are readily absorbed by the body include yogurt, sardines with bones, canned salmon with bones, oysters, broccoli, collard greens, dandelion greens, turnips, mustard greens, and kale. Some foods, such as spinach, chocolate, sorrel, swiss chard, and rhubarb, are high in oxalic acid, which may boost the body's ability to absorb calcium.

Scientists have found that vitamin D aids in calcium absorption, though its exact role is not clearly understood. Vitamin D is available from the ultraviolet rays of the sun and some foods. Fifteen minutes of exposure to the midday sun without sunscreen should provide a sufficient daily supply of vitamin D. The body's ability to manufacture vitamin D directly from the sun becomes less reliable as we age, and we must depend increasingly on getting this vitamin through our diet.

Most milk and some other calcium sources have been fortified with vitamin D. Check food labels to see if you are getting more vitamin D than you knew. If you don't get enough vitamin D in your food, ask your doctor if you need a supplement.

Two studies are being sponsored by the National Institute on Aging in hopes of alleviating osteoporosis. STOP/IT (Sites Testing Osteoporosis Prevention/Intervention Treatments) is due to continue until 1996. More than thirteen hundred men and women over age sixty-five are participating in the study, which will evaluate physical exercise, nutritional supplements, and hormone replacement in preventing, lessening, or reversing osteoporosis.

The other NIA study, FICSIT (Frailty and Injuries: Cooperative Studies of Intervention Techniques), is in progress, with results due in 1997.

Resources

A walking program and other physical activities are described in Part Three, "Staying Active."

Changes you can make in your home to achieve a safer environment are outlined in Chapter 12, "Adapting the Old Homestead."

Services

Calcium Information Center. Questions you pose relating to calcium will be answered by mail or phone. CIC, Division of Nephrology and Hypertension, Oregon Health Sciences University, 3314 Southwest Veterans Hospital Road, PP262, Portland, OR 97201, (800) 321-2681.

Dairy Ease Hot Line. Manufacturer of lactose-reduced products and caplets answers questions. Bayer Corporation, Consumer Relations, P.O. Box 5967, Parsippany, NJ 07054, (800) 331-4536.

Lactaid, Inc. Hot Line. The manufacturer of products for people who are lactose-intolerant will answer questions and provide information on its products. Brochure available. FREE samples. McNeil Consumer Products, Consumer Affairs, 7050 Camp Hill Road, Fort Washington, PA 19034, (800) LACTAID (522-8243).

Osteoporosis and Related Bone Diseases — National Resource Center. Information about the prevention, early detection, and treatment of osteoporosis. 1150 17th Street, NW, Suite 500, Washington, DC 20036, (800) 624-BONE (2663).

Publications

Preventing Osteoporosis by Kenneth H. Cooper, M.D. This book is comprehensive and suitable for a nonmedical audience. Enumerates risk factors for osteoporosis and offers a clever description of bone formation. Practical and detailed exercise and diet routines. Lists of substitutes or exchanges in different categories of foods. Recipes for calcium-fortified food, using powdered milk as a booster and keeping in mind a balanced diet and lowered calories and low-fat foods. The recipes have calorie, calcium, and cholesterol counts. 1989. Bantam Books.

"Preventing Osteoporosis," American College of Obstetricians and Gynecologists. This pamphlet provides an overview of the causes and treatment of osteoporosis and a list of foods containing calcium. FREE with SSE. ACOG Resource Center, 409 12th Street, SW, Washington, DC 20024.

"Boning Up on Calcium," American Dietetic Association. Overview of calcium in the diet and a list of calcium-rich foods. FREE. ADA, 216 West Jackson Boulevard, Chicago, IL 60606, (800) 745-0775.

"How Strong Are Your Bones?," National Osteoporosis Foundation. A discussion of tests that can measure the strength of your bones and an explanation of the effect of osteoporosis on your bones. FREE. NOF, Box 96173, Department BDT, Washington, DC 20077, (202) 223-2226.

"Stand Up to Osteoporosis," National Osteoporosis Foundation. Overview of the causes, prevention, and treatment of osteoporosis. FREE. NOF Hot Line, 1150 17th Street, NW, Suite 500, Washington, DC 20036, (800) 223-9994.

"Osteoporosis: The Bone Thinner," National Institute on Aging. An "Age Page" summary of osteoporosis, including other sources. FREE. NIA Information Center, P.O. Box 8057, Gaithersburg, MD 20898, (800) 222-2225.

"Osteoporosis," American College of Orthopedic Surgeons. A brief discussion of diagnosis and treatment. ACOS, 222 South Prospect Avenue, Park Ridge IL 60068, (708) 823-7186.

"Live It Safe! Prevent Broken Hips," American Academy of Orthopaedic Surgeons. An overview of dietary and lifestyle changes you can adopt that can help you avoid a broken hip. FREE. AAOS, 6300 North River Road, Rosement, IL 60018, (708) 698-9980.

Resources for Other Special Diets

American Parkinson's Disease Association Hot Line. Publications, referrals, and information. 1250 Hylan Boulevard, Suite 4B, Staten Island, NY 10305, (800) 223-2732.

"Nutritional Considerations of Parkinson's Disease," National Parkinson Foundation. A discussion of diet and Parkinson's disease, including a detailed diet plan with exchanges and alternative choices. NPF, Bob Hope Parkinson Research Center, 1501 Northwest 9th Avenue, Bob Hope Road, Miami, FL 33136, (800) 327-4545, or in Florida call (800) 433-7022.

Organizations

National Osteoporosis Foundation. Inquiries, referrals to services, resources, support groups, publications. NOF, 1150 17th Street, NW, Suite 500, Washington, DC 20036, (202) 223-2226.

Chapter 8

Home Cooking

"I don't have all the latest gadgets, and I'm not a gourmet, but I can make what I'm hungry for."

Being responsible for your own meals is an important goal for those who want to live independently. It can be made easier if you shop by phone, buy foods prepared by a local store, or sign up for Meals on Wheels. There are many simple modifications that will make your kitchen more accessible.

Small changes can be a big help in preparing and storing your food. When you need to stoop to the lowest drawer or reach the highest shelf, you limit the most effective use of the kitchen. A review of your kitchen equipment and your cooking methods may suggest safer and easier ways of preparing your meals.

Kitchen Safety Alert

DO NOT USE WATER ON KITCHEN FIRES. *SMOTHER* ALL FIRES IN THE KITCHEN. USE A POT LID, POUR SALT OR BAKING SODA ON FLAMES, OR USE A FIRE EXTINGUISHER.

KITCHEN DESIGN AND STORAGE

Kitchen designers describe the most efficient work space as a triangle where the sink, refrigerator, and stove are one or two steps from one another. The ideal kitchen has the dishwasher located on your dominant-hand side of the sink, with utensil drawers on the opposite side. A seated chef is most comfortable with a built-in cooktop installed with space rather than cabinets underneath and with a set of drawers to the side. An oven is accessible from both sitting and standing postures if it is thirty inches off the floor with room to approach from either side. (The fact that the oven door always pulls down, not to the side, to open makes it an obstacle when you approach the oven.)

Of course, most of us don't work in perfectly accessible kitchens, designed to match our special requirements, so we usually have to adapt kitchens already in place to suit us.

Storing Within Your Reach

For accessible storage, items must be within your reach — your effective reach — defined as an imaginary circle whose diameter is six inches less than your arm's length and whose center is your shoulder. To locate the most efficient place to store pots, pans, and pantry items, evaluate how frequently you use an item, and consider its weight. A heavy item, even if used rarely, should be stored closer than arm's length because you need to support it with your body when you lift it. The heaviest objects or the most frequently used items should be stored between twenty-eight and sixty-four inches from the floor. This enables a person of average height to reach them without stretching. Pots and pans stored above the waist or hanging from a rack can be retrieved without bending.

Your reach can be extended by lengthening your arm with a variety of reachers, poles with graspers to pick up boxes or utensils. A plastic child-size garden hoe is handy for sliding cans or other items from the back of a cabinet to within reach.

Small appliances, knives in a knife holder, or cooking spoons in a jar can be placed on the counter. Each item on the counter means one less drawer to open and one less utensil to reach for. Items can sometimes fit at a convenient height on hooks on the insides of kitchen and cabinet doors. Cabinet doors can hold shelves with elastic retainers or plastic containers mounted on the doors, so that items don't jar loose when you open the doors. A pegboard on the wall is convenient for hanging heavy pots, small utensils, spices, mugs, anything that will liberate a waist-high drawer for other storage

148

items. Magnetic tape or a magnetic knife strip on a wall within easy reach can be used for lightweight metal items. Plates are easier to pick up when they're stored upright in a rack, rather than in piles.

Organizing Cabinet Space

Cabinet doors may be just another obstacle in the kitchen; they open outward, creating a barrier, if not a danger. Items stored in doorless cabinets may get dusty, of course, but if you use them frequently, storing your dishes and equipment in plain view makes it easier to find just what you need; other people will also be able to find items easily and not worry about misplacing something when they help you in the kitchen. Sliding curtains, either fabric or matchstick, permit an entire closet to be completely opened and remain open without creating a hindrance.

To maximize the space in your most accessible cabinets, add shelves. The more shelves you have, the less stacking you need to do. A vinyl-covered wire stand can be placed on an existing shelf to create another level. If the hardware on your kitchen cabinets and drawers is difficult to grasp, loop a piece of cloth through it to grab and pull. Small knobs can be replaced with ones that more easily accommodate your whole hand.

Kitchen cabinets with roll-out shelves eliminate the need to reach for items at the back. A lazy Susan and a corner cabinet with shelves attached to the door render every item accessible. A lazy Susan in any cabinet will make stored items easier to find and reach. Your reach is enhanced if the upper shelves are deeper and the lower shelves are shallower, a sort of inverse pyramid that reduces interference from lower shelves. Shelves may be tilted slightly down toward the wall so that items are less likely to fall out when you replace them. To reach items stored in upper cabinets, use a kick stool that moves easily with casters but brakes under your weight when you step on it. A child's chair step with two small steps offers security because it is low, but be sure it is made for your weight. A kitchen stool that converts to a miniladder with a handhold is also useful.

Countertop Efficiency

An uninterrupted work space lets you slide pots full of liquid, mixing bowls, or hot casseroles along the counter from the stove to the sink, for example, rather than have to lift and move everything from place to place. The perfect kitchen would have work spaces at various levels — thirty to thirty-six inches high — to accommodate both those who sit and those who stand while cooking.

If you need one hand to hold on to the counter or a cane, leaving only one hand for kitchen work, you may find it more convenient to sit as you do kitchen tasks. For a standard thirty-six-inch-high countertop, a stool about twenty-four inches high is most convenient. A swivel seat, a backrest, and a footrest make a stool more comfortable. A glider chair has large casters that let you move from place to place by using your feet, while you remain seated. Even if you don't have a convenient place for your legs underneath a counter, you will save energy and reduce fatigue in your legs and hips if you sit as you work.

Counter extensions, like pull-out cutting boards or shelves, are handy for gaining additional space. One of these pull-out shelves might include a round cutout to hold a mixing bowl. An adjustable-height ironing board makes a convenient auxiliary work surface.

Resources

Products

Variety of Lengths and Styles of Reachers:
AfterTherapy catalog, (800) 235-7054
Smith & Nephew Rolyan catalog, (800) 558-8633

Reacher. Adds 30 inches to your effective reach, with rubber-tipped metal prongs and a wooden handle. $6. Carol Wright, (402) 474-4465.

Reacher with Hand-Brake Style Mechanism. 32 ½ inches long. $12. Independent Living Aids catalog, (800) 537-2118.

Lobel Food Markers. To help you identify contents of packages by touch with reusable plastic markers in food shapes, mounted on the box or can with elastic or magnets. Also large-print labels with magnetic or adhesive backs. Basic kit, fifteen popular fruit and vegetable shapes with elastics, $3.50. Fifteen large-print magnetic labels for vegetables, $6. Gladys E. Loeb, 2002 Forest Hill Drive, Silver Spring, MD 20903, (301) 434-7748.

Fold-Away Butler Cart. A two-tier rolling cart that folds to 3 inches wide and has a lip to keep items from slipping off. $50.

Enrichments catalog, (800) 323-5547.

Rolling Cart. Three shelves and two wire baskets on casters. 54 inches high by 19½ inches wide by 14½ inches deep. Includes electric outlets for appliances. $150. Chef's catalog, (800) 338-3232.

Versa-Table. Adjustable in height, tilting surface, heavy-duty folding table with casters. Good for food preparation or as a snack tray. $70. Vermont Country Store catalog, (802) 362-2400.

Leg-X-Tenders. To add 3, 4, or 5 inches to a chair or stool to work at the counter, these plastic extenders fit over the legs of a chair. $33. Enrichments catalog, (800) 323-5547.

Raising Blocks. Four wooden blocks to fit legs 1, $2^1/_{16}$, or 3⅛ inches in diameter to raise a table, chair, or bed 3⅛ inches. $38. Smith & Nephew Rolyan catalog, (800) 558-8633.

Roll-About Chair. Allows you to sit and move around on casters by moving your feet. This chair adjusts to your height and gives you 90 percent support, putting less strain on your feet, legs, and back. $60. Adaptability catalog, (800) 243-9232.

Two-Step Ladder. With a handrail. Folds. $50. Wooden Spoon Catalog, (800) 431-2207.

Safety Step Stool. Moves easily when nudged, brakes cleanly when you step on it. It has a 12-inch-diameter step. $40. Maddak catalog, (800) 443-4926.

Step Stool. Rubber wheels and antiskid bottom ring to stabilize stool when you stand on it. $45. Gaylord catalog, (800) 448-6160.

Tilt Rack Pantry Organizer. A three-level shelf that is slanted to allow a can to roll into the front space when one can is removed. $6. Signatures catalog, (909) 943-2021.

Three Tier Stand. Items on the rearmost levels are raised to be visible over the front ones, like a grandstand. $6. Signatures catalog, (909) 943-2021.

Door-Mounted Spice Shelves. For inside cabinet door. Mounts with adhesive strips or hardware. Set of six shelves to hold twenty-four jars or tins, with press-on labels. $14. Vermont Country Store catalog, (802) 362-2400.

Publications

"Reaching Aids," Health and Welfare Canada. A pamphlet that discusses various types and features of reachers and their uses. FREE.

Independent Living, Disabled Persons Unit, Health and Welfare Canada, Ottawa, Ontario K1A 1B5 Canada.

"Storage," Health and Welfare Canada. Suggestions for accessible storage of items in your kitchen, bedroom, and bathroom. FREE. Independent Living, Disabled Persons Unit, Health and Welfare Canada, Ottawa, Ontario K1A 1B5 Canada.

"Designs for Independent Living," Whirlpool Corporation. Design considerations for better accessibility in the kitchen, either complete renovations or simple modifications. Also some options to evaluate when selecting major appliances. FREE. Appliance Information Service, Whirlpool Corporation, Administrative Center, Benton Harbor, MI 49022.

KITCHEN EQUIPMENT AND APPLIANCES

There's no need to start from scratch to streamline your kitchen. Your ideal kitchen may include just a few favorite pots and pans and some frequently used gadgets and knives. Rather than simply add to your supply, consider donating to a neighbor some of your heavier, larger pots, as well as any you haven't used for a year. Ask some friends to join you in holding a garage sale for kitchen equipment you don't use regularly.

Some of your old cookware may need updating. Old pots may have lids with knobs too small to grip comfortably. The knobs can be replaced with ones large enough to accommodate four fingers. Many hardware stores carry a selection of kitchen drawer pulls that you can adapt for this use. An additional handle can be fitted over the edge of a pot to give you the security of a two-handed grip. An old top-of-the-stove potato cooker — really just a heat diffuser with a cover — can be requisitioned for use as a mini oven for cooking small items.

If you do need to replace pots and pans, look for lighter-weight, smaller cooking equipment. An electric wok is a handy frying pan because it can be used away from the stove and because it has high, slanted sides that make it hard for food to overflow.

New accessories can simplify life in the kitchen. If you ever ruined a kettle because you forgot you put water on to boil or you didn't hear the whistle and the water boiled away, consider purchasing an electric kettle with an automatic shutoff. An electric frying pan or a slow cooker gives you the flexibility of working at the counter or a table rather than at the stove. A toaster oven or a broiler oven can substitute for a broiler that requires awkward bending to floor level; microwave ovens can add to the ease and speed of meal preparation.

Small amounts of water, about two cups, can be boiled in an inexpensive electric hot pot, especially one with an interrupter on/off switch, which saves you from having to plug and unplug the pot every time you use it. A submersible coil is placed directly in the water and does a good job of boiling small quantities of liquid quickly. You can resurrect an old electric coffeemaker (minus the inserts) to use as an electric kettle. Two cups of water in a glass or plastic measuring cup will boil in a microwave oven in about five minutes.

If you need to fill a large pot with water, use the sink spray attachment to fill the pot on the counter and then slide it, if possible, to the stove, or fill it directly on the stove using measuring cups of water. When you boil spaghetti or vegetables, first place them in a strainer or fryer basket insert, which will contain the food as it cooks in a large pot. This allows you to remove the food, leaving the heavy pot full of boiling water to cool on the stove.

When you stir or add food to pots and pans, you can steady them on the stove with a stabilizer that blocks the pot handle between two small barriers attached with suction cups to the stove. You may be able to wedge a pot handle against the back of the stove or anchor it against a filled kettle or pot on a back burner.

Modern kitchen appliances have many features that make them easier to use, including better visibility and handier controls. The size and location of burner knobs can affect the safe use of the stove. Rear-burner controls are hard to reach, especially from a seated position, and your sleeve may dangle too close to the flame. Rear-mounted controls can be operated by reaching across the stovetop with a potato masher (a wire bent like a series of S curves with a handle) to turn the knobs.

Knob covers can convert smaller controls into ones that are easier to grasp, with a soft, larger gripping surface. A clothespin can extend the gripping area if it is placed over the projection on stove controls.

A small piece of sandpaper, a piece of toothpick, or a bean under a piece of tape can be a tactile marker for the off position or for certain temperature markings. Contact your local public utility companies to see if they have small raised dots to stick on the oven knob as indicators of specific temperature settings on the oven knob. Electronic controls offer touch pad convenience, eliminating the need to turn or push a knob.

The most practical refrigerator is a side-by-side model where freezer items are as accessible as those in the refrigerator compartment. The doors of a side-by-side model refrigerator are narrower and easier to open and close, and they protrude less into the kitchen space when they are open than do full-width doors. You can reorganize your refrigerator by rearranging shelves to locate beverage storage in the middle level, where heavier items are easier to handle, with less frequently needed items or lighter-weight foods stored on the top shelf. Extra shelves, partial shelves, or drawers can be added to the refrigerator. Small plastic baskets are convenient for storing onions, potatoes, and fruits.

For a refrigerator door that seals too tightly, break the vacuum with a pinch of electrical tape on the gasket at the bottom of the door in one or two places. Gain leverage over a too-tight refrigerator door by looping a dish towel through the refrigerator door handle and using your forearm rather than your hand to open it.

A microwave oven on the countertop is convenient for sliding dishes in and out easily. If the microwave is on a rolling cart, it may reach the level of the countertop for easy loading and unloading and then be rolled to an out-of-the-way corner when not in use.

Resources

Products

Guard Rail. To stabilize pots and pans on electric ranges. Either 6¼- or 8⅛-inch inside diameter. $14. Maxi-Aids catalog, (800) 522-6294.

Pan Stabilizer. Mounts on the stove with suction cups and blocks a pot or pan handle from moving. Folding pan stabilizer, $12. Nonfolding, $9. Enrichments catalog, (800) 323-5547.

Water Boil Minder. Place it in a pot, and it noisily vibrates if the liquid boils away. $3. Ann Morris catalog, (516) 292-9232.

Electric Kettle. Shuts off automatically if the water boils dry.

Optional whistle. $25. Maxi-Aids catalog, (800) 522-6294.

Glass Kettle. Has 2-cup capacity, with a plastic handle so that it can be used to boil water in the microwave. $10. Ann Morris catalog, (516) 292-9232.

Char-B-Que. An electric grill with a cool-to-the-touch terra-cotta base. $60. Community Kitchens catalog, (800) 535-9001.

Smoke 'N' Grill. A combination steamer, grill, smoker, and roaster that fits on a tabletop. This 16-inch-diameter and 26½-inch-tall utensil allows you the flexibility of cooking where it suits you best. Recipes and instructions included. $130. Williams-Sonoma catalog, (800) 541-2233.

Electric Fry Pan. 12 inches square, lined with nonstick surface, with a vented dome cover. $50. Ann Morris catalog, (516) 292-9232.

Solo Stir. An 8-inch-diameter wok with a flat bottom for good stability. $35. Calphalon. Chef's catalog, (800) 338-3232.

Pots with Locking Lids. Water drains through holes in the lid. The 3-quart version, with one long and one short handle, $21. The 6-quart, with two short handles, $27. Ann Morris catalog, (516) 292-9232.

Aluminum Pot Strainer. Locks onto the rim of pots from 5 to 10½ inches in diameter for one-handed draining, straining, or rinsing. $2. Maxi-Aids catalog, (800) 522-6294.

Steamer. A lift-out colander fits into a 3-quart stainless steel pot. $16. Signatures catalog, (909) 943-2021.

Knob Turner. The surface grips handles of any shape and uses lever action. $17. Enrichments catalog, (800) 323-5547.

T-Turning Handle. Pegs adjust to and grip odd-shaped handles, like stove knobs, up to 1¼ inches in diameter. Plastic pegs, $12. Aluminum pegs, $24. For a distributor near you, contact Maddack, Inc., 6 Industrial Road, Pequannock, NJ 07440, (800) 443-4926.

Door/Drawer Opener. For opening cabinet doors or drawers with hard-to-grip knobs or handles. This device hooks over a round knob or into a C-shaped drawer pull for added leverage. $20. For a distributor near you, contact Maddack, Inc., 6 Industrial Road, Pequannock, NJ 07440, (800) 443-4926.

Tactile Marks. A package of twelve stick-on acrylic dots and twelve dashes to mark appliances, on/off switches, etc. $4. Ann Morris catalog, (516) 292-9232.

Loc Dots. Six clear plastic adhesive-backed raised dots for oven controls. $1. Lighthouse Consumer Products catalog, (800) 829-0500.

Small Stainless Broiler Pan. 12 by 9 inches with rack. $16. Vermont Country Store catalog, (802) 362-2400.

Services

Replacement Parts. To keep older small appliances in working order. Culinary Parts Unlimited, 80 Berry Drive, Pacheco, CA 94553, (800) 543-7549, or in California call (800) 722-7239.

Publications

"Tools for Independent Living," Whirlpool Corporation. Illustrated ideas for easier use of major home appliances. Directions on how to use everyday items like clothespins and potato mashers to turn knobs and open doors. Also how to make a specialized cutting board. FREE. Appliance Information Service, Whirlpool Corporation, Administrative Center, Benton Harbor, MI 49022.

KITCHEN TOOLS

You don't have to mince parsley and chop onions like a professional when you're cooking for yourself or your family. Experiment with a pair of scissors for chopping or cutting up certain fruits and vegetables. Use them for cutting cooked or raw spinach and lettuce for salad, mincing herbs, cutting meat, and chopping tomatoes. Stainless steel kitchen scissors wash nicely. They are useful for opening boxes and cellophane bags that resist when you try to break the vacuum seal. If you have two pairs, one long and thin, one shorter, you will find uses for them both.

A spatula is perfect for flipping pancakes, but for turning meat, try long-handled tongs, a half tong and half spatula, or barbecue tongs. Barbecue utensils allow you to maintain distance from the stove and to avoid bending.

A lowly potato peeler pares many foods besides potatoes. Its handle can be built up with a foam hair curler, a piece of sponge, or wrapping for a tennis racket grip. The peeler also can be outfitted with a vise that attaches it to a counter, letting you move the potato against it.

Slicing and cutting chores can challenge your arm or hand strength. A knife with a bent handle provides better leverage, while a knife with a guide measures the width of the slices. Serrated blades "bite" into the surface of things more perceptibly than straight blades. A curved-blade knife, or a rocker knife, permits cutting without pressing down with wrist action, as you have to with a regular straight-bladed knife.

To scrape bowls, use your hands or a boomerang-shaped plastic scraper that is easier to hold than a spatula. Potholders or mitts should be well insulated and long enough to protect your hands and your forearms when you reach into the oven. Tubular potholders that fit over pan handles don't need to be wrapped and folded like regular ones.

Resources

Products

Loop Scissors. They squeeze to cut, then open automatically. No need to fit your fingers into little holes; just hold the outside of the large handles. $20. AfterTherapy catalog, (800) 235-7054.

Kitchen Scissors. Flexible handles and no restrictive finger slots. Dishwasher-safe. $15. Enrichments catalog, (800) 323-5547.

Self-Opening Shears. Broad handles for comfortable hold and to press against table for extra leverage. Stainless steel and dishwasher-safe. $17. Smith & Nephew Rolyan catalog, (800) 558-8633.

17-inch Oven Mitts. Scorch-resistant, Teflon-treated, $2. Flame-retardant, $3. Lighthouse Consumer Products catalog, (800) 829-0500.

16-inch Stainless Steel Tongs. Can be used as a reacher, to turn foods, or to pull out an oven shelf. $4. Heavy duty, $8. A Cook's Wares catalog, (412) 846-9490.

Deluxe Food Turner Spatula. Two stainless steel spatula tongs, 10½ inches long. $5. Lighthouse Consumer Products catalog (800) 829-0500.

Barbecue Food Holder. Foods are enclosed and can be easily turned to cook on the other side with long handles. For hamburgers, $8. For chicken or meat, $10. Ann Morris catalog, (516) 292-9232.

Combination Barbecue-Length Spatula-Tong. A 15-inch distance from pots when turning and grabbing food. $4. Campmor catalog,

Slicing Tongs. Hold eggs, tomatoes, onions, or potatoes, and slice through the slots. $11. Ann Morris catalog, (516) 292-9232.

One-Handed Potato Peeler. Attaches to the edge of a table or counter. $16. Maxi-Aids catalog, (800) 522-6294.

Dazey Stripper. Holds potatoes, apples, or other firm-fleshed fruits and vegetables and peels them automatically. Also slices. $35. Sears Home HealthCare catalog, (800) 326-1750.

EZ-Grip Vegetable Peeler. Swivel blade and a handle large enough for the whole hand to grip. $2. Maxi-Aids catalog, (800) 522-6294.

Power Peeler. Lightweight, electric vegetable peeler. Blade snaps out for cleaning. $30. Comfort House catalog, (800) 359-7701.

Handle Grip Serrated Bread Knife. Cut with the strength of your entire arm, rather than with only your hand and wrist. Suitable as an all-purpose knife, not just for bread. 8¾-inch blade. $30. Adaptability catalog, (800) 243-9232.

Slant Handle Slicing Device. 13½-inch serrated blade adjusts to cut at various thicknesses. $60. Enrichments catalog, (800) 323-5547.

E-Z Grip Knife. Handle is positioned over the blade, rather than extends from it, to avoid exerting pressure on your hands and wrist. $5. Support Plus catalog, (800) 229-2910.

Chopping Bowl and Chopping Knife. 10½-inch plastic chopping bowl and curved-blade knife. Dishwasher-safe. $15. Chef's catalog, (800) 338-3232.

Self-Contained Grater. Suction feet, two sizes of grater blades, and catch bin. $11. Enrichments catalog, (800) 323-5547.

See-Through Grater. One panel of the hexagonal grater is transparent and has measurement marks. A bottom cover contains the grated contents and slides to allow access. $10. Community Kitchens catalog, (800) 535-9001.

Mincer. Ten round blades cut as you roll the device back and forth over food, such as herbs. $5. Ann Morris catalog, (516) 292-9232.

Self-Holding Bowl. A 3-quart stainless steel bowl is held stable on a metal frame for mixing. When it's time for scraping, it can be supported on its side or lifted off for pouring. $50. Enrichments catalog, (800) 323-5547.

Double-Face Suction Holder. Double suction cups are activated when disk is twisted, so that one side grips tabletop, while the other holds a bowl or plate in place. $5. Smith & Nephew Rolyan catalog, (800) 558-8633.

Sugar or Ground or Instant Coffee Dispenser. Dispenses one teaspoon each time you pour. $2. Lighthouse Consumer Products catalog, (800) 829-0500.

Carton Gripper. For half-gallon juice and milk cartons. $3. Enrichments catalog, (800) 323-5547.

E-Z Pour Handle. For 2-liter plastic bottles. $2. Maxi-Aids catalog, (800) 522-6294.

Portable One-Hand Mixer. Compact, battery-powered stirring and whisking appliance. $10. Bruce Medical Supply catalog, (800) 225-8446.

Foam for Building Up Handles. Cut to size from a cylinder and insert utensil handle into the center of the cylinder. ¼-inch-diameter hole in ¾-inch-diameter foam by 1 yard. $6. AfterTherapy catalog, (800) 235-7054.

Say When Liquid Level Indicator. Hooks over the rim of a cup, and a loud buzzer sounds when the cup is full. $13. Also the Say Stop liquid level indicator with a musical chime indicator. $10. Maxi-Aids catalog, (800) 522-6294.

Liquid Level Indicator. Plays "There's No Place Like Home" when the liquid comes to within half-inch of the top. $12. Independent Living Aids catalog, (800) 537-2118.

Tactile Meat Thermometer. Stainless steel, with markers between 120 and 200 degrees. Dishwasher-safe. $15. Independent Living Aids catalog, (800) 537-2118.

No-spill Ice Tray. Actually it's a bottle to which you add a half cup of water and place on its side in the freezer. When it's frozen, you pour out the cubes. It can be used as a cold pack too. $3. Ann Morris catalog, (516) 292-9232.

Timers

Kitchen timers can always be used for more than just telling you when the food is done. Sophisticated ones can be programmed to remind you of appointments or television shows, and some can even turn appliances on or off. Digital timers are more flexible and are worth the trouble of learning how to operate them. They can be set once and will ring at the same times every day. Before purchasing, check timers with digital screens for legibility because glare from kitchen lights may interfere, and frequently they are just too small.

See if the knob on a timer is comfortable to grasp and turn and if the numbers are easy to read. You can set one timer to ring in the kitchen and keep one in your pocket as a backup, in case you don't hear the first one.

Of course, you must find a timer with an alarm that is easy for you to hear. Some ring for a few seconds, some for as long as one minute; the digital ones often have high-pitched beeps; others are more like bicycle bell ringers. Test the alarm carefully for loudness before you decide which one is best for you.

Resources

Products

Magnet Timer. An easy-to-program twenty-four-hour timer with a five-minute warning. Can also be used as a stopwatch or clock. Hangs on the refrigerator with a magnet or clips to your pocket. $17. A twenty-hour timer is also available, $11. Zabar's catalog, (212) 496-1234.

Talking Key Chain Timer. Announces the time and has a digital display and an alarm. $11. Lighthouse Consumer Products catalog, (800) 829-0500.

Easy-To-Read Timer. An 8-inch round timer with a long ring. Choose either a black face with white numbers or a white face with black numbers. $16. Maxi-Aids catalog, (800) 522-6294.

Compact Digital Timer. ¾-inch-high numbers. $20. Independent Living Aids catalog, (800) 537-2118.

2⅜-inch Round Timer. One-minute beep. Raised buttons for easy use by those with poor vision. Magnet for the refrigerator and loop for use as a key chain. $10. Independent Living Aids catalog, (800) 537-2118.

Eggtimer. Changes color according to the degree of cooking you prefer. Placed in pot with the eggs, the timer turns from yellow to orange or red to purple to show when eggs are soft, medium, or hard. $8. Community Kitchens catalog, (800) 535-9901.

Nondigital Timer. Long ring with vibrations that will attract your attention if you carry it in your pocket. Only 2½ inches in diameter, it can be worn around the neck with the lanyard that is included. $18. Independent Living Aids catalog, (800) 537-2118.

Tactile Timer. Single-, double-, and triple-raised dots for different intervals up to one hour help you set the right amount of time. $15. Ann Morris catalog, (516) 292-9232.

Long Ring Windup Timer. Has a magnifier for easy setting and viewing. $10. LS&S Group catalog, (800) 468-4789.

Openers

Sometimes a package puts up a struggle before it opens: unyielding milk and juice carton spouts, vacuum-sealed jars, the tiny top on a bottle of vanilla extract, boxes of soap, cellophane bags. The bags inside the boxes are often as hard to penetrate, such as those for cereal or cookies — just the ones you want to reseal to keep the contents fresh!

Many openers work on the principle of an adjustable wrench, allowing you to squeeze many different sizes of caps and force them open without using a lot of arm, finger, or wrist energy. A nutcracker might do just as well for some jars and bottles. Some vacuum-sealed jars can be opened with a rubber sheet that you place on the palm of your hand to provide traction to break the seal and turn the lid. Sometimes just the pressure of the palm of your hand pressing down straight-armed to add strength will open a vacuum-sealed lid.

Wedge openers for jars are installed under a cabinet or mounted on the wall. Positioning them about a foot over a counter leaves a safe distance for the can to be held and not too much distance should it drop. A sponge cloth strategically placed on the counter can cushion a falling jar. Jars slide into the wedge until they hold tight and then are forced open by turning. Using two hands, preferably the palms, avoids putting too much stress on a single hand. Openers with strong stainless steel teeth are the most durable.

Electric can openers require varying amounts of strength and dexterity to operate. Some openers release when the can is opened. The lid stays magnetized on the opener, and the can falls to the countertop. That's fine if the distance isn't too great. A pot under the can will catch it or any of its contents. Some openers remain attached to the can until you release them and avoid this problem. Electric openers may require two-handed operation, one to hold the can, one to press a button. The ideal opener operates either automatically or with an on/off switch rather than a button or a lever that needs to be held down continuously during operation.

While plastic containers like Tupperware are convenient for storing leftovers, they can be difficult to open and close. A clothespin may be easier to use than a twist tie as a seal for plastic bags. Very fat rubber bands can stretch to close a plastic bag filled, for example, with vegetables. Twirl the bag closed, holding the opening and using the weight of the contents; then stretch an elastic band around the contents and the twisted neck. Ziploc bags are now available with easier and more secure closings.

If you can't find an opener that performs well for you, ask a friend to help you transfer the contents of jars or cans to other containers when you bring them home from the store. Sometimes all it takes is breaking the vacuum seal once and reclosing a jar more loosely. You might transfer juices, milk, or other liquids to one or two small pitchers or covered plastic containers. Remember to store items in the refrigerator if necessary once they have been opened.

Resources

Products

Variety of Openers. AfterTherapy catalog, (800) 235-7054.

Openers for Vacuum-Sealed Jars and Bottles

Open Up. A battery-operated under-cabinet opener for jars and bottles from nail polish size to a 4-inch diameter. $35. Appliance Science Corporation. Williams-Sonoma catalog, (800) 541-2233.

Under-The-Cabinet Opener. Unscrews ⅜- to 3⅜-inch-diameter tops. $6. Enrichments catalog, (800) 323-5547.

Wall-Mounted Opener. Accommodates tops from ½ inch to 3 inches in diameter. Includes a pry-up opener and bottle hook. $8. Enrichments catalog, (800) 323-5547.

Un-Skru Opener. Mounted under a cabinet, it opens lids from ⅜ inch to 5 inches in diameter by wedging them inside an angle against a steel gripper. One-handed operation without the need for wrist action. $8. Multi Marketing & Mfg., P.O. Box 1070, Littleton, CO 80160.

Under Cabinet Jar Opener and Closer. Turn jar after fitting it into an angle that accommodates tops with ¼- to 4½-inch diameters.

$13. Bruce Medical Supply catalog, (800) 225-8446.

Faucet-Style Faceted Opener. For screw-top caps such as those on soda bottles. $5. Easy Street catalog, (800) 959-EASY (3279).

Jar and Bottle Wrench. Adjustable strap accommodates tops from ¼ inch to 4½ inches in diameter. $11. Easy Street catalog, (800) 959-EASY (3279).

Rubber Sheet Jar Opener. A 5- by 5-inch flexible textured rubber sheet that adheres to a lid so that it is easier to open. Three for $5. Bruce Medical Supply catalog, (800) 225-8446. Also a similar 5½-inch round Dycem material gripper, red or navy. $5. Enrichments catalog, (800) 323-5547.

Universal Jar Lid Opener. Any size lid can be squeezed between steel nutcrackerlike parts. $8. Real Goods catalog, (800) 762-7325.

Jar Opener. Viselike lever action for any size top. $6. Ann Morris catalog, (516) 292-9232.

Openers for Screw-Top Beverage Caps and Cans

Tab Grabber. $2. Independent Living Aids catalog, (800) 537-2118.

BEST BUYS. **Cans and Bottle Cap Opener.** A notch for beverage can stubs and a circle for bottle caps. Two for $5. Bruce Medical Supply catalog, (800) 225-8446. The same item with a magnetic back for hanging on the refrigerator door. Two for $4. Enrichments catalog, (800) 323-5547. $2 for one. Independent Living Aids catalog, (800) 537-2118.

Openers for Vacuum-Sealed Cellophane Bags

Slit-A-Bag. A sharp prong breaks the vacuum seal and opens a bag as it is pulled along. $1, or two for $1.80. Independent Living Aids catalog, (800) 537-2118.

Bag Opener. Concealed and recessed razor blade cuts as the bag is slid through a guide. Mounts with adhesive back under a cabinet or on a wall. $7. Enrichments catalog, (800) 323-5547.

Snippits. Two plastic razor holders for opening sealed plastic bags. Can be clipped to an apron or stored with a magnet on a refrigerator. Two for $3. Miles Kimball catalog, (414) 231-4886.

Openers for Boxes of Detergents, Small Boxes, and Boxes You Must Puncture and Pull Up to Create a Spout

Piercer. First pierces the box, then lifts it open. $3. Enrichments catalog, (800) 323-5547.

Box Topper. Opens boxes and has a built-up handle. $4. Lighthouse Consumer Products catalog, (800) 829-0500.

Can Openers

Electric Can-Do Can Opener. Attach it to can, and press to start; stops automatically. Rechargeable. $48. Adaptability catalog, (800) 243-9232.

Cordless Can Opener. Operates and stops automatically after the can is pierced. You don't need to hold it while it is operating. Rechargeable, it mounts on wall. $30. Enrichments catalog, (800) 323-5547.

Miscellaneous

Bag Clips. In place of twist ties to secure plastic, paper, or cellophane bags. Space to label contents. Safe for freezer, dishwasher, and microwave. Twelve assorted sizes, $7. AfterTherapy catalog, (800) 235-7054.

Cutting Boards

Variations on the theme of the simple wooden or plastic cutting board can do more than just provide a cutting surface. It can be as simple as a wooden board with stainless steel or aluminum nails protruding upward on which to skewer a vegetable or fruit for slicing or peeling. Rubber pads at the corners or a kitchen towel or a damp sponge cloth underneath will keep the board from slipping. A dampened large sponge cloth can be a good cutting board by itself and will contain cut-up food that would skitter off a slick board.

Resources

Products

Maple Paring Board. 11-inch square with holding pins, corner guards, and suction cup feet. $19. Or an 8- by 10-inch Formica board. $16. Enrichments catalog, (800) 323-5547.

Cutting Board with a Chute. Prepared food is guided down the chute into a bowl or pot, with handle. Dishwasher-safe. $7. Independent Living Aids catalog, (800) 537-2118.

Over-The-Sink Wooden Cutting Board. Handle moves to adjust to sink size. Corner rim for keeping food braced, two nails for holding food, also rubber feet for use on countertop. $22. Enrichments catalog, (800) 323-5547.

Spreadboard. Two lips to hold food in place and a rim to steady the board against the edge of the table or counter. $17. Adaptability catalog, (800) 243-9232.

BEST BUY. **Adjustable Cutting Board.** Fits over the sink, with a strainer segment for rinsing and draining. Adjusts from 13 inches to 19 inches. $13. Independent Living Aids catalog, (800) 537-2118.

Preparation Board. Designed for cutting food with one hand, a viselike mechanism stabilizes bowls, packages, bread, food, or other items. Also stainless steel spikes hold foods for cutting. $60. AfterTherapy catalog, (800) 235-7054.

Low Vision Cutting Board. Reversible cutting board, black or white, to provide high contrast for dark or light food. Dishwasher-safe. $25. Lighthouse Consumer Products catalog, (800) 829-0500.

The Kitchen Sink

Cleaning up after meals can seem as arduous as it is thankless. Even if you have an automatic dishwasher, there is still plenty of washing and rinsing to be done. A rolling cart can simplify cleanup chores by eliminating trips between table and sink. Fill a plastic dishpan directly from the table, put other garbage and kitchen items on a cart, and roll them all to the sink. Use a spray attachment to fill a dishpan or to rinse dishes, and let the dishes soak while you put away leftovers. If the sink is too deep for you to reach the bottom easily, place a dishpan on a plastic-coated rack or an upturned plastic box.

Rolling carts with several shelves can become permanent storage for silverware and dishes, easily rolled to set the table and used to transfer food to table. Carts are essential if your hands are occupied with a walker, a cane, or crutches.

Rubber matting at the bottom of the sink can protect glasses and dishes from breaking. Rubber gloves protect your hands against cold or hot water and provide traction to prevent items from slipping. Brushes designed for cleaning glasses and a nailbrush-size brush for cleaning vegetables are available with suction cups to attach to the side of the sink. A large car-washing sponge mitt is useful for washing or rinsing dishes, and a plastic spatula can be used to scrape food without damaging dishes. A windshield squeegee mop cleans up counters quickly. Air-dry everything except cast iron cookware. To reduce stress, keep your fingers extended rather than curled whenever you can; rather than grasp a sponge, work with it under the flat of your open hand. Likewise, when lifting a pot or platter, rather than grasp the handles, slide your entire hand on each side under the bottom and lift it using both hands. Pump-style liquid hand soap dispensers that can be pressed down with the flat of the hand are a convenient alternative to squeeze containers for dispensing dishwashing soap.

Single-lever faucets require less hand and arm effort to adjust water flow and temperature than two rotating faucets. The single lever may be shifted from side to side and back and forth by nudging it with the side of your hand or forearm, without grasping. If your kitchen has two rotating faucets, hold a sponge in your hand as you turn them. Some newer faucets are activated with buttons or switches. One variety responds electronically to the presence of your hands.

Several gadgets are on the market to protect you if you leave the water running and risk a flood in the kitchen. The drain plug commonly found in the kitchen sink has a mechanism for stopping the water from draining that is so delicate it is often difficult to determine when it is engaged and it can slip into place on its own. If the water is accidentally left running with the drain accidentally engaged, the sink can overflow in only a few minutes.

In order to be able to sit comfortably at the kitchen sink, you can make room for your legs by removing the base cabinet. Chances are your knees will bump against the plumbing, including the hot-water pipe, unless you install a new sink with the drain placed toward the rear of the sink to allow room for your legs. In the meantime, wrap the hot-water pipe with a towel, run the hot water into a dishpan, or fill the sink before you sit down.

Products

Water Detector. For placement under sinks, behind refrigerators, on the floor in front of dishwashers, or on basement floors to detect leaks or flooding. An alarm sounds when water touches two metal sensors on the detector. The device does not need to be mounted anywhere, just placed. Battery-operated. $8. For a dealer near you, contact Zircon Corporation, 1580 Dell Avenue, Campbell, CA 95008, (800) 245-9265.

Vinyl Sink Mat. 16″ × 13½″ mat with a drain hole and small feet. $4. Ann Morris catalog, (516) 292-9232.

Publications

"Dishwashing Aids," Health and Welfare Canada. Suggestions for simplifying dishwashing chores. FREE. Independent Living, Health and Welfare Canada, Ottawa, Ontario K1A 1B5 Canada.

Tableware

If you find your usual plates, glasses, and knives and forks inconvenient to use, you may need utensils that are easier to hold, ones that have built-up handles, or heavier-weight or lighter-weight ones.

If you want to build up the handles of your own silverware, try masking tape, tennis racket grip tape, or foam rubber tubing that comes with different-size interior holes to fit over various items, like toothbrushes and knife handles. Gauze, cheesecloth, or terry cloth can be secured around silverware, or a potholder taped into place. A dishrag or a terry washcloth can be taped on or slipped on. If you need a significantly larger diameter, try a bicycle handle grip. A liquid plastic, Plasti-Dip, available in hardware stores, can be used to build up handles: You dip the handle into the plastic, which hardens when it dries.

Various combination utensils can assist in cutting food. A "knoon" is a knife and spoon in one, a "knork" is a knife and fork, and a "spork" is a spoon and fork, or you can use a three-in-one utensil:

a spoon with tines and a sharpened edge for cutting.

If you are in the market for new dishes, consider plates that have deeper rims or lips to keep food from scooting off. Test the handles on cups or mugs to see if they are easy to grip, if the ear is large enough to accommodate a finger or two, and that you won't accidentally burn yourself on a hot cup because your fingers can't avoid touching the side. Glassware should be well balanced, both full and empty, and you should be able to reach to the bottom of the glass to clean it. Glassware with stems may not fit in a dishwasher. Try to select glasses that are not easily broken and are solidly stabilized as they stand.

If your plate tends to slide around or shifts in its place as you eat, use a cloth place mat. A slightly damp cloth, nonslip place mats, nonslip coasters, and suction cups provide good traction for plates.

Rather than depend on the strength of your fingers to grasp a bowl, use both hands on opposite sides, or your palms, squeezing the bowl and bracing it against your body.

Test your hand agility by making the okay sign with your thumb and first finger. If it's difficult, you shouldn't depend on only that hand to grasp items. The hand with the lesser strength can be used to hold or stabilize food or a bowl while the other one does the work of mixing, cutting, and so on.

Resources

Products

Utensils and Dishes for Various Needs:
Adaptability catalog, (800) 243-9232
AfterTherapy catalog, (800) 235-7054
Cleo of New York catalog, (800) 321-0595
Enrichments catalog, (800) 323-5547
Maxi-Aids catalog, (800) 522-6294
Smith & Nephew Rolyan catalog, (800) 558-8633
Support Plus catalog, (800) 229-2910
TASH ADL catalog, (416) 686-4129

Sporks. A combination stainless steel spoon and fork comes in small, medium, and large, 5, 6, and 7 inches. $4. Cleo of New York catalog, (800) 321-0595.

Combifork. A knife is incorporated into one edge of the fork. Specify right- or left-handed use. $26. TASH ADL catalog, (416) 686-4129.

Foam Tubing. Center holes of various sizes; different colors. Two foot-long pieces about $10. Maxi-Aids catalog, (800) 522-6294.

Easy Grip Tubing. To build up narrow handles. Three tubes 4 inches long and 1 inch in diameter with a ⅜-inch hole. $5. Support Plus catalog, (800) 229-2910.

Cookbooks

Experienced cooks probably have a collection of cookbooks and won't need to learn the basics of how to cook or what equipment to buy. Many of the older cookbooks rely heavily on outmoded habits of eating and food preparation and food fashions that are now considered less healthy. Often there is a heavy reliance on canned soups, intensive use of butter and other fats, and a focus on meat as the centerpiece of every meal. New appliances, new ingredients, and new products that have come on the market over the past fifty years give evidence of how radically cooking methods have changed.

Today's cookbooks tend to concentrate on specific topics, foreign cuisines, or special diets, either to control weight, use less sodium, or reduce fats. No single cookbook has everything for everyone, and few cookbooks directly address the problems of the mature cook. To follow the Food Pyramid guidelines, choose books that include a nutritional analysis of each recipe, which makes it easier to calculate how many calories come from fat, and so on. Many of these cookbooks can suggest ways of preparing foods that you can apply to your own recipes.

A Lucite holder will keep your cookbooks clean. A photo album or rotary photo holder with cellophane pockets can protect your own handwritten recipes.

Products

Adjustable Cookbook Stand. Acrylic covering. Backrest moves for best viewing angle. $21. Williams-Sonoma catalog, (800) 541-2233.

Recipe Album. Binder with plastic-covered pages, pockets. $17. Solutions catalog, (800) 342-9988.

Publications

BEST BUY. Jane Brody's Good Food Book: Living the High-Carbo-hydrate Way. This is two books in one: a nutrition guide and a source of 350 healthful recipes. Although written before the Food Pyramid appeared, Brody's book is philosophically in tune with the latest dietary thinking. A good adjunct to any kitchen library. 1985. W. W. Norton & Co.

"Celebrate Good Health: Recipes for Special Occasions That Follow the Dietary Guidelines to Lower Cancer Risk," American Institute for Cancer Research. A group of low-fat recipes with the amounts of fats, calories, and cholesterol and the percentage of calories from fats, as compared with traditional recipes. For example, a recipe for carrot cake cuts the fat from 32.8 grams to 8.9 grams. FREE. AICR, 1759 R Street, NW, Washington, DC 20009, (800) 843-8114.

For Goodness Sake: An Eating Well Guide to Creative Low-Fat Cooking by Terry Joyce Blonder. Each recipe has a nutritional break-down, and most recipes follow the government's dietary guidelines. A variety of recipes, including low-calorie desserts, are included in easy-to-read type. 1990. Camden House Publishing, Ferry Road, Charlotte VT 05445.

The Good Eating, Good Health Cookbook by Phyllis C. Kaufman. All 150 recipes have nutritional analysis, including total fat and poly-unsaturated, monounsaturated, and saturated fats. The author adheres to a low-fat diet, no red meat or shellfish recipes, and none overly difficult. 1990. Consumer Reports Books.

The Four-Course 400 Calorie Meal Cookbook: Quick and Easy Recipes for Delicious Low-Calorie Low-Fat Dinners by Nancy S. Hughes. You don't have to count calories in this book if you choose any main course, plus any vegetable dish, salad, and dessert; they all add up to four hundred calories, with the grams of fat per serving listed. Two hundred recipes are included, plus some no-cooking ways of serving low-calorie and low-fat foods. 1991. Contemporary Books.

"Dietary Guidelines and Your Diet," "Making Bag Lunches, Snacks and Desserts," "Shopping for Food and Making Meals in Minutes," and "Eating Better When Eating Out." These four pamphlets include recipes and advice on ways to carry out the new low-fat recommendations. HG-232 38-11. Human Nutrition Information Service, U.S. Department of Agriculture, Hyattsville, MD 20782.

"No Time to Cook: Quick and Easy Meals that Follow the Dietary Guidelines to Lower Cancer Risk," American Institute for Cancer Research Information Series. This brochure suggests how to reduce the time used for planning and preparing meals. It includes recipes and menu suggestions. FREE. AICR, 1759 R Street, NW, Washington, DC 20009, (800) 843-8114.

"Sneak Health into Your Snacks: Snacking and the Dietary Guidelines to Lower Cancer Risk," American Institute for Cancer Research Information Series. This brochure contains suggestions for low-fat substitutions for common snack foods. FREE. AICR, 1759 R Street, NW, Washington, DC 20009, (800) 843-8114.

"Fresh, Light & Fast." Tips, recipes, and menus for low-fat cooking; also a list of suggested cookbooks. FREE. Williams-Sonoma catalog, (800) 541-2233.

Shortcuts and Tips

If you cook, you probably have developed a repertoire of easy methods for making certain recipes. Sometimes the need for efficiency clashes with what's desirable for your diet. You end up relying on canned foods, prepared frozen foods, or takeout meals from a supermarket or deli.

When you are limiting salt or trying to prepare healthful foods, try to keep a supply of homemade broths on hand. To make homemade broth or stock without doing all the work yourself, invite a friend or two and ask each of them to bring one or two ingredients all ready for the pot. Socialize together as the pot simmers slowly during the afternoon. Play cards or do mending as you wait, and then share the results. Each participant can bring a half-gallon container in which to take home some broth.

When your energy is limited or if you dislike cooking, you have to depend more on shortcuts. Think of ways to simplify supermarket trips. Avoid the confusion of a crowded store and the jostling and motion of a crowd by getting to the store when it opens, shopping early in the week, and asking about special services, especially during the year-end holidays. A food processor saves a lot of effort and time, but you may need a little practice to feel comfortable using it. Ask a friend to lend you one and give you a lesson or two so that you can experiment and develop some confidence.

If you tire easily, schedule your cooking with frequent rest periods, preparing recipes in steps. Get your meals ready early in the day so that you don't use up all your energy by mealtime.

Modern shopping relies as much on the postal service and the telephone as on a personal visit to a store. Catalogs can simplify shopping by saving energy and time for other things. New services, including drugstores and supermarkets that encourage you to order by phone, are springing up to fulfill this need. One such phone service facilitates banking, paying bills, and shopping for such products as books, flowers, and kitchen supplies.

If supermarket displays, reaching toward high shelves, and constantly looking around create visual confusion, find a store that fills orders by phone and delivers.

Consumer laws protect you when you shop by mail or phone. Problems about items you receive by mail that fall short of your expectations or are faulty may be resolved by recourse to a public agency with the responsibility for enforcing consumer protection laws.

Resources

Catalogs that offer food delivered by mail are mentioned in Chapter 6, "Choosing Foods for a Healthy Heart."

Products

A Folding Carry-All With Wheels. More versatile than a shopping cart, this opens from a tote bag size to twenty-one inches tall. $14. Independent Living Aids catalog, (800) 537-2118.

A Cane/Seat. When you need a place to sit while waiting on line or if your legs get tired, use this lightweight aluminum folding seat that doubles as a cane. $30. Lighthouse Consumer Products catalog, (800) 829-0500.

Services

Home-Cooked, Mail-Order Meals. For less than $10 a day you can receive a week's worth of complete dinners, including desserts and breads, frozen and ready to put in the oven. The cost varies, depending on the menu from $60 to $65 for one person or $95 to $100 for two people, plus shipping charges. Special diets may be ordered. Extended Family, Falls Road, RD 3, Hudson, NY 12534, (800) 235-7070.

Personal Chef Service. Hire a chef to provide two to four weeks of cooked meals to store in your freezer. The chef will plan the menu, shop for groceries, and prepare and package the meals. For a personal chef near you, contact United States Personal Chef Association, 7200 Montgomery, NE, Suite 241, Albuquerque, NM 87109, (800) 995-2138.

Shoppers Express and Pharmacy Express. These services deliver your grocery and drugstore orders to your home. Deliveries cost about $2 per order for pharmacies, $10 for supermarkets. To find out if a supermarket or pharmacy near you offers this service, call Shoppers Express, Pharmacy Express, (800) 999-1387.

ScanFone. Shop by phone with a bar code reading pen and phone supplied FREE. Can be used for Shoppers Express and Pharmacy Express, described above. Also has services including banking, bill paying, and shopping from a variety of catalogs for various products, books, flowers, kitchen supplies. To find out if it is available in your area, call (800) 876-2099.

Publications

"Shopping by Phone and Mail," Federal Trade Commission. This fact sheet describes what to expect when you shop by phone or mail and how to resolve problems that may arise. FREE. Federal Trade Commission, Washington, DC 20580.

Staying Active

Chapter 9

Achieving the Four Elements of Mobility

"Sure, I don't get around like I used to, but I still go to the library once a week and stop at my stores on the way home. My shopping cart is full by the time I'm done. Without my neighbor's help, I couldn't get everything up the stairs to my apartment. It's a struggle, but if I had to give it up, I might as well just give up."

"I used to take an umbrella with me rain or shine for years because I didn't like the idea of a cane. It struck me as the beginning of the end if I had to use a cane. Now I don't mind so much. A cane is really the least of my worries — and so many of my friends can't get out even with a cane — so a cane adds up to nothing at all."

"I see young people jogging around, and it seems so undignified, bare legs and all. That's what I think of when I hear the word 'exercise.'"

Maintaining or improving your *strength, endurance, flexibility,* and *balance,* the four elements of mobility, is a prerequisite for being able to walk and remain active. In maturity we become more acutely aware of how greatly our independence is facilitated by our mobility. To shop, bank, or socialize, we need to get around the house, the block, the neighborhood. We must be strong enough to perform our daily tasks. Of course, we can use some help. If the supermarket delivers, if there is a nearby bus or someone to carry packages, these are welcome assistance. Whatever we need to help us get around — for example, a walker or cane — should be willingly accepted as a means of prolonging our independent lives.

Research on mobility challenges traditional ideas of the "natural process of aging," a concept that now is just short of being self-contradictory. One at a time, items have been eliminated from the list of complaints that were once assumed to be the inevitable result of long life. Researchers have found that muscle mass, heart capacity, and lung capacity can improve with exercise, regardless of a person's age. Frailty is not the natural result of growing older, but it *is* the result of inactivity. The watchword of the nineties is a prescription for people as old as their nineties: Be active and thrive.

Despite these findings, shocking statistics about people over age seventy-five living at home were highlighted in a 1991 report to Congress by the National Institute of Aging (NIA). It found that 32 percent had difficulty climbing ten steps, 40 percent had difficulty walking a quarter of a mile, 22 percent couldn't lift ten pounds, and 7 percent couldn't walk across a small room.

As a measure of mobility these deficiencies make it difficult for individuals to prepare meals, clean their homes, visit stores, socialize, or dress themselves. Yet the NIA commented that "we are learning that people are never too old to prevent or reduce physical frailty." Being active should be part of a health program designed to allow you to continue to accomplish your daily needs; exercise is a drug-free prescription for maintaining mobility.

The exercise boom of the eighties exploded the notion that a rocking chair awaits us all. Now we hear that we should blame that rocking chair for our trouble. While the new ideas make sense, we may have to change our attitudes toward energetic activity, as well as relax our reluctance to use canes or other aids to help us get around. It's not easy to put aside the customs of a lifetime, but you can choose from many different ways of becoming and remaining physically able. Sweat and physical exertion are not necessary to improve your abilities. According to new research, a total of thirty minutes a day of light activity may improve your physical condition. Of course, further fitness will result from more intense activity.

THE REWARDS OF AN ACTIVE LIFE

Some call it exercise, but we prefer to think in terms of activity. Only recently has the connection between activity and independent living been noted. The benefits now claimed for activity are so many that the list resembles the claims for Mother's Cure-All Elixir sold from the back of a truck.

The Benefits of Activity

- Reduces the risk of heart disease, tension, and the effects of arthritis
- Ameliorates osteoporosis, diabetes, and overweight
- Improves lung capacity, digestion, and hypertension, circulation, flexibility, muscle tone, mood, mental acuity, self-image, stamina, energy, and ability to sleep
- Lowers blood cholesterol levels
- Aids in weight control

Not every activity improves equally each of the items in the box above, but some activity will be effective for your specific needs. Precisely why activity is such a panacea is not clear in every case, but the beneficial effects have been documented. In 1992 the American Heart Association declared lack of exercise to be a major risk factor for heart disease. According to the association, 20 to 30 percent of American adults — thirty-five to fifty million people — are inactive enough to be at significantly increased risk for heart disease. Inactive people are found to have nearly twice the risk of developing heart disease as active people, the same risk as that caused by smoking a pack of cigarettes a day. In addition, active people are more likely than the sedentary to survive a heart attack. Activity has a positive impact on several of the other risk factors for heart disease: raising "good" cholesterol levels in the blood (Chapter 6, "Choosing Foods for a Healthy Heart," has a detailed discussion of cholesterol), helping control weight, lowering blood pressure, and even reducing stress.

Certain types of activity are thought to play a part in strengthening bones by placing enough stress on them to stimulate the process that leads to increased bone density. These activities all involve "weight-bearing exercise" as an antidote to osteoporosis, a disease that results in brittle bones that break under minimal stress, causing disability. A 1994 study of postmenopausal women found women who were in the habit of walking about a mile each day had reduced their risks of developing osteoporosis; they had denser bones and slower rates of bone loss in their legs. Loss of bone mass can be limited by involving the muscles in an activity, causing them to bear the weight of the body and in turn stress the bones to which they are connected. Exercise *in combination* with hormone replacement therapy and/or calcium supplements may help prevent excessive bone loss in postmenopausal women.

When muscles are in use, they require glycogen, the sugar found in the blood. Thus the more muscle tissue, the more sugar is likely to be withdrawn from the blood. This process reduces the risk of diabetes and may lessen its severity.

Exercise is diet's partner in weight control. When you cut back on calories in your diet, your body responds by burning both fat and muscle; exercise increases muscle mass while burning fat. In addition, since muscle cells need more energy — or calories — to function than do fat cells, having more muscle will help you lose weight by burning more calories.

Lung capacity is dependent on the strength of the diaphragm and abdominal muscles and can be increased by activity. After activity, blood cholesterol levels show an increase in high-density lipoproteins (HDLs), which remove cholesterol from the bloodstream. Hypertension has been found to respond favorably to exercise, which is often preferred to medication as an initial treatment. Physical movement of muscles and joints lessens the effects of arthritis and enhances flexibility, muscle tone, and stamina. Activity speeds digestion and reduces the incidence of constipation.

People who are active often experience positive emotional results: an improved self-image, reduced tension, a more cheerful mood. Most active people report increased energy and mental alertness, attributable, perhaps, to the increased flow of blood to the brain. Fewer sleep problems may be a result of your being more relaxed and more tired after exercise.

Only you and your doctor know your current level of activity and your physical needs, so consult your doctor *before* beginning an activity program. Together you must decide on an exercise routine that's right for you. Performing an activity at low intensity but for increasingly longer duration often carries the least potential for injury and the greatest chance of fulfillment.

Now let's examine in detail each of the four elements you need for an active life.

STRENGTH

To carry grandchildren, groceries, and gardening tools, you need to use the muscles in your arms, shoulders, back, and legs. The stiffness in your shoulders or arms after the first spring day of digging in the garden is a message that your muscles are strengthening. As the days go by, you won't feel as sore, unless you increase the amount of time you work or the intensity of your work. If you stop working in the garden and don't engage in other activities that require your arm muscles, they will diminish in size and ability over a relatively short time. This is true regardless of your age.

By age twenty our muscles reach a peak of capacity and, without proper exercise, thereafter begin to deteriorate. Over a lifetime muscles tend to decline in size and strength by 30 to 40 percent; a sedentary person loses about six and one-half pounds of lean body mass, mainly muscle, every ten years. To counteract this trend, we must do activities that involve using the muscles.

In order to strengthen arm muscles, leg muscles, or stomach muscles, you must use them. Muscles don't retain their size without use. One extreme of muscle development is personified by Mr. and Ms. America, the body builders. We are at the other extreme, simply needing our muscles to help us perform our daily tasks. Strong muscles also reduce stress on weakened joints and strengthen the bones to which they are connected.

In the past loss of muscle mass during aging was thought to be irreversible as well as inevitable. Research has proved otherwise: We can become stronger if we are active. In one study ten nursing home residents ages eighty-six to ninety-six, all described as frail and inactive, gained an *average* of 174 percent in strength after lifting leg weights three times a week. After eight weeks the participants were able to increase the average weight they could lift from fifteen to forty-three pounds. A mere four weeks after resuming an inactive life, however, they experienced a 32 percent loss in muscle strength. In 1994 a follow-up study discovered that strengthening muscles with weight training was more important to increasing muscle strength than was improving nutrition. Nursing home residents improved their walking speeds, climbed stairs more easily, and were able to do more activities after a three-day-a-week weight program. Clearly, making exercise a habit is essential to any strengthening plan.

Anyone with a medical condition should be sure to consult a doctor to determine activities that will strengthen muscles without interfering with treatment or aggravating their symptoms.

Walking is less jarring than high-impact sports; still, it strengthens the muscles around joints and improves mobility and stability.

Stretching muscles before an activity is not the same as warming muscles up. In fact, muscles should first be warmed up by walking slowly, then gently stretched. The purpose of stretching is to make muscles as flexible as possible so that they withstand your activity and will be less likely to tire or be injured. Abruptly stopping an activity can cause cramps in your muscles, so you should cool down the same way you warmed up and stretch again.

Strengthening Activities

For leg muscles: walking; walking up and down hills; pedaling, either a stationary or moving bicycle; dancing; calisthenics; swimming

For arm muscles: swimming; using arms to pull, push, or lift

People with low energy levels may require longer periods for rest and recovery after activity. Rather than one day of recuperation from muscle soreness, perhaps two or three will be necessary at first, but over time one or two probably will be enough.

Aches and Pains

Pain is not a legitimate part of activity. If any activity is painful, do not continue it.

On the other hand, try to make a distinction between pain and the soreness or achiness that is an indicator that a muscle is being used and strengthened. Expect mild soreness or ache to develop a day or two after you use a muscle, not during an activity. Pain while performing an activity is a signal to stop. If postactivity soreness persists, consult your doctor.

Tips for Strengthening Leg Muscles

Increasing your muscle mass by 10 percent corresponds to a 200 percent increase in strength. This is a more significant gain at age ninety, when the thigh is 30 percent muscle, than at age twenty, when it is 90 percent muscle.

Strengthened leg muscles provide numerous benefits:

- You can stand longer — for example, while cooking, taking a shower, or waiting in line at the bank or supermarket.
- Your walking ability improves, as does your confidence while walking, safely negotiating curbs, and enjoying outdoor excursions.
- Getting out of chairs is easier.
- Going up and down stairs is easier.
- Balance is improved, and the chance of a fall is reduced.

Strategies to Aid in Sitting Down and Standing Up

Gravity makes it easy to sit down in a chair and can make it impossible to get up. Movement problems or muscle stiffness, such as those that accompany Parkinson's disease, can make even sitting down a trial. Strengthened leg muscles will help you get out of bed and chairs.

One technique for sitting down on a chair is to back up until you feel the chair behind you and then to bend forward as if you were going to touch your toes and slowly sit down. To get up, place one foot forward and the other back, under the chair if possible. Now, bending your torso forward, put your weight onto your front foot, and push yourself up vigorously

183

with your arms. To gain momentum, rock your torso back and forth a few times if necessary.

Raising the back legs of a comfortable armchair or all four legs of your bed with four-inch wood blocks can give you a natural boost onto your feet. If someone offers to help you rise from a chair, ask for a push on your back as you lean forward, rather than be pulled from the front by your arms. A knotted rope or towel attached to the foot of your bed also can be used to pull yourself to a sitting position.

There are devices available that boost you out of a chair: either cushions with mechanisms that push you up or chairs that tilt forward until your weight is almost entirely on your feet. Adjustable beds that facilitate getting up are also available.

It is primarily the lower leg muscles that are strengthened by walking. Adding hills to your walk, either by using a treadmill that adjusts for inclines or by walking on hilly routes, can involve the muscles of the upper leg too.

Another activity that improves thigh muscles (as well as the use of hips and knees) is pedaling, either on a stationary bicycle, a recumbent bike, or a regular bike or with a set of pedals. Of course, like all indoor equipment, stationary bikes provide you with an opportunity for activity even in inclement weather. It's a great way to exercise, but be sure to guard against losing the habit of going outside altogether so that you don't risk isolation and lack of stimulation.

Before you purchase a stationary bicycle, try the seat for comfort, size, and stability. Be sure you feel secure in the riding position and both holding and not holding the handlebars. Check whether the pedals revolve on their own even without your feet in position; if so, they might hit your legs if you stopped pedaling suddenly. A recumbent stationary bike has pedals on a level with your pelvis. This eliminates the pressure or numbness some people experience in the groin after sitting on upright bikes. Since the chair is contoured, your back is supported, in contrast with bikes with seats that you perch on. A pedal set allows you to sit in any comfortable, secure chair as you pedal. A stationary bicycle or pedal set is beneficial even if one leg is weaker than the other. If you choose pedaling as your exercise, continue until your legs feel heavy, gradually working up to a continuous ten- to twenty-minute session every other day.

Swimming is an ideal activity to avoid aggravating a knee or hip condition or to strengthen leg muscles. Problems finding a pool, transportation to and from a pool, or handling dressing and undressing logistics may make swimming seem inconvenient. A weekly class would be a good starting point; you could share some locker room assistance with the other participants. The benefits of swimming, especially for symptoms of arthritis, can be far greater than the minor inconveniences involved.

Tips for Strengthening Arm Muscles

It's easy to incorporate arm-strengthening movements while walking. Swing your arms loosely but purposefully, or bend them at the elbow to add energy to your walk. Pumping arms bent at the elbow as you walk provides a more vigorous outing. The mild ache you feel afterward indicates that your muscles have been activated. Arm swing provides balance and energy to your walking motion. When the arm swing is shortened, as may happen with arm weakness or loss of range of movement in the shoulder, your gait becomes less steady, and you need to take smaller steps.

You can gain muscle strength by lifting a weight a limited number of consecutive times. If you have high blood pressure, a heart condition, tender joints, or diabetes, your doctor may not recommend working with weights, so be sure to consult him or her before beginning any work with weights. A physiotherapist, a physiatrist, or a health club assistant with experience in the use of weights may devise a program suited to your individual needs. You can improve your muscular endurance by repeatedly lifting a light weight — that is, one you can lift and lower ten times in a row without straining or discomfort. It's time to add a small amount to that when it still feels light even on the tenth time you lift and lower it. Lifting and lowering one pound ten times twice a week will build muscle. Never hold your breath as you lift a weight. Practice exhaling at the maximum exertion and inhaling when the muscles relax.

To fashion homemade weights, fill a plastic container with two cups of water to create a one-pound weight. A sixteen-ounce can that is comfortable to hold in your hand can serve the same purpose. A gallon container weighs about eight pounds if filled with liquid; more if you fill it with sand.

People with arthritis can benefit from muscles warmed from lifting a weight, but they shouldn't overdo. In this case using a weight machine under supervision may be better than using handheld or free weights.

Resources

NOTE: Manufacturers of electrical muscle stimulators and passive exercise machines claim that their products provide all the benefits of exercise without the effort. Although these devices are used to advantage in rehabilitation clinics, they have been found by the Food and Drug Administration to be the equivalent of no exercise for a healthy person. The machines do not help weight loss, increase aerobic capacity, or help tone muscles, and they can even cause electrical shocks or burns if they are used inexpertly.

Products

Pedal Exerciser. You sit in a chair and use the stand-alone pedal device. Tension control changes pedal resistance. $55. Sears Home HealthCare catalog, (800) 326-1750.

Chairs and Beds
Leg-X-Tenders. Plastic items that add 3, 4, or 5 inches to straight-leg chairs without damage to the chair. Four for $37. Enrichments catalog, (800) 323-5547.

Lift Chairs. Touch a button and the mechanism moves to standing, seated, or fully reclined positions and others in between. Side pocket holds magazines and newspapers. Lifts up to 350 pounds. Also has a vibrator unit and a heater unit that maintains a temperature between 140 and 150 degrees. Med-Lift & Mobility, Inc., P.O. Box 189, Highway 8 East, Vardaman, MS 38878, (800) 748-9438.

Recliners. From $800 to $1,000. Electric Mobility, 1 Mobility Plaza, Sewell, NJ 08080, (800) 662-4548.

Portable Foam Cushion. Adds 4½ inches to chair seat. Removable cover and carrying handle. $40. Comfort House catalog, (800) 359-7701.

Pneumatic Lifter. Boosts you up from a seat when you lean forward. For people who weigh up to 300 pounds. $330. Enrichments catalog, (800) 323-5547.

Automatic Lifter Seat. Portable. For up to 150 pounds, $120. For up to 250 pounds, $140. Independent Living Aids catalog, (800) 537-2118.

Seat Lifter. Portable spring-activated chair lift. You operate a lever that opens the lifter to a 45-degree angle to help you out of a chair. For 150 pounds to 220 pounds, $210. For under 150 pounds, $200. Sears Home HealthCare catalog, (800) 326-1750.

Buddy Bar. A portable device to assist you in sitting or standing. When you step on the platform, your own weight stabilizes the Buddy Bar, which you can hang on to in front of you as you rise from or lower yourself onto a chair or bed. Available with a side bar for use at the toilet. $175. Health and Community Living, Inc., 9833 Whetstone Drive, Gaithersburg, MD 20879, (800) 736-6617.

Bed Pullup. A 40-inch-long loop that you use to pull yourself to a sitting position attaches to the end of the bed or bed frame. $15. AfterTherapy catalog, (800) 235-7054.

Weights

Dumbbells, Wrist Weights, and Other Types of Weights:
    AdaptAbility catalog, (800) 243-9232
    Fitness Wholesale catalog, (800) 537-5512

Heavyhands Weight Handles. The handles weigh 1 pound. Additional weights may be added. Handles, $17. Weight sets: four ½-pound weights, $9. Fitness Wholesale catalog, (800) 537-5512.

Heavy Balls. Handholds carved out of a sphere make these easier to use than dumbbells. Filled with water, sand, or lead shot, they can weigh from 2 to 30 pounds. Equipment Shop, P.O. Box 33, Bedford, MA 01730, (617) 275-7681.

WalkWeights. Adjustable strap, easy-to-hold foam grip, with instructions. Not only for use when walking, of course. Two 1½-pound weights, $25. Two 2½-pound weights, $27. For a dealer near you, contact Aspire, 3545 Scarlet Oak Boulevard, St. Louis, MO 63122, (800) 264-1990.

SoftHands. Dumbbells with large-diameter, ridged-foam grips for ease of holding. Two 1½-pound weights, $20. Two 3-pound weights,

$22. For a dealer near you, contact Aspire, 3545 Scarlet Oak Boulevard, St. Louis, MO 63122, (800) 264-1990.

Water Weights. Wrap around the wrist or ankle with a Velcro tab. When water is added, the weight increases from 1 to 3 pounds. $16. Enrichments catalog, (800) 323-5547.

Adjustable Wrist or Ankle Weights. Velcro closing. 1 pound, $9. Fitness Wholesale catalog, (800) 537-5512.

Gel Weights. These pound weights for wrists or ankles look like wristbands and have washable terry cloth covers. $20. Enrichments catalog, (800) 323-5547.

Dyna-Bands. 6-inch-wide stretchable latex bands are available in four levels of resistance to incorporate in a strengthening workout, usually used in 3- or 4-foot lengths. A sample comes with an instruction card describing fifteen exercises. Lengths, $3 to $5. Samples: one, $5, four, $13. Fitness Wholesale catalog, (800) 537-5512.

Thera-Band Plus. A kit with three 6-inch-wide stretchable rubber strips with grips. Each strip has a different resistance. Exercise book and instructions included. $20. Enrichments catalog, (800) 323-5547.

Thera-Band Supplies. 6- or 50-yard packages and handles sold separately. Stretchable tubing or bands also available. 6-yard light resistance, $9. Handles, $5 a pair. AdaptAbility catalog, (800) 243-9232.

Videotapes

Armchair Fitness. Three 20-minute stretching and strengthening workouts. Large-print instructions included. $40. CC-M Productions, P.O. Box 15707, Chevy Chase, MD 20815, (301) 588-4095.

Firm at 40 with Jan Burke, M.A. An upper-body workout with light weights. Demonstrates correct positioning and proper technique for using weights. Includes cardiovascular, strength, and flexibility exercises. 30 minutes. $10. Simitar Entertainment, 3850 Annapolis Lane, Plymouth, MI 55447, (800) 486-8273.

Video Cycle: Switzerland. View scenes from the Swiss Alps as you exercise on your stationary bicycle. 60 minutes. $20. Collage Video Specialties catalog. (800) 433-6769.

Audiotapes

The Exercise Program. A toning and strengthening workout, plus manual. 60 minutes. $35. Demos Publications, 386 Park Avenue South, Suite 201, New York, NY 10016, (800) 532-8663.

Publications

"Fitness: A Way of Life," American Physical Therapy Association. Several guidelines for fitness from a physical therapist's perspective. FREE. APTA, 1111 North Fairfax Street, Alexandria, VA 22314, (703) 684-2782.

ENDURANCE

Having enough energy to do sustained activity means we have the endurance to do what we need every day. This energy is a reflection of the fitness of our cardiovascular systems, our hearts and lungs. If we are fit, we are able to supply our muscles with oxygen, enabling us to do our daily tasks. Only aerobic activity, demanding that your heart and lungs work near their highest levels, will improve the cardiovascular system. To benefit your heart and lungs requires vigorous and sustained activity: raising your heartbeat above its usual level for at least twenty minutes. *For cardiovascular benefits, sporadic activity doesn't count.*

The ability to perform an activity is predicated on the amount of oxygen the body can utilize, another instance in which age is not an accurate prognosticator of physical condition. An active person, age sixty, can breathe in more oxygen than a sedentary twenty-year-old. In order to maintain aerobic capacity, you must be active. This circular reasoning sounds like an oversimplification, but it is the simple truth: To be active, you must be active.

Without activity the body's utilization of oxygen declines. A person whose maximum oxygen use falls to one liter per minute is in jeopardy of losing the ability to carry out daily activities. Someone whose maximum oxygen usage is high can do more activities without feeling tired than a person the same age who has a lower breathing capacity.

Aerobic activity can improve oxygen use even in people who were previously sedentary.

Just as a marathon runner tailors a training program for the distance of the race, so too must we define our goals before selecting an activity program. A statement of modest, nonathletic goals might be as follows: "I want to be able to get around my home, climb a few stairs when I need to, and walk a couple of blocks."

These unassuming objectives can signify independence for the person who attains them. Your activity level will depend on your goals and your body's condition. The 60 percent of Americans who are sedentary (active for less than twenty minutes three times a week) will have to begin some activity in order to improve or maintain their cardiovascular capacities. Many have found walking is a sensible beginning point.

One researcher has calculated that every mile covered by someone who previously was not active would add twenty minutes to that person's life.

People with arthritis can derive aerobic benefits from activities that place the least stress on the joints, such as bicycling, swimming, rowing, low-impact dance classes where one foot is always on the floor, or walking. Jogging and running put too much pressure on the joints, but brisk walks provide adequate aerobic activity. Running

---

A Graduated Walking Plan

New walkers. Walk any distance, any duration, any speed. Walk as much as feels comfortable, indoors or outdoors.

The next step. Do not stroll as you walk, but concentrate a bit on your footwork. Step on your heel, and roll your foot forward until you push off with the toes. Let your arms relax and swing comfortably at your side. Stop whenever you feel you are losing your balance or your breath. If you feel unsteady at all, walk with a friend or walk indoors. Walk any distance, any speed, but work up to walking as much as ten minutes at a stretch.

Another step. If you feel comfortable, walk outside, purposefully, without stopping, working up to twenty minutes. Go any distance, any speed, every day. Even if you only walk around your home for twenty minutes three times a week, you are out of the sedentary category and can consider yourself an active individual.

in place in waist-deep water or walking in thigh-deep ocean water also activates the cardiovascular system.

Walking in a mall can be a solution for people who are sensitive to air pollutants, live in climates with extremes of heat and cold, and prefer a secure atmosphere.

Heart Rate

Your pulse, or resting heart rate, is an indicator of your endurance. The stronger your heart is, the lower your pulse will be, the longer and harder you can work — or walk. Doing any activity can strengthen your heart, as long as you raise your pulse rate.

A stronger, more efficient heart will send more oxygenated blood through your system with each beat and will beat fewer times. Check your resting heart rate against the categories in the box below to evaluate your current fitness level.

How to Take Your Pulse

Feel your pulse either at your wrist — in the depression on the inside of your wrist, just under your radial bone as it extends from your thumb — or on the side of your neck — at the midpoint between your ear and your chin, behind the larynx.

Resting Heart Rates

70-75 beats or less per minute: very good
76-90 beats per minute: average
91-100 beats per minute: poor

Reducing your resting heart rate by ten beats per minute will save the heart three weeks of work over a year, according to the President's Council on Physical Fitness and Sports.

In order to improve your endurance level, you have to push your heart muscle just as you push your skeletal muscles to become stronger by doing more work. As you walk, your heart will beat faster than usual, but gradually your resting heart rate will be lower.

How to Add Intensity to Walking to Improve Heart Function

- Don't vary the distance, but actively swing your arms or lengthen your stride.
- Vary your speed by walking more quickly for one minute (or less) and then at a more normal pace for the next minute.
- Add hills to your walking route.
- Try to cover more ground in the same amount of time.
- Walk briskly, a pace of three to four miles an hour.
- If you already are walking at a brisk pace, walk more vigorously, a pace of four to five miles an hour.
- Use a pedometer to measure the distance you cover.
- Check your heart rate with a pulse meter to sustain a certain intensity or to vary effort during an activity session.

A minimum benefit can be obtained by raising your pulse above ninety beats per minute and keeping it there for ten minutes. Of course, while you want to exert yourself enough to benefit your heart, you don't want to exercise so much that you exhaust yourself. An indicator of a healthy level of exercise is your awareness that you are breathing more deeply and that your heart is beating more quickly than usual, yet that you can converse reasonably well, without panting or gasping for breath. If you break into a light sweat, you are exerting yourself sufficiently.

A study by the Institute for Aerobics Research in Dallas found that exercise capacity and cholesterol levels in women may show improvement with a regimen of slow but regular walking, though more benefits resulted from more aerobic activity. Regardless of walking speed, higher HDL cholesterol levels, a sign of reduced risk of heart disease, were measured in participants. Those who walked three miles a day, five days a week, had a 6 percent increase in HDL levels, regardless of whether they walked a mile in twelve minutes or twenty minutes.

To monitor your fitness level, learn to take your pulse as you walk or do other activity, so that you know if you are maintaining adequate intensity. Heart rate monitors provide instant readings during activity. Vary your walk or jog routine over a week's time, including some sessions at a faster pace and other workouts at a longer distance but slower tempo. Concentrate on a fast walk or run on one day, a long walk or run another day, and a loping walk or comfortable jog the days in between. If you can't last the allotted time at a fast pace, do intervals, speeding up for a spell, followed by a slower recovery period. If your legs become heavy and tired, slow down for the remainder. This idea can be applied to other activities as well.

Precautions

Because heart disease does not always manifest symptoms, you should consult your doctor before embarking on an aerobic activity program. A stress test can be given to determine your maximum heart rate — the rate your heart beats when you are working as hard as you can. Your doctor then calculates your target heart rate — the rate you should achieve during exercise to benefit your heart, a percentage of your maximum heart rate. Moderate activity is defined as working out at 30 to 40 percent of your maximum heart rate. Although you can arrive at a target heart rate by using a chart or subtracting your age from 220 and using a percentage, the stress test will be more accurate for your particular level of conditioning. Alternatively, you can exercise at a rate twenty beats per minute faster than your resting heart rate.

Breathing Capacity

The nine million Americans who suffer from breathing difficulties can adapt walking programs for their needs. You can increase the amount of oxygen your lungs can hold if you breathe by expanding your diaphragm. Be careful to distinguish your diaphragm from your abdomen; the diaphragm is the muscle above your waist, just under the place where your rib cage separates. If you are short of breath, concentrate on exhaling more than you inhale, by taking two steps on each inhale and four steps on each exhale, keeping the rhythm steady and comfortable.

An informal way to test your lung ability: Hold a lit match a foot away from your mouth, take a deep breath, and exhale to extinguish the flame. You should be able to blow it out easily.

If lung capacity is a problem for you, consider dividing your walk into two widely spaced sessions to avoid overdoing — for example, fifteen minutes morning and evening. When you can cover a certain distance or walk for a certain amount of time without stress or being out of breath, add a few steps or a few minutes to the session.

If walking continuously is not possible at first, try this: Stop, take a breath, and as you exhale, take a step or two. Stop again and inhale before taking a few more steps. Apply this strategy to all your activities, breaking them into small portions, resting in between, standing as little as possible, and *always exhaling during the moment of exertion.* Think *Exhale on exertion.* In addition, since it takes more effort to use tense muscles than relaxed ones, do what you can to be relaxed, mentally and physically, by trying meditation or other stress reduction techniques.

Cold air can constrict airways, so try to warm winter air by breathing through your nose. Covering your nose and mouth with a scarf on the coldest and windiest days can help. The Environmental Protection Agency considers the period between April 1 and September 30 to be ozone season: More sunlight and higher surface temperatures cause chemicals in polluted air to combine to produce ozone, the major ingredient in smog. Ozone reacts with lung tissue and can cause breathing problems even in apparently healthy people. Ozone levels are usually noted in newspaper weather reports. If you already have trouble breathing, stay indoors in ozone season, during peak hours and on the worst days, and do most activities during the early morning.

Being short of breath can be a self-perpetuating condition; the first indication of a breathing problem can create anxiety, which in turn can exacerbate the condition. Pursed-lip breathing may relieve this anxiety, calm you, and restore your regular breathing rhythm. To do pursed-lip breathing, sharply inhale two breaths as if you were drinking from a straw and exhale four breaths the same way. Practice this breathing technique a few times when you are breathing normally, and then try it to alleviate your next attack of shortness of breath.

The air in your home may contain pollutants that exacerbate breathing problems. The by-products of tobacco smoke affect people who have allergies or breathing difficulties. To keep your home smoke-free if you have breathing problems, display a No Smoking sign in your home, and throw out all the ashtrays.

194

Clues to the Presence of Irritants in the Air at Home

- Unusual odors
- A high humidity level
- Moisture on the windows or elsewhere
- Seemingly stale air
- Noticeably warm or cold house temperature
- Little air movement or ventilation
- Obvious dust accumulation
- Dust or dirt on walls, ceilings, upholstered furniture, or drapes

Of course, this is not a housekeeping or cleanliness lecture. The problem with dust is that it contains dust mites, minuscule bugs whose excrement in the air can hamper breathing. One way to control the dust mite population is to adjust the humidity; the mites do not survive when the humidity is below 50 percent.

Controlling Dust Mites and Bacteria, Mold, and Pollen in the Home

- Maintain a humidity level between 30 and 50 percent; in the summer, use air conditioning to keep the humidity below 50 percent.
- Install exhaust fans vented to the outside in kitchens, bathrooms, and clothes dryers.
- Ventilate the attic to prevent the buildup of moisture.
- People with breathing problems shouldn't vacuum and shouldn't be in the house when vacuuming is done, since vacuuming itself may increase the number of mites and pollutants in the air.
- Cover pillows, mattresses, and box springs with dust-proof covers.
- Use hot water — at least 130 degrees — to wash all sheets and blankets.
- Remove curtains, carpeting, upholstered furniture, and stuffed toys from the bedrooms.

If breathing problems limit your activity, ration your energy. Sit at every opportunity rather than stand in the kitchen, bathroom, and so on. To conserve energy, become either more organized or more relaxed. Make one trip upstairs with accumulated items, not many trips; keep duplicate necessities upstairs and downstairs or in different rooms. Get help with chores if you need it; ask to have groceries and other items delivered.

Certain houseplants can absorb some pollutants while adding oxygen and moisture to the air. A ten- to twelve-inch potted plant is adequate for the air in a room about ten by ten feet. Some species thought to be particularly effective are: reed palm, English ivy, peace lily, snake plant, Chinese evergreen, dracaena, aloe, and banana tree.

Resources

NOTE: A portable oxygen tank with twenty minutes of oxygen, marketed for athletes, is not effective. The American Lung Association says there is no evidence that taking oxygen makes a healthy person feel better, and it may be harmful to people with cardiovascular illness or chronic lung disease.

Products

Polar Accurex. A wireless heart rate monitor that provides a continuous heart rate readout. It beeps when you are above or below your targeted range. Chest transmitter and wristwatch monitor, water-resistant for swimming. $250. Other models available. Polar Electro, Inc., 99 Seaview Boulevard, Port Washington, NY 11050, (800) 227-1314.

Pulse Watch II. Counts heartbeats by means of an infrared beam of light through the thumb. Press the monitor button with your thumb until the reading registers (about three seconds). The monitor can be clipped to clothing or an exercise machine. Includes a chart with suggested heart rates. The monitor is within 2 to 5 percent of accurate and operates without a chest strap transmitter. $50 to $60 at sporting goods stores. Precise International, 15 Corporate Drive, Orangeburg, NY 10962, (800) 431-2996.

Heart Rate Chart. A laminated chart from which you can determine the target heart rate for ages up to sixty-five. The chart also includes an explanation of how to take your pulse. A Velcro clip is included for hanging near the TV, for use as you follow exercise videos. $3. Collage Video Specialties catalog, (800) 433-6769.

Earlobe Clip Pulse Monitor. Readout may be mounted on the handlebar of a bicycle. $120. Cleo of New York catalog, (800) 321-0595.

Perforated Mask. To filter outdoor pollution, the mask fits over the nose and mouth and traps airborne fumes and pollen. It has a replaceable charcoal filter. $50. Real Goods catalog, (800) 762-7325.

Dust and Pollen Disposable Masks. Three for $3. High-efficiency respirator, $9. Allergy Clean Environments, 125 3rd Avenue, Haddon Heights, NJ 08035, (800) 882-4110, or in New Jersey call (609) 546-1101.

Non-Electric Sweeper. This may disperse dust less than electric vacuums as you clean carpet or floors. $45. Seventh Generation catalog, (800) 456-1177.

Nilfisk Home Allergy Vacuum Cleaner. Retains 99.97 percent of all particles 0.3 microns in size and larger. Attachments, filters. With Goretex filter, $500. With HEPA (high-efficiency particulate air) filter and microfilter, $550. Allergy Clean Environments, 125 3rd Avenue, Haddon Heights, NJ 08035, (800) 882-4110.

Electronic Air Cleaner. Mounted on the ducts of a central heating/cooling system, it removes 95 percent of pollutants. For a dealer near you, contact Honeywell, 1985 Douglas Drive North, Golden Valley, MN 55422.

Electrostatic Air Cleaner. A furnace filter that installs without wiring or other changes to the existing heating/cooling system. It operates on the principle of static electricity and is cheaper than electronic systems. The filter is permanent and requires cleaning every sixty to ninety days. $150. For a dealer near you, contact Newtron Products, Inc., 3874 Virginia Avenue, Cincinnati, OH 45227, (800) 543-9149.

Home Comfort Station. Monitors indoor temperature and humidity. Memory retains maximum and minimum temperatures and humidity readings. Battery-operated, either self-adhesive wall mount or desktop stand. $40. Safety Zone catalog, (800) 999-3030.

Pillows and Mattress Covers. Made to be "impermeable to allergens" such as dust mites. Standard pillow size, $11. Allergy Control Products, Inc., 96 Danbury Road, Ridgefield, CT 06877, (800) 422-DUST (3878).

Services

National Indoor Air Quality Information Clearinghouse, U.S. Environmental Protection Agency. Fact sheets, brochures, and referrals to other sources, (800) 438-4318.

Lungline. Provides information, publications, and answers to medical questions about pulmonary diseases. National Jewish Center for Immunology and Respiratory Medicine, Attention: Lungline, 1400 Jackson Street, Denver, CO 80206, (800) 222-LUNG (5864).

Videotapes

Let's Get Fit. A 1-hour program set to music. $20. Shepherd's Center, 5200 Oak Street, Kansas City, MO 64112, (816) 444-1121.

Armchair Aerobics. $25. Also audiotape, $10. The Fitness Firm, P.O. Box 367, Port Washington, WI 53074, (414) 375-2502.

Keep Fit While You Sit. An aerobic program using the arm, torso, neck, and shoulders for those who want to be active while sitting. 33 minutes. $30. Disability Bookshop, P.O. Box 129, Vancouver, WA 98666, (800) 637-2256.

Anybody Can Sit and Be Fit by Martha Rounds. 20 minutes of exercises involving arms and upper body and some leg lifts. $20. Accent on Living catalog, (800) 787-8444.

Dancin' Grannies. Designed specifically for mature women in three levels: beginner, active, or trim and tone. 45-52 minutes. $20 each. Dancin' Grannies Video, 370 Yarnell Parkway, Clinton, TN 37717, (800) 848-3200.

Sit and Be Fit Series. Four stretch and flexibility programs designed for specific physical conditions: stroke, pulmonary disease, multiple sclerosis, Parkinson's disease. 22 minutes each. $16 per tape. Collage Video Specialties catalog, (800) 433-6769.

Audiotapes

Jacki Sorensen's Prime of Your Life Aerobic Program. Includes illustrated guide with diagrams of all exercises and a heart rate guide. Also available on a long-playing record. 30 minutes. $11. Kimbo Educational catalog, (800) 631-2187.

Seatworks. A musical workout done while sitting. 35-minute audiocassette or long-playing record, with instructions and illustrations of each exercise. $11. Kimbo Educational catalog, (800) 631-2187.

Sittercise. Includes stretching, warm-up, and aerobic activities to be done from a chair or bed. Manual describes and illustrates all movements. 35-minute audiocassette or long-playing record, $11. Kimbo Educational catalog, (800) 631-2187.

Publications

Fitness Without Exercise: The Scientifically Proven Strategy for Achieving Maximum Health with Minimum Effort by Bryant A. Stamford, Ph.D., and Porter Shimer. A personal account by two individuals who kept fit without strenuous workout programs. Deemphasizes target heart rates and repetitive activities that may discourage participants from continuing in favor of daily activities that can keep you fit and accomplish needed chores or hobbies. 1990. Warner Books.

"Exercise and Your Heart: A Guide to Physical Activity," American Heart Association and the National Heart, Lung, and Blood Institute. A pamphlet with tips to encourage more physical activity. Includes a suggested walking program. FREE. NHLBI Information Center, P.O. Box 30105, Bethesda, MD 20824, (301) 251-1222.

"Silent Epidemic: The Truth About Women and Heart Disease," American Heart Association. Discusses risk factors and other aspects of heart disease that concern women. FREE. AHA, National Center, 7272 Greenville Avenue, Dallas, TX 75231, (800) AHA-USA1 (242-8721).

"An Older Person's Guide to Cardiovascular Health and Disease," American Heart Association. Describes various heart and vascular conditions and some treatments and preventions. FREE. AHA, National Center, 7272 Greenville Avenue, Dallas, TX 75231, (800) AHA-USA1 (242-8721).

BEST BUY. "Help Yourself to Better Breathing," American Lung Association. Suggested exercises and strengthening routines. Very comprehensive. Discusses medications. FREE. ALA, 1740 Broadway, New York, NY 10019, (800) LUNG-USA (586-4872).

"Breathe Easy Relaxation Exercises," American Lung Association of California. A brochure that suggests ways of strengthening the breathing mechanism and how to relax by using the technique of deep breathing. FREE. ALA of California, 424 Pendleton Way, Oakland, CA 94621, (800) LUNG-USA (586-4872).

BEST BUY. "The Inside Story: A Guide to Indoor Air Quality." This booklet describes the variety of pollutants in the air and what steps can be taken to combat them. FREE. Indoor Air Quality Information Clearinghouse, P.O. Box 37133, Washington, DC 20013, (800) 438-4318.

"Use and Care of Home Humidifiers," Indoor Air Facts No. 8. FREE. Indoor Air Quality Information Clearinghouse, P.O. Box 37133, Washington, DC 20013, (800) 438-4318.

"Residential Air-Cleaning Devices: A Summary of Available Information." An extensive description of different types of air cleaners to enable you to compare different units. FREE. Indoor Air Quality Information Clearinghouse, P.O. Box 37133, Washington, DC 20013, (800) 438-4318.

Organizations

American Heart Association. Publications, inquiries, referrals to resources and cardiac rehabilitation centers, support groups for people who have had strokes or have cardiovascular disease. AHA, 7272 Greenville Avenue, Dallas, TX 75231, (800) AHA-USA1 (242-8721).

American Lung Association. Publications, information, referrals, and support services for those with asthma and breathing problems, including Better Breathing clubs. Also stop smoking clinics. ALA, 1740 Broadway, New York, NY 10019, (800) LUNG-USA (586-4872).

American Academy of Allergy and Immunology. Provides the name of an allergist near you as well as pollen information. AAAI, 611 East Wells Street, Milwaukee, WI 53202, (800) 822-ASMA (2762).

National Institute of Allergy and Infectious Disease. Information and publications available. NIAID, Building 31, Room 7A-50, Bethesda, MD 20892, (301) 496-5717.

Asthma and Allergy Foundation of America. Information about symptoms, causes, and ways to control asthma and allergies; referrals for support groups, equipment. Offers publications. AAFA, 1125 15th Street, NW, Suite 502, Washington, DC 20005, (800) 7ASTHMA (727-8462).

American Allergy Association. Provides information and self-help for people with food and chemical allergies. AAA, Box 7273, Menlo Park, CA 94026, (415) 322-1663.

FLEXIBILITY

The natural ease of movement that makes youngsters fun to watch slowly declines during the more sedentary lives of young adults and adults. The degree of movement we used to have can't be maintained if we don't regularly extend our joints to their fullest. You may notice limitations in small ways. As you glance quickly around to check oncoming traffic from the driver's seat, for example, if your neck doesn't respond with a full rotation, you may not be able to drive safely.

In order to be active, your muscles and joints must permit movement of your limbs and body. Tight muscles restrict mobility. After an initial warm-up by a bit of pacing or walking in place, the muscles you intend to use should be stretched so that you can achieve the best performance. Similarly, joints need to be activated to keep them at maximum function.

Exercises for the joints are called range-of-motion exercises, referring to the degree of movement a joint can perform. Attempting the following test can provide a minimum idea of how well your joints are functioning.

The One-Minute Range-of-Motion Test

1. Sit with your knees together. Lean forward, and touch your toes.
2. Bend your elbows and place your hands in front of your mouth.
3. Place your hands behind your neck with your elbows extended to the side.
4. Reach both hands behind to the middle of your back.
5. Place your palms on your upper buttocks.
6. Place your hands on top of your head, making a diamond-shaped space with your elbows outstretched to the side.

Stiffness caused by arthritis may worsen the less you use your joints. An indication of this phenomenon is the amount of stiffness you feel in the morning, after your joints have been immobile during sleep; when you use them, they move better. You may find your movements enhanced if you begin the day with a warm bath to soothe the joints, followed by a period of activity to maintain your range of motion. Alternating rest periods and activity periods throughout the day may help you function with less discomfort.

Although you may choose walking for its convenience, other low-impact activities, such as swimming, bicycle riding, and rowing, are beneficial for flexibility and range of motion. The buoyancy of water relieves pressure on joints, making swimming a favored activity. Water reduces the body's weight to 10 percent of its land weight and offers four times the resistance of air. All water activities present much less risk of injury than bicycling or higher-impact activities.

Many public pools offer water exercise classes, most of which are not conducted in deep water or dependent on a knowledge of swimming, but are simply movements done in water. A variety of flotation devices are designed to give you confidence in the water even if you can't swim, without interfering with the movement of your joints. Water has a cooling effect (even in heated pools, where a water temperature in the range of eighty to eighty-four or even eighty-six degrees can soothe sore joints). Keeping your body's temperature down may allow you to swim for longer periods without tiring than you could do other activities. If you don't have access to a pool or the ocean, you can flex your legs and rotate your ankles as you sit in the bathtub.

If certain swimming strokes aggravate neck or shoulder problems, they can often be modified. For example, if the breaststroke strains neck muscles as you lift your head, turn your head to the side, rather than lift it up for a breath, or try the sidestroke.

Riding a bicycle, pedaling a stationary bike, or just using a set of pedals provides movement for the large leg joints as well as leg muscles. Upright, or touring-style, handlebars may be less stressful on the back than racing-style handlebars that require you to lean forward. The bicycle seat height should allow your leg to extend fully when the pedal is down. Cross-country skiing machines are also easy on the joints and provide a workout as well for the lungs, heart, and muscles.

Products

AquaJogger. A flotation jacket that allows you to jog upright in a pool. Comes with explanatory booklet. $39. Video available also. Fitness Wholesale catalog, (800) 537-5512.

Exercise Pedals. An alternative to an exercise bicycle, these are just the pedals. Sit in a regular chair and pedal. Adjustable tension. $60. Easy Street catalog, (800) 959-EASY (3279).

Pedal Exerciser. For use on a table to exercise arms or on the floor as pedaler. Adjustable tension. $10. Dr. Leonard's Health Care Products catalog, (800) 785-0880.

Digi-Flex. A way to exercise each finger independently to develop grasp and finger extension and promote flexibility and coordination. It can strengthen the hand and forearm as well as the fingers. Five different strengths from 1½ to 9 pounds, $10 each. Cleo of New York catalog, (800) 321-0595.

Videotapes

Chair Dancing. Three levels of intensity for range of motion and flexibility. 42 minutes, including warm-up and cooldown. $20. Collage Video Specialties catalog, (800) 433-6769.

Angela Lansbury's Positive Moves. Includes stretches and toning exercises. 46 minutes. $20. Collage Video Specialties catalog, (800) 433-6769.

Exercise SeniorStyle. Both seated and standing exercises done to music. For flexibility, range of motion, coordination, and more. Two different 30-minute tapes. $30 for both. Cottonwood Press, 305 West Magnolia, Suite 398, Fort Collins, CO 80521, (800) 864-4297.

BEST BUY. *Water Workout.* A 45-minute instructional video about using water's resistance and buoyancy for the greatest health benefits. $16. Fitness Wholesale catalog, (800) 537-5512.

Audiotapes

Fitness for Seniors by Stephanie Sorine. With explanatory guide. 36 minutes. Cassettes or long-playing record, $11. Kimbo Educational

BALANCE

A prerequisite to mobility is maintaining your balance, something you don't think about until you've lost it.

Statistics reveal that between 20 and 40 percent of adults over age sixty-five who live at home fall each year. Balance-related falls are blamed for more than half of the accidental deaths among the elderly. A sedentary lifestyle that leads to poor muscle strength and joint mobility may in turn lead to a deteriorated sense of balance and a reluctance to be active for fear of falling, which, unfortunately reinforces a sedentary lifestyle.

Balance is to some degree a skill that can be relearned and practiced. The body's balancing system can be retrained to compensate for sensory or other deficits by slowly combining head movements with body movements a little at a time.

An Exercise for Balance

As you stand on one leg, tighten your thigh muscle and stand for thirty seconds. Repeat with the other leg. Increase the time until you can stand on one leg for one minute. Do the same thing first with one eye closed; then with both eyes closed.

A rowing machine can improve your coordination of arm and head movements. A treadmill provides an opportunity for walking while holding on, for a secure feeling. Activities that include head movements, such as swimming, tennis, or other racket sports, can be used for balance training.

The Chinese movement routine called tai chi, which means "highest reach" in Chinese, is a combination of philosophy, psychology, meditation, physical exercise, and martial arts. For nearly a millennium the Chinese have been performing this series of positions that gently flow into one another. The National Institute of Aging is investigating how tai chi can help people over age seventy improve their balance. Learning the meaning of the exercises, rather than just doing the motions, may yield additional benefits, such as stress reduction and relaxation.

To keep your balance, try to avoid changing your position too rapidly when you stand after lying down or when you turn from side to side. Sudden head movements, such as looking up, bending over, reaching up, or turning your head quickly, can cause dizziness. In addition, walk with a stride that is long enough to allow you to see your feet.

Resources

Ideas for changing your home environment to reduce your chances of falling are discussed in Chapter 12, "Adapting the Old Homestead."

Videotapes

Staying Even, Vestibular Disorders Association. A dramatization of balance problems, diagnosis, and treatment. 30 minutes. Two-week rental; you pay return postage. $7. $35 to purchase. VDA, P.O. Box 4467, Portland, OR 97208, (800) 837-8428.

Publications

Balancing Act: For People with Dizziness and Balance Disorders by Mary Ann Watson, M.A., and Helen Sinclair, R.N., M.S. A comprehensive resource for handling dizziness problems: how to compensate and how to get help. 1992. $8. Vestibular Disorders Association, P.O. Box 4467, Portland, OR 97208, (800) 837-8428.

Organizations

Vestibular Disorders Association. Physician referrals, information, newsletter, support system, and publications. P.O. Box 4467, Portland, OR 97208, (800) 837-8428.

Chapter 10

On the Move

YOUR ACTIVITY PROFILE

"I believe each person has an exercise personality. It took me a long while to find the style of exercising that really suited me. I hated walking because it was too easy. I needed more incentive. Finally I bought a cheap stopwatch and I got interested. Trying to go faster than I did the previous time kept me in a perpetual race against myself."

People without a habit of regular activity will be more comfortable if they devise programs that accommodate their natural style. For clues to your own, examine the way you organize your life. For example, do you clean house a little bit each day, or do you leave everything for a one-time session? Do you wash, dry, and put away each meal's dishes as you go along, or do you let them accumulate? Do you have several projects going at once and follow a different pattern every day, or do you like a fairly established routine? Adopt an activity program that feels closest to your natural pattern, which may be one of the following:

Self-competitive. A self-competitive person likes to set personal goals and derives satisfaction from reaching them. Choose activities you can do alone, such as walking, using exercise machines, or swimming, and keep records of your progress.

Social/competitive. A social/competitive person's motivation comes from being able to exercise with others or comparing his or her performance to that of others. A health club setting, activity partners, and being active in a group context may be most gratifying for you.

Spontaneous. If you resent the enforced discipline of a regular time schedule or the regimentation of needing to accomplish a certain number of laps or repetitions, you should look for diversified activities. Change walking routes, follow different exercise routines, and alternate activities to make exercise more enjoyable.

Steady and steadfast. If you look forward to similar routines each day, chances are you are organized and can accommodate your schedule to include a half hour activity session, such as a regular video workout period, a walk along a favorite route, or a visit to a health club.

The large choice of activities makes it unlikely that you will fail to find one that suits your own style. No single activity program is good for everyone; pick and choose elements of various activities or alternate them for variety. Try to do activities that address the four elements of mobility.

Activity for Weight Control

To lose weight, you need not participate in an aerobic, high-intensity activity; you can simply increase the number of calories you burn each day. Researchers continue to argue about why it is more difficult for some people to lose weight than for others. Still, being active — burning calories — is essential to any weight loss regimen.

Moderate activity can help control your weight and reduce body fat. A two-hundred-pound person can lose about fourteen pounds in a year without changing his or her diet merely by walking a brisk mile and a half per day. The *duration* of an activity, rather than its intensity, is important in controlling body fat, because after glycogen supplies are depleted, the body calls upon fat for energy.

Although our bodies burn calories even when we are inactive, one study calculated that expending two thousand calories a week in activity, a mere one hour per day, would add one year to your life span. Exercising for twenty to thirty minutes can burn calories (about two hundred for vigorous exercise, about one hundred for moderate), reduce fat, and increase muscle (increasing muscle mass can help burn more calories: Muscle burns thirty to fifty calories per day, even when you are at rest; fat does not). The trend has moved away from measuring pounds in favor of describing body composition as a measure of fitness: the amount of fat compared with the amount of muscle. Since muscle weighs more and is more desirable than fat, experts say that the standardized height/weight charts may be misleading. You may weigh more than the chart indicates for your height, but if your body is mainly muscle, with little fat, your weight may be healthy.

Counting calories, both those in the food you eat and the ones you burn during activity, is tedious. If you count on activity for losing weight, you may prefer to keep a record for a week of all your activity, approximate the calories you burn, and adjust your exercise schedule according to the calories you consume in your diet over a week's time. To lose weight, of course, the balance must lean toward burning extra calories from activity.

Examples of Calories Burned During Certain Activities

Light house or office work for 30 minutes — 200 calories
Gardening for 30 minutes — 200 calories
Walking a mile, regardless of how fast — 100 calories
Sitting for 1 hour — 90 calories
Raking the lawn for 30 minutes — 50 calories
Climbing 10 to 12 stairs — 4 calories
Pacing back and forth for 15 steps — 1 calorie

While the number of calories you burn varies depending on your weight and how energetically you do an activity, you can approximate yours from the examples in the box.

Swimming is an effective activity for weight control because extra weight is less of a factor in the water, enabling you to do activities in the water longer than you might be able to do on land.

Resources

Information on nutrition and weight control is detailed in Chapter 7, "Following a Special Diet."

Services

ElderCamp. A ten-day stay at a health resort with advice on nutrition, fitness, and staying healthy. About $3,500. Canyon Ranch,

8600 East Rockcliff Road, Tucson, AZ 85715, or 91 Kemble Street, Lenox, MA 01240, (800) 726-9900.

Publications

BEST BUY. "Pep Up Your Life: A Fitness Book for Seniors," American Association of Retired Persons. Specifically designed for adults over age sixty. Exercises for strength, flexibility, and endurance at different intensity levels. FREE. AARP Publications, 601 E Street, NW, Washington, DC 20049.

BEST BUY. *Getting Fit Your Way: A Self-Paced Fitness Guide*, Maryland Department of Health and Mental Hygiene and Maryland Army National Guard. A well-structured design for developing your own fitness program, with charts, explanations, and pep talks. The program builds slowly: two weeks for setting goals, three weeks to begin, and nine weeks to get into the habit. It also includes a workbook for controlling smoking and weight. $3.25. Superintendent of Documents, U.S. Government Printing Office, Washington, DC 20402.

Taking Control of Your Health and Fitness, National Center for Women. Preventive measures for staying healthy and ways of integrating a nourishing diet and invigorating exercise into your life. $11. NCW, Long Island University, Southampton, NY 11968, (800) 426-7386.

Preventing Osteoporosis by Kenneth H. Cooper, M.D. A detailed exercise program is included with specific time, distance, and frequency prescriptions for various age groups for walking, cycling, rope jumping, jogging, stair climbing, aerobic dancing, swimming. 1989. Bantam Books.

ACSM Fitness Book, American College of Sports Medicine. A simple-to-follow color-coded fitness program. You adjust the program according to the results of a self-test. Covers the four elements of mobility, plus body composition. 1992. $12. Leisure Press, Box 5076, Champaign, IL 61825, (800) 747-4457.

Organizations

Aerobics and Fitness Foundation of America. Hot line, fitness information, and product evaluation. AFFA, 15250 Ventura Boulevard, Suite 200, Sherman Oaks, CA 91403, (800) BE-FIT-86 (233-4886).

President's Council on Physical Fitness and Sports. Publications available. 450 5th Street, NW, Suite 7103, Washington, DC 20001, (202) 272-3430.

National Heart, Lung, and Blood Institute. Publications and information available. National Institutes of Health, P.O. Box 30105, Bethesda MD 20824, (301) 251-1222.

American Physical Therapy Association. Publications on fitness available. APTA, 1111 North Fairfax Street, Alexandria, VA 22314, (703) 684-2782.

American Podiatric Medical Association. Publications, referrals to state association for members in your area. APMA, 9312 Old Georgetown Road, Bethesda, MD 20814, (800) FOOTCARE (366-8227).

WALKING, THE UNIVERSAL ACTIVITY

"When I started walking, I wouldn't buy any sweat suits or fancy running shorts. I just wore raggedy stuff my kids had outgrown. I wanted to be incognito. Then people started telling me how they admired my commitment, and my friends told me they had seen me walking around town. Gradually I got used to it myself."

It's hard to find fault with walking as an activity. After all, being able to walk is itself an objective of being active.

Attributes of Walking

- It needs no special skills.
- It requires no special equipment other than comfortable shoes.
- It can be done indoors or outdoors.
- It can be varied in location, speed, and duration.
- It builds muscles.
- It burns calories.
- It helps improve balance.
- It activates the leg muscles and joints, the cardiovascular system, and metabolism.
- It's a weight-bearing activity and helps increase bone mass.
- It's the best exercise for your feet.

A very impressive accounting indeed! Walking is activity's ace in the hole. Even people who are resistant to the idea of being active and risk a future of reduced mobility and reduced ability to perform daily tasks have little ammunition in an argument against walking.

Repetitive activities, such as walking, swimming, bicycling, and stair climbing, may strike you at first as being boring. The trick is to let your mind wander while your body does the activity. After a while the repetitions lull the brain, similarly to what happens when you meditate on a sound or thought, providing restorative mental relaxation and stress relief. Of course, you can also wear a cassette player and headphones and listen to music or learn a language.

How Much Walking?

You can measure walking in terms of time spent, distance covered, number of steps taken, or speed. You can include the walking you do around your home, the distance you walk to the store, or add it up however you like.

The unstated premise of activity is that you begin at a certain level and slowly improve over time. This is the reason for the odometer on the exercise bicycle, the stopwatch, the pulse meter, etc. These all are measures of performance. Many people are bothered by this approach because it focuses on an ulterior motive for walking, not just to walk but to walk faster, farther, or longer.

In a way this is true. If you are walking for some of the advantages listed earlier, there is no finish line, only a continuing quest to improve, but improvement is defined not as achieving increasingly difficult athletic goals but, as continuing to profit from the activity.

If you now can walk one step, one block, or one mile, after a while you can add another step, another half block, or a few more yards to increase your benefits. Your own beginning point provides the measure, and the goal remains the same: to be able to accomplish daily tasks. Walking a step, a block, or a mile becomes easier and easier each day you do it, as your muscles, heart, and lungs improve. It's natural to go to the next step, and the progress should bring with it satisfaction and the motivation to continue.

The beauty of walking is that it is adaptable to any schedule and any weather condition. You can walk alone or with others, in a mall, on a treadmill, in the woods, or on city streets. Walking can be fiercely aerobic or just a stroll; you can avoid or seek out hills. You can walk five minutes one day and thirty the next. Walking is the "no-excuses" activity; you can't claim you don't have time, money, or the equipment. If you aspire to independent living and you have never been active, take a walk.

Warm-ups for Walking

Gently arch and flex your back.
Turn your head from side to side.
Slowly march in place, raising your knees as high as possible.
Bending at the waist, gently rotate your upper body in a
   slow circle.

Tips and Techniques for Better Walking

Your body needs at least a quart of water for each hour you exercise, so drink a glass or two before starting out and again when you finish. Even in winter, though you sweat less, you still can become dehydrated. The air in winter is colder and drier than in summer, so your body expends energy to heat the air and hydrate it as you breathe before it can be absorbed by the lungs. Wearing a face mask will hydrate the air more quickly. The vapor you breathe out is moisture, but although you are losing water, your thirst mechanism is not as functional in cold weather. Frostbite is more likely if you are dehydrated because dehydration lowers blood volume so that not enough blood may be reaching your toes, fingers, and face.

Walking on a hard, even surface optimizes balance and promotes a secure step. The first choice should be a concrete walkway, such as a bicycle path; a second choice would be a gravel or dirt path, like a running track. The worst surface is grass or any uneven, pebbly path. Walking in traffic or in low-light conditions, such as at dusk or dawn, can be distracting and dangerous.

Walking is considered a low-impact activity, since each step exerts a force on joints and muscles a half or a quarter of that exerted by running. Still, the force of one step is 50 percent greater than your body weight. Walking, which doesn't jolt the body, is a good activity for people with joint problems, people who are overweight, someone with eye or nerve damage, or anyone who needs to avoid jarring movements. Walking has been found to be beneficial and safe for arthritis patients. The act of moving the joints tends to facilitate more ease of movement. A warm morning bath can precede a period of walking, as a means of loosening joints that are stiff from overnight inactivity. You may try alternating periods of activity and rest to keep your joints loose throughout the day.

If you have a low energy level or tire easily, you can budget your walking to periods of the day when you feel most alert.

Improvement in leg muscles can be measured in the length of your stride, the height each foot reaches as you step forward, and the rotation of your hips.

Walking is also a beneficial activity for those with tremors or poor control of leg muscles. In these cases rubber-soled sneakers may grip too well on the floor and cause you to trip, so leather-soled shoes may be preferable. You may get good results from using a large stride. If your legs don't respond, tap the hip of the leg you want to start with, bend your knees, and straighten up, or rock from side to side to begin.

If you monitor your blood glucose levels, do so before you take a walk, and ask your doctor what a safe level is for you. Eat one to three hours before activity, and take a source of sugar with you as a precaution. If you have diabetes, monitor your feet for blisters, and walk in mild, not extreme, weather for about twenty minutes three times a week.

Circulation problems also can be helped if you keep your legs in motion, rather than sit or stand still. When you do sit, jiggle your legs to keep them moving, and don't cross one leg over the other. Resting with your feet elevated to a position above the level of your heart will help circulation and ameliorate varicose veins. Raising the foot of your bed may improve circulation and reduce nighttime swelling of your legs and feet.

Walking and Your Feet

As mentioned in the box on page 210, the best exercise for your feet is walking. Naturally you can't improve your mobility if your feet hurt. Warm foot baths, gentle massage, and walking all increase the circulation of blood to the feet. Diabetics should be especially attentive to foot care since their condition may make them prone to foot sores and may lessen their ability to feel pain from a foot infection; regularly examining your feet can keep them fit for walking or other activities. Keep your feet warm and dry; if you have trouble bending down to towel-dry your feet after bathing, use a hair dryer on the coolest setting. Carefully trimming your toenails and smoothing away dead skin with a towel can help keep your feet healthy.

Tips for Healthy Feet

- Keep your feet clean and dry, especially between the toes.
- Whenever possible, let your feet get air and sun.
- Fit shoes properly so they will not rub or squeeze the feet.
- Cut toenails straight across to avoid ingrown toenails.
- Use moisturizer on your feet to prevent dry skin.

Tight shoes or socks tend to restrict circulation. Before buying your next pair of shoes, measure your foot in case your shoe size has changed. Feet tend to get wider, not longer, over time.

At night, socks can keep your feet warm. Electric blankets and heating pads may lead to burns if you have little feeling in your feet, so it's advisable to avoid them. You can stretch out cramps in your feet at night by leaning into a wall with your feet flat on the floor for a count of ten, by walking around with an exaggerated heel-to-toe motion, or by using your hands to flex your toes toward your knee.

Arthritis often occurs in the balls of the feet. Soaking your feet in warm water and Epsom salts or in a whirlpool before a walk tends to loosen the joints and make walking easier.

Resources

Opportunities for organized walking tours in America and abroad are listed in Chapter 18, "Continuing to Learn."

Measures to consider for a safe walk are discussed in Chapter 15, "Feeling Safe on the Road."

Products

Shoes, Foot Care Products, Stockings, and Panty Hose. Support Plus catalog, (800) 229-2910.

Heavy Duty Toenail Trimmer. 5-inch-long handles with a curved blade for trimming and shaping. $20. Bruce Medical Supply catalog, (800) 225-8446.

Easy Grip Manicure Scissors. They close with gentle pressure and open automatically by means of a spring. Short blade, $25. Long blade, $20. Bruce Medical Supply catalog, (800) 225-8446.

Maniquick System. Motorized manicure and pedicure system with callus smoother, cuticle trimmer, nail file, toenail smoother, and buffer. Battery-operated. $80. Support Plus catalog, (800) 229-2910.

Giant Nipper. Toenail clipper with 5½-inch-long handles and ¾-inch blade. $9. Dr. Leonard's Health Care Products catalog, (800) 785-0880.

Super Nail Scissors. Toenail scissors with long shank and 1-inch blade. $7. Dr. Leonard's Health Care Products catalog, (800) 785-0880.

Battery-Powered Nail Filer. For quicker, easier filing of fingernails or toenails. Eliminates the need to move your hand back and forth. $8. Miles Kimball catalog, (414) 231-4886.

Easy-Reach Foot Care Scissor. 6-inch-long scissors make it easier to cut your toenails. $4. Carol Wright Gifts catalog, (402) 474-4465.

Foot Shock Absorbers. Insert in your shoes to help absorb the foot strike as you walk. Can provide relief from foot pain, lower-back pain, heel spurs, shin splints, leg fatigue. One size fits all. $4. Carol Wright Gifts catalog, (402) 474-4465.

Cushioned Walking Socks. Support for instep and arch, cushion for instep, sole, and heel. $9. Campmor catalog, (800) CAMPMOR (226-7667).

Gel Insoles. Insert gel-filled insoles into shoes to cushion your feet. Washable. $17. Comfort House catalog, (800) 359-7701.

Oversized Socks. Nonconstricting socks meant for swollen feet or for use over bandages. $9. Comfort House catalog, (800) 359-7701.

Lectra-Sox. Thermal knit socks with a heating element in the toe area. Batteries provide four to five hours of heat. Heat control snaps off for hand washing. Sizes S, M, L. $18. Campmor catalog, (800) CAMPMOR (226-7667).

Ice Treads. Straps slip over your shoe or boot to position metal spikes under the sole to give you better traction on ice. For men or women, $10. Ann Morris Enterprises catalog, (516) 292-9232. Also, Miles Kimball catalog, (414) 231-4886.

Hot Pockets. Disposable hand warmers are activated by contact with the air, then are inactive when replaced in pouch. The flexible packets fit into mittens or pockets and provide a total of about twenty-four hours of use. Box of six, $6. Independent Living Aids catalog, (800) 537-2118.

Hand Warmers, Toe Warmers. One-time-use packets keep warm five to seven hours; merely press each packet and warmth is generated. Hand warmers, four pairs, $8. Toe warmers, four pairs, $10. Safety Zone catalog, (800) 999-3030.

Safe-T-Vest. Similar to vests worn by school crossing guards; a reflective stripe across the chest provides safety when walking on the road at night. $8. Independent Living Aids catalog, (800) 537-2118.

Manual Treadmill. A treadmill with computer, adjustable tension belt, side rails. Folds for storage. $200. Sears Home HealthCare catalog, (800) 326-1750.

Automatic Pedometer. Digital display shows distance covered, stores last seven walks and total miles. Can keep the tally for two walkers. $40. Sharper Image catalog, (800) 344-4444.

Videotapes

Walk-Aerobics for Seniors. A variety of aerobic walking exercises, not complicated or strenuous. The 33-minute program using four low-impact steps is equivalent to a brisk two-mile walk. $15. Collage Video Specialties catalog, (800) 433-6769.

Audiotapes

Walking Tapes. Songs from the sixties and seventies and classical music at different walking speeds. $13. Collage Video Specialties catalog, (800) 433-6769, or Fitness Wholesale catalog, (800) 537-5512.

Fit for Life Walk Series. Choose ragtime, jazz, or other music for 1 hour of instrumental walking accompaniment. Includes warm-ups and cooldowns. $10. Collage Video Specialties catalog, (800) 433-6769.

Publications

"Your Feet: An Owner's Manual," National Council on the Aging and the American Podiatric Medical Association. A general summary of foot problems and tips for foot care. $1. APMA, 9312 Old Georgetown Road, Bethesda, MD 20814, (800) FOOTCARE (366-8227).

"Foot Care and Diabetes," a bibliography from the National Diabetes Information Clearinghouse. Besides informational publications, includes sources for special shoes, some custom-made from molds of your feet, and other resources. FREE. NDIC, 1 Information Way, Bethesda, MD 20892-3560, (301) 654-3327.

Walking Medicine: The Lifetime Guide to Preventive and Therapeutic Exercisewalking Programs by Gary Yanker and Kathy Burton. Discusses walking for various health purposes. Includes comparison of walking shoes and a directory of doctors who advocate and practice walking as exercise. 1990. McGraw-Hill.

"Walking for Exercise and Pleasure," President's Council on Physical Fitness. Illustrated warm-ups and suggested walking programs. $1. Consumer Information Center, P.O. Box 100, Pueblo, CO 81002.

"Health Alert: Exercise," National Council on the Aging. Brief discussion of exercise, suggested ten-week walking program, target heart rate chart. FREE. NCOA, 409 3rd Street, SW, Washington, DC 20024, (202) 479-1200.

Walking, the Complete Guide to the Complete Exercise by Casey Meyers. Everything you need to know about walking. Argues that fast walking is more aerobic and burns more calories than jogging or running, with less danger of injury. 1992. Random House.

Organizations

National Organization of Mall Walkers. Awards given for personal distance achievements. Logbooks available for recording progress. Membership available, but not necessary to participate in award program. NOMW, P.O. Box 191, Hermann, MO 65041, (314) 486-3945.

Chapter 11

Overcoming Obstacles to Being Active

Sometimes, despite your best intentions, circumstances conspire to keep you at home and obstacles interfere with your active life. A sedentary existence might result from pain from arthritis, a sore back, or any chronic pain; problems created by incontinence; embarrassment at your need for assistance; difficulties hearing or seeing; awkward speech; or tremors.

LIVING WITH PAIN

"Pain," like "beauty," eludes simple definition. We all know what it means, yet it means something different for each of us. Whatever form it takes, pain can restrict mobility and be a deterrent to activity, but there are methods of circumventing or accommodating it to pursue an active life.

Arthritis

Although there are more than a hundred types of arthritis, most of the thirty-five million Americans who experience it would describe it generically as "painful joints."

Researchers have been frustrated in their attempts to seek a cause or cure for arthritis, which usually announces its presence with morning stiffness, joint swelling or pain, or the inability to move a joint. Most commonly it attacks the hips, knees, feet, and spine and sometimes the finger joints, the joint at the base of the thumb, and the big toe.

Arthritis Statistics

More than half of people over sixty-five will experience some symptoms of arthritis.

By age sixty-five 80 percent will have arthritis in the knee.

More than 5,400,000 Americans over seventy-five have limitations in mobility caused by arthritis.

Pain and limitation of movement are the main complaints about arthritis. Until a cure is discovered, doctors can only recommend ways of "managing" the pain and restricted movement, often with physical therapy.

Ideas for Alleviating Arthritis Pain

- Relieve pressure on the knees by walking with a cane.
- Heat may relieve pain from arthritis, so exercise in or just after a warm, not a very hot, bath, or walk in a warm pool.
- When possible, try to use the largest joints — the wrist or shoulder — rather than the smaller finger joints.
- Conserve energy by resting your joints frequently during an activity or by stopping and resuming later.
- If you get relief by sleeping with pillows under your knees but find it causes stiffness the following morning, use the pillow once in a while, not two nights in a row, and be sure to exercise the following day.
- To provide warmth at night without the weight of heavy blankets, try a down comforter or an electric blanket on a low setting.
- Many people prefer the support of a water bed to a regular mattress and box spring.
- Raising your bed one or two inches with blocks may make it easier to get out of bed.
- Control your weight to avoid extra pounds that may add stress to your leg joints and your back.

New Developments

• As a disease without a cure that affects a large number of people, arthritis attracts the attention of drug companies, quacks, medical researchers, writers, and physical therapists, each of whom has a concept about how to deal with it. Before trying anything new, check with your physician first and foremost, as well as with the Arthritis Foundation, the Food and Drug Administration, or the National Institute of Arthritis and Musculoskeletal and Skin Diseases to substantiate any claims. Some products may be harmful; others are simply a waste of money.

• New medications and treatments are being explored — for example, hyaluronic acid, a natural substance currently used to improve mobility and reduce pain in the knees of racehorses; a combination of oil derived from shark liver, garlic, and soybeans; and a cream containing capsaicin, the active ingredient in hot peppers, such as chili and cayenne.

Watch Out!

• If you take aspirin to relieve arthritis pain, keep in mind that all aspirin is the same; you may save money if you buy a generic aspirin. Check the label of any medication billed as being arthritis strength; it may simply be aspirin with caffeine or an antacid added.

• Alternative methods of dealing with arthritis pain and inflammation may be needed by people who rely on aspirin or ibuprofen for relief. For maximum effectiveness the drugs must be used continuously, but after about four weeks of use these medications can cause ulcers. The arthritis pain returns about a week after use is discontinued.

• DMSO, an industrial solvent, has been publicized as a "wonder" drug for arthritis, but for some people it may be fatal. The FDA has approved it for use only in treating a bladder disorder and, under some circumstances, for animals.

Hip and knee replacement can restore mobility to people whose joints have deteriorated severely. More than 150,000 older Americans annually receive hip replacements, a procedure that is becoming more common and refined each year. Technological advances in the type of materials used and the methods of bonding the new joint to existing bone will continue to improve the results obtained by these operations.

Resources

Products

Infralume Heat Therapy Massager. Curved handle allows you to reach all areas of your body. $30. Maxi-Aids catalog, (800) 522-6294.

Mini Vibrator. A ball, spot, or flat disk attachment for use on small muscle areas. Battery-operated. $15. AfterTherapy catalog, (800) 235-7054.

Thermal Warmers. Soft stretch laminated jersey warmers provide warmth by retaining body heat. Washable. Available in different shapes for use on back, joints, hand, $7. For spine, $10. Maxi-Aids catalog, (800) 522-6294.

Heated Mitts and Booties. Adjustable heat with a plastic liner for use with creams. Mitts, $60. Booties, $70. Solutions catalog, (800) 342-9988.

Folding Blanket Support. Keeps the weight of a blanket off the feet. $14. Enrichments catalog, (800) 323-5547.

Hot or Cold Pack. A portable, reusable pack to freeze or microwave for about half an hour of use. No leaks, pliable even when frozen to wrap and attach with Velcro. Four different shapes for different uses: multiuse wrap, neck wrap, lumbar wrap, and shoulder wrap. $35 to $60. Self Care catalog, (800) 345-3371.

Herbal Remedies. A source for herbs as medicinal remedies if your doctor approves. FREE catalog. Health Center for Better Living, 6189 Taylor Road, Naples, FL 33942, (813) 566-2611.

Videotapes

People with Arthritis Can Exercise (PACE), Arthritis Foundation. Level one offers gentle exercises for those with significant joint problems; level two is geared to those with milder joint problems. Exercises are intended to facilitate activities of daily living by improving joint flexibility, range of motion, and muscle strength. Most PACE exercises are designed to be performed in a straight-back chair. An illustrated manual describes each exercise and the area of daily life it may benefit. About 30 minutes. Each tape, $20. AF, 1800 Robert Fulton Drive, Reston, VA 22091, (800) PACE-236, (722-3236) or in Virginia call (703) 391-7896.

Feeling Good with Arthritis. Two workouts covering every joint area. Medical information from the American College of Rheumatology. 56 minutes. $20. Collage Video Specialties catalog, (800) 433-6769.

Exercise Can Beat Arthritis. Ten mini workouts, lasting 2 to 5 minutes. Includes information booklet. $25. Collage Video Specialists catalog, (800) 433-6769.

Publications

"Arthritis: Unproven Remedies," Arthritis Foundation. An evaluation of current unproved remedies for arthritis and in what ways they may be dangerous. FREE. Order through your local chapter, which you can locate by contacting AF, P.O. Box 19000, Atlanta, GA 30326, (800) 283-7800.

Exercise and Arthritis, National Institute of Arthritis and Musculoskeletal and Skin Diseases. Resource material available. FREE. NAMSIC, 1 AMS Circle, Bethesda, MD 20892-3675, (301) 495-4484.

BEST BUY. "Coping with Pain," Arthritis Foundation. Provides a variety of strategies for dealing with the pain of arthritis and instructions for several heat and cold treatments. FREE. Order through your local chapter, which you can locate by contacting AF, P.O. Box 19000, Atlanta, GA 30326, (800) 283-7800.

"Arthritis." A brochure with a brief explanation of symptoms of and some treatments for arthritis. FREE. American Academy of Orthopaedic Surgeons, 222 South Prospect Avenue, Park Ridge, IL 60068.

"Osteoarthritis," Arthritis Foundation. A brochure explaining the diagnosis, treatment, and ways of living with arthritis. FREE. Order through your local chapter, which you can locate by contacting AF, P.O. Box 19000, Atlanta, GA 30326, (800) 283-7800.

"Total Joint Replacement." A small pamphlet with explanatory diagrams and a summary of the advantages and disadvantages of replacement joints. FREE. American Academy of Orthopaedic Surgeons, 222 South Prospect Avenue, Park Ridge, IL 60068.

"Understanding Paget's Disease," National Institute of Arthritis and Musculoskeletal and Skin Diseases. FREE. Osteoporosis and Related Bone Diseases — National Resource Center, 1150 17th Street, NW, Suite 500, Washington, DC 20036, (800) 624-BONE (2663).

"Assistive Devices for People with Arthritis," ABLEDATA Fact Sheet. A list of catalogs and other publications that can help you find products you may need. FREE. National Rehabilitation Information Center, 8455 Colesville Road, Suite 935, Silver Spring, MD 20910, (800) 346-2742.

"Exercise and Your Arthritis," Arthritis Foundation. An informational brochure explaining the importance of a regular exercise program for people with arthritis. An illustrated description of nine range-of-motion exercises. FREE. Order through your local chapter, which you can locate by contacting AF, P.O. Box 19000, Atlanta, GA 30326, (800) 283-7800.

Organizations

The Paget Foundation. Information and referrals. PF, 200 Varick Street, Suite 1004, New York, NY 10014, (212) 229-1582.

National Arthritis and Musculoskeletal and Skin Diseases Information Clearinghouse. Educational material, inquiries, list of publications. NAMSIC, 1 AMS Circle, Bethesda, MD 20892-3675, (301) 495-4484.

Arthritis Foundation. Information, publications, support groups, self-help courses, water exercise programs, arthritis fitness classes, referrals to a rheumatologist. For the chapter nearest you, contact AF, P.O. Box 19000, Atlanta, GA 30326, (800) 283-7800.

Back Pain

Ironically, the main source of back pain is often the abdomen. A sedentary job and lifestyle, inadequate exercise, poor posture, poor sleeping habits, and weakened muscles, particularly abdominal muscles, are contributing factors to developing back pain. It may also be a consequence of osteoporosis or arthritis. In addition, excess weight in the abdomen exerts extra pressure on the spine, deepening the spinal curve and causing the buttocks to sway out in compensation. Ten extra pounds on the abdomen mean a hundred extra pounds of pressure on the disks of the spine.

The positions we assume during the third of our lives we spend asleep, specifically sleeping on the stomach, can exacerbate back problems.

Sleeping Positions to Alleviate Back Pain, in Order of Preference

Preferred. On your side — the fetal position. Curve the back to stretch the muscles and ligaments. Place a pillow between your knees to keep the upper hip from falling forward.

Satisfactory. On your back. Raise your knees and place your feet flat against the mattress, or place a pillow under your knees (not for people with arthritis). An adjustable bed can be positioned to support bent knees.

Least preferred. On your stomach. If you can't avoid this position, at least minimize the discomfort it may cause by placing a pillow or your arm under your abdomen to straighten your back. Bend one leg to reduce back strain.

The principal treatment for acute low back pain is a day or two of relieving pressure on the spine with rest, aspirin, and either a hot-water bottle or an ice bag. Spinal manipulation may work only in the short run and is not advisable if you have disk problems or osteoporosis. More extreme diagnostic and treatment options may not be necessary, according to a 1994 federal health panel that evaluated them. Lower back problems were found to improve without extended bed rest, prescription medication, or surgery in 90 percent of cases. In fact, more than four days of bed rest may delay recovery — by weakening muscles and bones.

Compensating for weak abdominal muscles often makes the back ache, so exercises to strengthen these muscles should bring relief. Effective exercises include modified or bent-leg sit-ups, leg lifts, and stomach curls. For maximum value these movements should be done slowly, and you should feel the tension on your abdominal muscles. To warm up for abdominal exercises, lie on your back with your legs straight. Bring one knee at a time toward your chest, and hold that position for five seconds.

Back muscles can be strengthened by using a rowing machine,

preferably one with a flywheel — a spinning wheel that provides a smoother resistance than those machines that operate with pistons. A machine with a seat that moves as you pull activates the correct muscles while putting the least stress on your back. Position the seat as far forward as possible before beginning your pull, bend forward, and hold the oars close to your chest. Then push your feet against the stirrups to move the seat backward. As the seat moves, bend your body backward at hips. Finish the stroke by pulling the oars close to your torso. First activate your feet, then your back, then your arms.

Protecting Your Back

- Walking, swimming, bicycle riding, and walking in chest-deep water are low-impact activities that can protect your back.
- Support the small of the back with a pillow or rolled-up towel when driving or sitting for extended periods. Use a low footstool and a work surface at a comfortable height.
- Lift objects with the help of your leg muscles. Bend your knees when you pick up something, and lift it with both hands as you straighten your knees.
- Don't stand in one position for long. If you must stand, shift your weight from one leg to another.
- Avoid twisting at your waist, lifting objects only when they are directly in front of you.

Resources

Items that may help you sleep comfortably are included in Chapter 17, "Getting Enough Sleep."

Products

Pillows, Massagers, Backrests, and Other Products for the Back:
Pillows for Ease, Inc., 4225 Royal Palm Avenue, Miami, FL 33140, (800) 347-1486
Sears Home Healthcare Catalog, (800) 326-1750.

Automatic Massage Pillow. Use on any area of your body for gentle massage. Battery-operated. $20. Maxi-Aids catalog, (800) 522-6294.

The Shape of Sleep. Pillows that provide back support. Mail Order Medical, 35 West Main Street, Smithtown, NY 11787, (800) 743-7176.

Comfort Foam Wedge. A pillow that can be used to raise the knees and lower legs to relax the spine. $25. Enrichments catalog, (800) 323-5547.

Obus Forme Backrest. A portable backrest that can be used at home or in the car. It is not just for the lumbar area but to rest the whole back. 22 by 17 inches. $95. Enrichments catalog, (800) 323-5547.

BackCycler with Continuous Motion. Device gently exercises the lower back by inflating and deflating at intervals to prevent discomfort or stiffness from sitting in one position while driving or in an office. Plugs into car's lighter or a wall socket. $200. Ergomedics, Inc., 15 Tigan Street, Winooski, VT 05404, (800) 959-3746.

The Flat-Back. Portable, foldable, lightweight back support. Slats covered with padded vinyl. 15 by 11 inches, 14 ounces. $20. The Flat-Back Corporation, 42 Main Street, P.O. Box 125, Bedford Hills, NY 10507, (800) 945-0699.

Comfort Curve. A lower back massager, with a remote control that permits only massage, heat and massage, or only heat. $40. Sears Home HealthCare catalog, (800) 326-1750.

Crunch-Master. A device to avoid neck, shoulder, and lower back strain when performing abdominal crunches, movements that require the simultaneous flexing of upper body and legs toward each other. It's a support cushion that you hold behind your head during sit-ups. $25. Flex Care Industries, 224 Birmingham Drive, Suite 1A2, Cardiff, CA 92007, (800) 536-FLEX (3539).

Adjustable Foot Rest. Carpeted, with a foot lever to change and lock a comfortable angle. $60. For a dealer near you, contact Ergodyne, 1410 Energy Park Drive, Suite 1, St. Paul, MN 55108, (800) 225-8238.

Videotapes

Back Pain Relief, by Dr. Art Ulene and the American Academy of Orthopedic Surgeons. Includes an instructional segment, plus 20 minutes of toning and stretching exercises. Also a seventy-two-page booklet. $20. Collage Video Specialties catalog, (800) 433-6769.

Say Goodbye to Back Pain. YMCA six-week program. 94 minutes. $40. Collage Video Specialties catalog, (800) 433-6769.

Publications

"Back Talk: Advice for Suffering Spines" by Evelyn Zamula. A lucid discussion of the anatomy of the back, various problems and treatments. FREE. FDA, Office of Public Affairs, 5600 Fishers Lane, Rockville, MD 20857.

Chronic Pain

Continuous, unrelenting pain can quickly become the focal point of your existence. Such pain affects your concentration and your appetite, interferes with proper sleep, and makes physical activity impossible. Some methods of relieving pain actually involve learning to replace thoughts of the pain with other thoughts. The goal of these methods is not to eliminate the pain but to refocus energy elsewhere. Some of these methods include psychotherapy, relaxation and meditation, hypnosis, biofeedback, behavior modification, and support groups. Other methods involve massage or physical techniques to lessen pain, including acupuncture, acupressure, and reflexology. All have worked in various cases and may be worth trying. A new division of the National Institutes of Health was established in 1992 to begin clinical studies to determine scientifically the benefits of alternative medicine. Some of these treatments may become more accepted by the medical profession if controlled studies prove their value.

The new approaches enumerated below are only a few of those being used to help the eighty-six million Americans each year who suffer severe pain and the twenty-one million people who experience more than a hundred days of pain in a year. Pain clinics, either in a hospital setting or on an outpatient basis, are organized to offer a variety of these techniques in an environment that provides the support you need to learn and use them successfully:

Flotation. The equivalent of eight hours of rest may be derived from floating for an hour in a special tank of body-temperature water in which Epsom salts have been dissolved to provide special buoyancy. Either total silence or background music can facilitate meditation, self-improvement, or problem solving.

Relaxation. Whether you adopt formal meditation, such as Zen, or use massage or another means of achieving relaxation, you may find your pain reduced. When the body tenses in the expectation of pain, the stiffness can lessen the body's ability to resist the pain. Among the techniques that have been used successfully in mind control are hypnosis and visualization.

Massage. Swedish massage stimulates the body through manipulation of the soft tissue. Shiatsu is based on the same principles as acupuncture, but gentle pressure is used instead of needles. Reflexology, a kind of foot massage, is an Asian methodology in which certain areas of the foot are thought to correspond to specific parts of the body and are manipulated accordingly.

Acupuncture and acupressure. These Asian treatments are successful for many people. The former uses needles, and the latter finger pressure, to relieve pain.

Postural adjustment. The Alexander Technique and Yoga involve achieving comfortable postural positions and mental control of the body.

Resources

Products

Mini Whirlpool. Provides a hot or cold massage or soaking to soothe muscles and joints, feet, hands, wrists, ankles, and elbows. $63. Enrichments catalog, (800) 323-5547.

Pollenex Whirlpool Spa. For the bathtub. $110. Sears Home HealthCare catalog, (800) 326-1750.

Hitachi Massager. For massage of large areas. Foam head cover and two-speed vibration. $37. AdaptAbility catalog, (800) 243-9232.

Seven-in-One Heat Massager Kit. A two-speed massager, with or without heat. $32. Sears Home HealthCare catalog, (800) 326-1750.

Electric Massage Cushion. Massager for feet, back, neck, etc. $38. Enrichments catalog, (800) 323-5547.

Kneading Fingers. This motorized portable massager has two large thumb-shaped massagers. Rather than vibrate or oscillate, it kneads rhythmically. $200. Waterloov, 210 Broad Street, Red Bank, NJ 07701, (800) 841-PAIN (7246).

Jet Stream Massage. Adjustable, pressurized water directed toward sore spots with handheld hose massages and stimulates circulation. HydroTone. $130. Innovative Health Products, P.O. Box 2868, Westport, CT 06880, (203) 227-4897.

Videotapes

Practical Yoga Videos. Three tapes for different needs. *Beginner:* step-by-step instruction in relaxation, breathing, flexibility, and strengthening postures. *Yoga Breaks:* for use when you want quick stress relief. *Therapeutic Yoga Course 1:* to relieve stiff joints or sore muscles. Each tape, $25, three for $65. Expect Miracles Productions, 515 Madison Avenue, Suite 1910, New York, NY 10022, (800) GET-YOGA (438-9642).

Publications

Books on Mind/Body Health. Also audiotapes and a newsletter to help you do what you can to be healthy. Institute for the Study of Human Knowledge Book Service, P.O. Box 176, Los Altos, CA 94023, (800) 222-4745.

The Alexander Technique by Judith Leibowitz and Bill Connington. A body awareness course that may help with pain control, as well as provide philosophical and psychological self-help and self-esteem building. Provides ways to break bad posture habits through awareness of body positioning. 1990. Harper-Collins.

Mind/Body Medicine: How to Use Your Mind for Better Health, edited by Daniel Goleman, Ph.D., and Joel Gurin. A compilation of experts' advice regarding what you can do to maintain good health. 1993. Consumer Reports Books.

Easy Does It Yoga for Older People by Alice Christensen. Illustrated, easy-to-follow exercises that can be done while sitting in a chair; standing and floor exercises too. Introduction to all aspects of Yoga, including meditation, nutrition, proper breathing. $13. American Yoga Association, 513 South Orange Avenue, Sarasota, FL 34236, (800) 226-5859, or in Sarasota call (941) 953-5859.

"Chronic Pain, Hope Through Research," National Institute of Neurological Disorders and Stroke. A comprehensive summary of causes, treatments, problems, and research developments. FREE. NINDS, Building 31, Room 8A16, NIH, Bethesda, MD 20892, (301) 496-5751.

Freedom from Chronic Pain by Norman J. Marcus, M.D., and Jean S. Arbeiter. A course of pain management that deals with physical and emotional aspects of pain. Techniques that can help you live a normal life even if you can't eliminate the cause of your pain. 1994. Simon & Schuster.

Chronic Pain Letter. A bimonthly newsletter with current research results, new treatment modes, and resources. Sample issue FREE. CPL, Old Chelsea Station, Box 1303, New York, NY 10011.

Organizations

National Chronic Pain Outreach Association. An information clearinghouse, providing publications, audio- and videotapes, newsletter, referrals to professionals and clinics, and support groups. NCPOA, 7979 Old Georgetown Road, Suite 100, Bethesda, MD 20814, (301) 652-4948.

American Chronic Pain Association. A self-help group that seeks to help members deal with pain by altering their self-images and learning coping techniques. Relaxation tapes. ACPA, P.O. Box 850, Rocklin, CA 95677, (916) 632-0922.

American Pain Society. List of pain control clinics in your area. APS, 5700 Old Orchard Road, Skokie, IL 60077, (708) 966-5595.

EMBARRASSMENT

There are times when embarrassment is a serious threat to an active life. Bladder problems, hearing deficiencies, speech or tremor difficulties, or needing a walking aid may keep you from maintaining the four elements of mobility. These conditions are not disgraceful or signs of weakness and shouldn't have priority over a rich social life, participation in activities, and being independent.

Continence

The social consequences of incontinence can be serious threats to an active life. Many people are admitted to nursing homes because of bladder problems, and most of those with such problems who remain in their own homes restrict their activities outside until they become, in effect, housebound. Since 30 percent of incontinence is temporary and about 80 percent can be cured or improved, these consequences are severe indeed and needlessly restrict life's pleasure for many.

When incontinence is untreated out of shame or ignorance, reclusiveness and inactivity can virtually eliminate social contact and reduce mobility to the point of frailty. Discarding the pleasures in life can lead to depression and loss of purpose.

Statistics on Incontinence

- At least twelve million Americans are incontinent.
- Of the people with bladder problems, 85 percent are women.
- Almost 40 percent of women over age sixty experience incontinence.
- From 15 to 30 percent of people with bladder problems live in the community.
- Half the residents of nursing homes are incontinent.

Stress incontinence, the most common type, can almost always be cured. This kind of incontinence occurs when small amounts of urine leak during exercise, while coughing or lifting, or in the course of other straining. Bladder training — urination according to a schedule — has been found to effect improvement. Pelvic floor, or Kegel, exercises, involving repeated contraction of the muscles surrounding the bladder outlet, have been found, in some studies, to be as effective as medication. Success in preventing leakage has resulted from the injecting of collagen, a component of skin, to add bulk to the tissues of the urethra.

Urge incontinence, the inability to hold urine until you reach a bathroom, and stress incontinence account for 85 percent of all incontinence cases. Some people experience overflow incontinence — the leakage of small amounts of urine when the bladder cannot empty because of blockage or the inability to contract — or functional incontinence, in which a person can't make it to the bathroom in time because of arthritis or other mobility problems.

Women experience more bladder problems than men because of the diminution of hormones after menopause, which results in the thinning and weakening of the urethral lining that should keep the bladder closed except during urination. Men's urinary problems are often due to benign prostate enlargement, which results in the constriction of the urethra.

Oddly, the most successful noninvasive cure for incontinence may be publicity. Many people fail to discuss bladder problems with their physicians because they believe the problems are an inevitable result of age or because they feel ashamed. A higher profile for incontinence is emerging in the wake of an advertising campaign by the manufacturers of adult disposable diapers and pads. A private organization is planning a public education campaign to spread the message that incontinence need not be a natural consequence of aging and is treatable in many cases.

Resources

Products

Incontinence Supplies:
Active Living catalog, (800) 522-3393
Home Delivery Incontinent Supplies Company catalog, (800) 2MY-HOME (269-4663)
Mail Order Medical Supply Catalog (800) 232-7443
Maxi-Aids catalog, (800) 522-6294
National Incontinent Supplies catalog, (800) 228-2718
Support Plus catalog, (800) 229-2910
Woodbury Products catalog, (800) 879-3427

SuperKegel Exerciser. Used by women and men to strengthen pelvic muscles to improve bladder control. A description of the exercises is included. $35. Home Health Products catalog, (800) 284-9123.

Services

Bladder Health Council and Prostate Health Council. Information on urologic diseases and disorders. Brochures available FREE. Contact the councils c/o American Foundation for Urologic Disease, 300 West Pratt Street, Suite 401, Baltimore, MD 21201, (800) 242-2383.

Audiotapes

Pelvic Muscle Exercise Training, Help for Incontinent People. Audiocassette and manual for people with mild to moderate urge and stress incontinence. 15 minutes. $7. HIP, P.O. Box 544, Union, SC 29379, (800) BLADDER (252-3337).

Publications

"Urinary Incontinence," National Institute on Aging. An "Age Page" overview, with resources. FREE. NIA Information Center, P.O. Box 8057, Gaithersburg, MD 20898, (800) 222-2225.

Staying Dry: A Practical Guide to Bladder Control by Kathryn L. Burgio and others. Provides a dietary approach, behavior modification, and exercises. 1989. Johns Hopkins University Press.

"Controlling Urinary Incontinence," National Institute on Aging Clinical Bulletin. Brief explanation of bladder training. FREE. NIA Information Center, P.O. Box 8057, Gaithersburg, MD 20898, (800) 222-2225.

Bladder Retraining. An informational brochure that describes a six-week program of bladder control. Includes a Uro-Log to keep track of your progress. $3. Help for Incontinent People, P.O. Box 544, Union, SC 29379, (800) BLADDER (252-3337).

"Urinary Incontinence in Adults: A Patient's Guide," Agency for Health Care Policy and Research. Brochure describing guidelines for treating incontinence. FREE. AHCPR Publications Clearinghouse, P.O. Box 8547, Silver Spring, MD 20907, (800) 358-9295.

"Incontinence: Everything You Wanted to Know but Were Afraid to Ask," Alliance for Aging Research. Brochure with resources and a brief discussion. FREE. AAR, 2021 K Street, NW, Suite 305, Washington, DC 20006, (202) 293-2856.

The Prostate Sourcebook by Steven Morganstern, M.D., and Allen Abrahams, Ph.D. A comprehensive discussion of the prostate gland's function, treatments for prostate problems, and related information. 1993. Lowell House.

Organizations

Simon Foundation. Information, referrals, publications. Organizes support groups, an educational program, "I Will Manage," to teach bladder scheduling, and pen pals. P.O. Box 835, Wilmette, IL 60091, (800) 237-4666.

Help for Incontinent People. Information about self-help groups, newsletter and resource guide, informative fact sheets, and a six-week, self-directed bladder-retraining program, with a continence chart included. HIP, P.O. Box 544, Union, SC 29379, (800) BLADDER (252-3337).

Sensory Needs

Hearing deficits do not physically interfere with an active life, but some people may reduce their activities because of difficulty in hearing. For example, if you have trouble hearing instructions in a swimming class or in a group aerobics session, it's hard to participate. Hearing aids may be uncomfortable to wear when you exercise, or the reception may be unpleasant because of an echo or noise in certain gymnasium types of halls. Instead of becoming sedentary, however, do your activities at home, either with a video or an audiotape.

Seek out secure areas for walking if you worry about not hearing traffic or feel confused in a crowd. Mall walking or using a treadmill in a health club or at home offers a protected environment.

If reduced vision restricts your activities, you still can find alternative ways of maintaining your mobility. For activities at home, clear an area and use an exercise mat or well-secured carpet with clearly defined borders that will help you avoid bumping into walls or furniture as you move. If you are reluctant to walk outside, seek out designated paths, running tracks, or other well-marked areas. A fenced-in area, such as a playground or tennis court, can be adapted as a walking path if you walk alongside the fence or on the painted lines.

If you keep your body strong and maintain the four elements of mobility, your feelings of security will increase. An adequate activity program can increase your balance, your overall strength, and endurance, all of which can help you compensate for vision loss.

You may be restricting your activity because of tremor or neurological problems, but you may find that activity will help you feel better.

A discussion of strategies for improving your hearing is in Chapter 3, "Keeping in Touch."

Pedestrian safety is discussed in Chapter 15, "Feeling Safe on the Road."

Advice on maximizing your vision is provided in Chapter 16, "Enhancing Your Memory and Vision."

Videotapes

Parkinson's — Get Up and Go. Exercises that can be done while seated, for balance, coordination, and body awareness in daily activities. 59 minutes. $40. Collage Video Specialties catalog, (800) 433-6769.

Multiple Sclerosis Workout Tape, New York City Chapter, National Multiple Sclerosis Society. 30 minutes of exercises that will benefit people with various neurological problems. $15. MS, 30 West 26th Street, 9th Floor, New York, NY 10010, (212) 463-7787.

Publications

"The Parkinson's Patient: What You and Your Family Should Know," National Parkinson Foundation. This brochure includes special exercises for people who have Parkinson's disease. NPF, 122 East 42nd Street, New York, NY 10017, (800) 327-4545.

Organizations

International Tremor Foundation. Information, referrals, newsletters. ITF, 833 West Washington Boulevard, Chicago, IL 60607, (312) 733-1893.

Parkinson's Disease Foundation. Supports research and provides information, counseling, and referral services. Newsletter with medical information and new findings about medication, treatment, and causes. 710 West 168th Street, New York, NY 10032, (800) 457-6676.

Parkinson's Educational Program. Information and support groups available. PEP, 3900 Birch Street, No. 105, Newport Beach, CA 92660, (800) 344-7872, or in California call (714) 250-2975.

National Parkinson Foundation, Inc. Information, referrals, educational materials, publications. NPF, 1501 Northwest 9th Avenue,

Miami, FL 33136, or 122 East 42nd Street, New York, NY 10017, (800) 327-4545.

United Parkinson Foundation. Referrals, exercises, and information. UPF, 833 West Washington Boulevard, Chicago, IL 60607, (312) 733-1893.

American Parkinson Disease Association. Information about support groups, referrals, publications, and centers for free examinations. APDA, 1250 Hylan Boulevard, Suite 4B, Staten Island, NY 10305, (800) 223-2732.

Walking Aids: If You Need One, Get One

"I resisted getting this cane until I realized I couldn't make it to the stores without it. If truth be told, I could barely make it to the kitchen without it. At first I felt apologetic, as if I really didn't need it. I thought people would feel sorry for me or think of me as elderly. Now I've gotten used to it and take it with me out of habit, like a pocketbook. I don't even think about what other people's opinions may be."

"When I really needed a walker, I got a cane. When I would have been more mobile with a wheelchair, I struggled with a walker."

Although no one is pleased about having to depend on a walker or wheelchair to get around, practical devices that allow you to be more active should be viewed with the most pragmatic attitude.

The freedom that a cane or a walker can provide should give you the incentive to use it; the security and the broadened horizon you will experience will be worth it. A walking aid relieves stress on the joints of the legs and hip and improves balance. A cane, walker, or wheelchair enhances, rather than diminishes, an active, independent life.

Canes

With a cane you can be active for longer periods each day, extending the time you can spend on your feet and the distance you can walk. A walking stick or cane is useful for balance, providing a stable point of reference, particularly if you must walk on uneven surfaces.

The correct height for a cane is the distance from the floor to your wrist when your arm is at your side. Many people find the best cane to be an adjustable metal one. A doctor or therapist can advise you about proper fit and give you guidance in learning how to use it. If you use a cane regularly, alternate canes with different grips, particularly if you have hand problems or want to avoid developing them. Try one with a forearm rest, a T-shaped handle, or a pistol grip. You may find certain canes more convenient for specific situations.

There is a knack to using a cane that involves the rhythm of your feet and the swinging forward of the cane, always held on the side opposite a weakened leg or foot. Allow plenty of time for practice after you get a cane for it to be most useful.

Walkers

A walker is a more stable cane. Rather than a single foot or four feet on one stick, a walker provides stability on both sides with four feet widely spaced for additional balance. Depending on your needs, how heavily you lean on the walker, how inconvenient it feels to pick it up and move it forward for the next step, you may be able to use a walker with wheels, similar to a grocery cart, that you can push ahead of you. Of course, a walker with wheels does not provide maximum stability.

A variety of carrying baskets or pouches are available to attach to a walker to help you to carry things. Some walkers have seats incorporated in the design, so that you can rest when you need to; some fold easily for portability.

Wheelchairs and Scooters

A wheelchair or a motorized scooter can help you move around when a cane or a walker is not enough support. The wheelchair may also be motorized or hand-operated, and both can be used indoors or outdoors. A scooter, also called a power-operated vehicle, a cart, or a three-wheeler, uses a motor powered by batteries that last about five hours. It travels from three to nine miles per hour as you sit on a seat perched on a platform with three or four wheels and a handlebar for steering.

Aside from a psychological distinction between using a wheelchair and a scooter, the scooter's greater versatility makes it more appealing to more users than a wheelchair. Many also find scooters easier to manipulate and maneuver than motorized wheelchairs. The use of scooters is growing, and more opportunities for them may be created as more buildings become accessible under the Americans with Disabilities Act.

Not surprisingly, scooters are more expensive than wheelchairs, with a basic model beginning at about a thousand dollars and going up to thirty-five hundred dollars for the largest, the ones with the longest-lasting batteries, and the most sophisticated models. Private health insurance may include coverage for some of the cost of a scooter. Purchase of a scooter by a person over age sixty-five may be covered by Medicare if he or she needs a wheelchair and cannot operate a manual wheelchair. Coverage is more likely if the scooter is called a power wheelchair.

Resources

Ideas for safe walking are offered in Chapter 15, "Feeling Safe on the Road."

Products

Canes:
   Independent Living Aids catalog, (800) 537-2118
   Maxi-Aids catalog, (800) 522-6294
   Sears Home HealthCare catalog, (800) 326-1750
Accessories for Walkers and Wheelchairs:
   AfterTherapy catalog, (800) 235-7054
   Smith & Nephew Rolyan catalog, (800) 558-8633

NextStep Rolling Walker. A four-wheel walker with a basket just above the wheels and a seat, similar to luggage carriers at airports. It folds, has two hand brakes or a one-handed brake, adjustable height. $375 to $475. NobleMotion, Inc., 5871 Centre Avenue, P.O. Box 5366, Pittsburgh, PA 15206, (800) 234-WALK (9255).

Care Covers. Synthetic sheepskin covers for walker handgrips. Attach with Velcro; machine-washable and dryable. $15 per set. Care Products, 158 North Main Street, Florida, NY 10921, (800) 446-5206.

Superwalker. Has a seat and basket, three wheels, hand brakes, and it folds. $360. Other models available, such as Roll About, which has four wheels and hand brakes, $225. For nearest dealer: Rajowalt by Temco, a Graham-Field Company, 400 Rabro Drive East, Hauppauge, NY 11788, (800) 645-8176, or in New York call (800) 632-8390.

Personal Travel Chair. Folds to the size of a briefcase, fits through fifteen-inch-wide doorways, airplane aisles, airplane bathrooms. Waterproof, not self-propelling. $550. Seatcase. For a dealer near you, contact SeatCase Inc., 6108 Dedham Lane, Austin, TX 78739, (800) 221-SEAT (7328).

Rascal. A scooter available in models with various features. Economy model, $2,500. Deluxe model, $4,600. Electric Mobility, 1 Mobility Plaza, Sewell, NJ 08080, (800) MOBILITY (662-4548).

Services

National Rehabilitation Information Center. Resource guides, directories, and referrals. Bibliographic information and abstracts available on disability and rehabilitation literature, including assistive devices, from REHABDATA. Up to one hundred citations, $10. NARIC, 8455 Colesville Road, Suite 935, Silver Spring, MD 20910, (800) 346-2742.

ABLEDATA. A national database of information on assistive technology. Includes detailed descriptions, including price, of more than eighteen thousand products. Up to twenty citations, FREE. Twenty-one to one hundred citations, $5. NARIC, 8455 Colesville Road, Suite 935, Silver Spring, MD 20910, (800) 227-0216.

Project LINK. A single source that will provide catalogs and brochures describing products for your specific needs. FREE. 515 Kimball Tower, 3435 Main Street, Buffalo, NY 14214, (800) 628-2281.

Assistive Technology Program. Information and referrals to help you find assistive devices and services for your needs. Some states have recycling services that can help you find used equipment, such as wheelchairs, ramps, closed-captioned televisions, text telephones. To locate the program that serves your area, contact RESNA Technical Assistance Project, Suite 1540, 1700 North Moore Street, Arlington, VA 22209, (703) 524-6686.

Secondhand Assistive Equipment. The following publications have classified advertisements that offer used wheelchairs and other devices for sale:

Access USA News, P.O. Box 1134, Crystal Lake, IL 60039, (800) 255-3778

Able Newspaper, P.O. Box 395, Old Bethpage, NY 11804, (516) 939-ABLE (2253)

Publications

"Walkers," American Association of Retired Persons Product Report. How to buy and use a walker. Includes manufacturers, features, and prices. FREE. AARP Publications, 601 E Street, NW, Washington, DC 20049.

"Canes, Crutches and Walkers: Product Comparison and Evaluation," REquest Rehabilitation Engineering Center. Specifications (including prices) of products for comparison, and evaluation after testing for safety and convenience. $6. 1990. National Rehabilitation Information Center, 8455 Colesville Road, Suite 935, Silver Spring, MD 20910, (800) 346-2742.

"Canes," AARP Product Report. How to fit and use a cane. Descriptions of various canes, features, and prices. FREE. AARP Publications, 601 E Street, NW, Washington, DC 20049.

"Wheelchairs," AARP Product Report. Description of different features of wheelchairs, available options, how to fit one to your body and your needs. FREE. AARP Publications, 601 E Street, NW, Washington, DC 20049.

"Scooters, Product Comparison and Evaluation," REquest Rehabilitation Engineering Center. Features of scooters, comparisons according to specific types and brands, and results of evaluations after testing. $5. 1991. National Rehabilitation Information Center, 8455 Colesville Road, Suite 935, Silver Spring, MD 20910, (800) 346-2742.

"Powered Scooters," ABLEDATA Fact Sheet. Describes features and types of scooters and lists manufacturers. FREE. National Rehabilitation Information Center, 8455 Colesville Road, Suite 935, Silver Spring, MD 20910, (800) 346-2742.

A Sense of Safety

Chapter 12

Adapting the Old Homestead

"In my lifetime I've had to get used to a lot of changes. There was the airplane, the refrigerator, the washing machine. We didn't always think these were improvements, but after a while we got used to them. I wouldn't be surprised to find newfangled inventions that make life easier than it is now; I could get used to them too."

Part of the American dream is owning one's home, as much for the continuity it represents as for the financial security it implies. Once our "roots" are established, we develop a special attachment to the place we live in. Only a small number of us want to move; according to a 1989 study of housing preference by the American Association of Retired Persons (AARP), 86 percent of people age fifty-five and older said they wanted to stay in their present home and never move.

Housing Preferences

- Nearly one third (28 percent) of older people live alone. Of these, 41 percent wanted to continue to live alone.
- Three quarters of older people prefer to live in a neigh-

- One half of older people wanted to live within a fifteen-minute walk or a half mile of a grocery, pharmacy, the doctor's office, and a hospital.
- Only 13 percent of respondents to the AARP survey wanted to move from their homes, 22 percent expected to move, but 70 percent expected to remain where they are.

SOURCE: *Understanding Senior Housing for the 1990s: An American Association of Retired Persons Survey of Consumer Preferences, Concerns, and Needs.*

The pivotal issues in deciding whether to move, apart from finances, are frequently safety and security. If your home is adapted to fit your specific physical needs and you have the means of calling for help in emergencies, then chances are you will be safe and sound and can avoid a move. Many intangibles should be weighed when you consider whether to adapt your home or move. The idea of moving away from friends, neighborhood stores, familiar surroundings, and reminders of the past may provide a strong inducement to modify your home. Adapting your home may turn out to be not only the most economical decision but also the wisest one emotionally.

Some estimates indicate that more than one million older persons nationwide need home modifications. If conditions in your home make it unsafe or inconvenient, rather than put yourself at risk, it is urgent to modify your home or to move to a residence where you will be safe.

Accidents — mainly falls and burns — are the third leading cause of death among all ages of Americans, following cancer and heart attacks. The leading cause of accidental death among older adults is automobile accidents, followed by accidents in the home. Despite these statistics, AARP learned that older Americans were more concerned with protecting themselves from crime than with safety from accidents or fire in the home.

AARP found that the following were the most common problem areas in the homes of older people:

- Stair railings and grab bars were either unstable or absent.

- Wires that could be tripped over were present.
- There was a lack of working smoke detectors.
- Loose bath mats threatened to cause a fall.
- Emergency numbers were not near the telephone.

Physical Conditions That May Lead to Home Accidents

Physical Condition	Potential Hazard
Loss of sensation in the fingers	Failure to detect errors when using switches on heating pads or toasters, which may result in fires or electrical problems
Reduced perception of pain	Breakdown in the body's alarm system for burns
Irregular sleep patterns	Napping or nodding off during the day, which may lead to inadvertently dropped cigarettes or failure to monitor cooking processes
Reduced alertness	Slower reaction time in response to emergency situations
Loss of concentration, sometimes interpreted as forgetfulness, which can occur when you attend to more than one activity at a time	Overflow of the kitchen sink as you answer the telephone
Loss of balance and physical vigor; instability because of dizziness or grogginess from sedatives, other medications, or combinations of medications	Falls when avoiding obstacles, recovering from stumbles, or climbing and descending stairs
Visual deficits caused by the eye's difficulty adjusting to different light intensities, different distances, glare, and colors	Missteps and misjudgments based on faulty perception

Other easily corrected problems include overloaded electrical outlets, poor visibility as a result of dim lighting, and outdated fixtures in the bathroom.

Falls and other accidents in the home can result from a combination of your physical condition and everyday household situations.

Our normal daily activities sometimes put us at risk for a fall: going up and down steps; reaching for items on high closet shelves; walking on unsecured area rugs, in poorly lit rooms, or where electrical cords can be tripped over; wet and slippery bathrooms (see later). Fortunately there are many low-cost ways to eliminate so many opportunities for a fall. For example, products are available to organize electrical cords and secure loose rugs to protect against tripping or slipping.

Ideally homes of the future will feature attractive design elements that facilitate living for people of all ages and all needs. These homes will incorporate "universal" design features, elements that are easy and safe for residents of all ages to use. For instance, twenty-first-century homes may include antiscald mechanisms on hot-water faucets, sprinkler systems to douse fires, doorways wide enough to

---

Falling Statistics

- More than 280,000 people fracture one of their hips each year, and 87 percent of these are 65 years old or older.
- Each year one third of people age 65 and older fall.
- A woman over age 65 has a one in five chance of breaking a hip if she falls because of the likelihood she has brittle bones (osteoporosis).

Safety Features of the Future

- Water heaters preset at 120 degrees F with a maximum temperature of 150 degrees F
- Safety designs and features incorporated into building codes, such as stair risers shortened to 7 inches from the current 8 inches and treads deepened from 9 to 11 inches; doorways widened to 32 inches rather than 26 or 29 inches
- Smoke detectors and sprinkler systems required in new home construction
- Odorants detectable by older people used in liquid propane gas

permit convenient walker and wheelchair access, rear drains on sinks to accommodate seated users, roll-in showers to simplify bathing, and other amenities that are uncommon today.

Until these items are in general use, however, your home will have to be adapted as your needs change. You may need to make alterations so that you can move easily from room to room or from level to level. If you have ever groped your way to the bathroom in the middle of the night, you know how a footstool can become an obstacle in the dark. Doorways seem the right size until you need to use a walker and have to slither through them sideways. Any one of the items mentioned in this section might make the difference between being able to remain at home and having to move elsewhere.

Altering your home to provide a safe environment does not have to be complicated or costly. Adding a light switch, fixing a doorbell, or adjusting a smoke alarm is not an expensive modification. Modern technology has created battery-operated devices and plug-in apparatus that can be installed without ripping out walls or rewiring a whole house.

A supportive home environment provides touch points always within arm's reach, be they heavy items of furniture, grab bars, or doorframes. You need to feel confident as you move about your own home, despite weakness, fatigue, or imperfect balance. Furniture can be positioned to allow unobstructed walkways within a room. Large, steady items of furniture can be contact points throughout a room. For example, a magazine rack, a hassock, a rickety telephone table, and the telephone cord all should be outside the boundaries of the walking route of a room. A sturdy armchair, sideboard, or large table can be strategically placed to offer a handhold for support.

Grab bars can be positioned wherever you need them, not just in the bathroom. An unobtrusive grab bar can be a godsend in a hallway, in an entryway, in a large room that has little furniture for that purpose. You may gain balance from touching a wall, but a flat wall can't provide support.

Small modifications often make a large difference in terms of convenience and ease of use. A rotary doorknob can be changed to a lever-action opener by replacing current doorknobs or by using an adapter. With a lever-style knob you can open the door using pressure from an elbow, an open hand, or one or two fingers. A regular rotary knob can be easier to use if you add treads or grippers that require less force to turn than a smooth-surfaced knob.

Finger and wrist strength can be maximized in turning a key in a lock if the key is inserted in a longer, larger extension, allowing you to use more than just the force of two fingers to turn it.

If double-hung windows are adapted to open with crank handles, you eliminate the exertion often necessary for sticky, resisting windows or windows you need to reach across a sink to operate.

A service dog, specially trained to assist people who have physical limitations, hearing problems, or limited energy or those who use wheelchairs, can help you at home. Dogs can be trained to retrieve objects, open doors, and operate light switches or elevator buttons. Of course, even untrained dogs can be protective escorts and a most effective home security "system."

Resources

Adaptations you can make to your home environment to enhance your hearing and programs that train dogs to alert you to household sounds are mentioned in Chapter 3, "Keeping in Touch."

Nutritional changes that may promote bone strength are mentioned in Chapter 7, "Following a Special Diet."

Suggestions for organizing your kitchen pantry and ideas for products to improve your cooking efficiency are discussed in Chapter 8, "Home Cooking."

Physical activity for keeping bones strong, strengthening leg muscles, tips for improving your balance, techniques and products to assist you in getting out of your bed or chair, and ideas for improving the quality of your home's air to enhance your breathing capacity are examined in Chapter 9, "Achieving the Four Elements of Mobility."

Financial aspects of housing are explored in Chapter 20, "Managing Your Finances."

Products

Opening Doors and Windows

Key Gripper. Slips onto a key to create a larger turning surface for better leverage. Three for $8, including a supply of super glue for installation. Adaptations catalog, (800) 688-1758.

Key Turner. An extended handlelike key holder to provide a larger grip for turning. Holder for one key, $5; for two keys, $8. AfterTherapy catalog, (800) 235-7054.

Rubber Door Knob Extension. Snaps on to create a 2½-inch lever type of handle. Two, $5. Enrichments catalog, (800) 323-5547.

Rotary to Lever Converter. Door opener attaches to a round doorknob, converting it to a lever-style opener. Beige or glow in the dark. Two for $25. AfterTherapy catalog, (800) 235-7054.

Door Knob Extender. A 3-inch steel handle fits over the doorknob. Brass finish. Two for $14. Enrichments catalog, (800) 323-5547.

Easy Grip Door Opener. A rubber grip that stretches over the knob and has star-shaped protrusions that facilitate turning. Two for $6. Support Plus catalog, (800) 229-2910.

Knobbles. A soft, cushioned gripper fits over doorknobs and faucet handles. Brown or glow-in-the-dark white. Two for $4. Independent Living Aids catalog, (800) 537-2118.

Door Knob Opener. A lever that hooks around the doorknob. It can also be used to open drawers and cabinets that have C-shaped hardware. $15. Independent Living Aids catalog, (800) 537-2118.

Push Lock Door Knob. No turning motion necessary to open door; simply push down the large button on top of the knob. Available in various finishes and colors. $45 to $85. Adaptations catalog, (800) 688-1758.

Swing Clear Hinge. Allows extra clearance to accommodate wheelchairs and walkers by swinging the door completely clear of opening. Different sizes and finishes. $12 to $30. Adaptations catalog, (800) 688-1758.

Automatic Door Closer. Replace hinge pin with this closer that swings the door closed after it has been opened. $10. Improvements catalog, (800) 642-2112.

Electrical and Telephone Cords and Plugs

Plug Puller. These plugs have two finger holes so that less effort is required for removing the plug from a wall socket. $3 for three. Easy Street catalog, (800) 959-EASY (3279).

Safety Wall Plate/Plug Ejector. A lever forces the plug out without your needing to pull on the wire or grip the plug. $3. Maxi-Aids catalog, (800) 522-6294.

Retractable Phone Cord. A 25-inch retractable cord for wall or desk mounting allows you to place the phone near you. $15.

Accessolutions catalog, (800) 445-9968.

Cord-Minder. A 16-foot cord that replaces the telephone handset cord and reels in and out as you move around. $16. Hello Direct catalog, (800) 444-3556.

Cord Control. Hides cords and wires by collecting all the cords from one outlet in a 1-inch-diameter plastic tube. Cut 6-foot length to size. $15. Safety Zone catalog, (800) 999-3030.

10-foot Cord Control Kit. Resembles a vacuum cleaner hose; holds all wires in one easily visible white cylinder. Also comes in black. $20. Hold Everything catalog, (800) 421-2264.

Flat Plug. An extension cord designed for use behind furniture, with a pull ring for removal. It converts one plug to three. Three for $20. Solutions catalog, (800) 342-9988.

Space Saver Plug. Extension cord that doubles the capacity of a two-receptacle outlet. Plugs are on the sides so that they are nearly flat to the wall. $10. Solutions catalog, (800) 342-9988.

Securing Rugs

Hug-a-Rug. A liner that keeps area rugs in place. Comes in two models: Ever-Grip deluxe and standard Hug-a-Rug. 3 by 5 feet, $20 to $25. 10 by 14 feet, $110 to $189. There is also a Hug-a-Rug for use with rugs on carpets. Solutions catalog, (800) 342-9988.

Dycem Non-Slip Netting. Trim to size to use under rugs, cushions, etc. 23½ inches wide on 6½-foot roll. $25. Enrichments catalog, (800) 323-5547.

Lok-Lift. A mesh tape that holds rugs in place. 2½-inch-wide roll, $10. 6-inch-wide roll, $16. Miles Kimball catalog, (414) 231-4886.

Pad for Rugs on Wood Floors. Underpad to keep rugs from skidding, slipping, or bunching on hard floors. 4 by 6 feet. $15. Comfort House catalog, (800) 359-7701.

Pad for Rugs on Carpets. Keeps rugs from moving when they are on carpeted surfaces. 4 by 6 feet. $25. Comfort House catalog, (800) 359-7701.

Super Grip Nonskid Spray-On Coating. Sprays onto the rug to keep it from slipping. $5. Independent Living Aids catalog, (800) 537-2118.

Services

Product Search Service. Advice on products that can solve specific mobility or safety problems. You get information on a minimum of three devices per category, $2 per product, or 50 cents per manufacturer or distributor. Institute for Technology Development, Advanced Living Systems Division, 428 North Lamar, Oxford, MS 38655, (601) 234-0158.

Accessible Housing Information Service. Information and referral for financial, architectural, or design aspects of accessible housing. Technical assistance with a specific design problem is available for a fee. Center for Accessible Housing, North Carolina State University, School of Design, P.O. Box 8613, Raleigh, NC 27695, (919) 515-3082.

Publications

A Consumer's Guide to Home Adaptation. Provides a method for determining what changes your home needs, setting priorities, and carrying out the practical aspects of construction. $10. Adaptive Environments Center, 374 Congress Street, Suite 301, Boston, MA 02210, (617) 695-1225.

"Easy Access Housing for Easier Living," by National Easter Seal Society. A room-by-room survey of ways to facilitate access in a home. FREE. NESS, 230 West Monroe, Suite 1800, Chicago, IL 60606, (800) 221-6827.

"The Doable, Renewable Home," American Association of Retired Persons. Suggestions for ways of adapting a home if you have physical limitations. FREE. AARP Publications, 601 E Street, NW, Washington, DC 20049.

"Living with Osteoporosis," National Osteoporosis Foundation. A brochure of tips for avoiding falls in the home and while you perform daily chores and activities. FREE. NOF, 1150 17th Street, NW, Suite 500, Washington, DC 20036, (202) 223-2226.

Safety Checklists

BEST BUY. "Safety for Older Consumers, Home Safety Checklist," U.S. Consumer Product Safety Commission. Room-by-room suggestions for ways to avoid falls, fires, and other accidents in the home. FREE. CPSC, 5401 Westband Avenue, Bethesda, MD 20207, (800) 638-2772.

"Home Safety Checklist for the Elderly," National Safety Council. A room-by-room inventory of safety features you can use to decide which areas in your home may need to be fixed. $1. NSC, 1121 Spring Lake Road, Itasca, IL 60143, (800) 621-7619.

"Home Eye Safety Guide," Prevent Blindness America. A series of checklists that may suggest ways of preventing eye injuries at home. FREE. PBA, 500 East Remington Road, Schaumburg, IL 60173, (800) 331-2020.

"A Safe Home Is No Accident: A Family Checklist," National Easter Seal Society and Century 21 Real Estate Corporation. Questions about home safety that will help you determine ways your home can be made more safe. FREE. NESS, 230 West Monroe, Suite 1800, Chicago, IL 60606, (800) 221-6827.

"How to Modify a Home to Accommodate the Needs of an Older Adult," Hartford House. One hundred twenty tips for adapting a home for various needs; lists of products, manufacturers, and catalogs. FREE. Hartford House, c/o The Hartford Insurance Group, Hartford Plaza, Hartford, CT 06115.

Home Safety Guide for Older People: Check It Out, Fix It Up by Jon Pynoos and Evelyn Cohen. A thorough room-by-room checklist for hazards and tips for remedying them. $14. Serif Press, 1331 H Street, NW, Suite 110, Washington, DC 20005, (202) 737-4650.

"Architectural Accessibility Resources," REquest Rehabilitation Engineering Center. List of organizations and publications with information about adapting a home for easier access. FREE. National Rehabilitation Information Center, 8455 Colesville Road, Suite 935, Silver Spring, MD 20910, (800) 346-2742.

HOME DESIGN

Steps

A flight of steps can be an insuperable obstacle and a source of danger unless you improve the lighting and update the tread covering. Stairs and steps are the fourth most common contributor to cause of death annually among persons age fifty and older. More than ninety-three thousand injuries a year among persons age sixty-five and older requiring treatment in an emergency room stem from falls on steps. Some of these falls are due to diminished depth perception, difficulty holding on to banisters, or poor balance. The greatest danger occurs when descending a flight of steps; your visual adjustment may be slow and can create a feeling of insecurity, even when you're standing still.

Most people are either right- or left-handed and right- or left-legged when it comes to going up or down steps. Either one foot or the other takes the lead, and one side or the other feels stronger. A flight of stairs can be made safer with a few small changes:

Distinguish the top and bottom steps so that you know when to start down the stairway and when you have finished. Mark the top and bottom steps with tape or a neon orange strip of tape, or position a night-light so that it illuminates the landings. You could also use a slightly different shade of carpeting on the first and last treads.

Avoid dark carpeting or patterned carpeting that makes the steps appear to blend into one another so that the entire flight of stairs seems a paisley or brown ski slope.

Install hand railings on both sides of the stairs so that your weaker side will be supported going up *and* down the steps.

Extend the railings beyond the top and bottom steps to keep a handhold until you are secure on level ground.

Position lights to bring the steps into relief, or use different shades of carpeting on the tread and riser to be able to distinguish the tread better. Light switches should be at both ends of the staircase.

Remember ideal tread and riser dimensions when you replace your porch steps or an inside staircase. Allow eleven inches for the tread, to accommodate your entire foot flat on it, and seven inches for the riser, to relieve demands on your flexibility or physical agility in stretching to the next step.

Improve lighting and safety for outside steps. Check for secure railings. Benches for seating at the bottom and top of the steps would offer a resting place and an opportunity to set down packages or pocketbook while locating the front-door key. A pebbly, non-slippery surface can be created on wooden porch steps by sprinkling a light coating of sand before the paint has dried. Rubber treads or matting will help make footing more secure.

A porch light outfitted with a motion sensor will illuminate as you approach your home, allowing you a good view of your front porch. You will be able to see the steps, any strangers, or a suspicious situation. Motion sensors can be operated by remote control so that you can activate them by telephone or from your car. Most motion-sensor light switches can be preset to turn off automatically between five minutes and thirty minutes after you go inside, and they can be programmed to operate only at night.

If you no longer feel safe navigating the stairs, an electric lift can carry you up or down seated in a chair. The lift can turn corners, cross landings, and provide the simplicity of living in a ranch house. An elevator is a more elaborate option that may become a commonplace amenity in newer homes.

Resources

Products

Stair Treads. Thirteen treads made of synthetic carpeting with foam backing to attach to steps. 7 by 22 inches, brown tweed. $12. Miles Kimball catalog, (414) 231-4886.

Rubber Stair Tread. 24 by 10¼ inches, trimmable with scissors; can be tacked or glued on; can overlap step lip. $4 each, or ten or more for $3.50 each. Vermont Country Store catalog, (802) 362-2400.

Non-Skid Safety Tape for Steps. Self-stick, black tape for secure footing or to wrap around handles or banisters for better grip. Cut to size 2 inch by 60 foot roll. $50. Independent Living Aids catalog, (800) 537-2118.

Motion Sensing Adaptor. Outside or indoor lights turn on when sensor, mounted nearby, detects someone approaching the house, $40. Brookstone catalog, (800) 926-7000.

Wireless Wall Switch. Adds a new switch without electrical wiring. Any lamp or appliance may be attached to the unit at the existing plug and the wall switch sticks onto the wall up to fifty feet away, at the other end of a staircase or even in another room. $45. Brookstone catalog, (800) 926-7000.

Stair Lifts, Elevators, and Wheelchair Lifts. Prices vary according to installation costs and choice of unit. Lifts for straight staircases,

$3,500 to $4,500; rentals available. Residential elevators, $14,000 to $17,000, plus $10,000 construction costs. Wheelchair lifts, beginning at $5,000. For a dealer near you, contact the manufacturer:

American Stair-Glide Corp., 4001 East 138th Street, Grandview, MO 64030, (800) 925-3100

Cheney, 2445 South Calhoun Road, P.O. Box 51188, New Berlin, WI 53151, (800) 568-1222

National Wheel-O-Vator Co., P.O. Box 348, Roanoke, IL 61561, (800) 551-9095

Residential Elevators. To connect two levels, about $18,000, depending on options and installation, plus additional construction costs. Otis Elevator Company, 1 Farm Springs Road, Farmington, CT 06032, (800) 441-6847.

Publications

"Stair Lifts," ABLEDATA Fact Sheet. Profiles types of lifts, specific products, and manufacturers. FREE. National Rehabilitation Information Center, 8455 Colesville Road, Suite 935, Silver Spring, MD 20910, (800) 346-2742.

"Installers and Manufacturers of Stair Lifts and Wheelchair Lifts," Information Center for Individuals with Disabilities. A list of manufacturers. Fort Point Place, 27-43 Wormwood Street, Boston, MA 02210, (617) 727-5540.

Lighting

Good indoor lighting is a source of comfort as you approach your home, a deterrent to burglars, and a boon to the eyes of people age sixty-five and older. Since pupils at that age do not dilate as widely as younger people's do, it can take six to eight times longer for the eye to respond to changes of light intensity.

The need for brighter lighting levels for mature eyes is buttressed by statistics.

Eye-Opening Facts

- At age thirty the size of the pupil begins to decrease, allowing less light to enter the eye.
- After age fifty the eye's ability to perceive fine detail is reduced and it becomes even more pronounced after age seventy.

- After age fifty-five the visual field narrows, and after age seventy-five it is markedly reduced.
- A seventy-year-old person takes three times longer to adjust to the dark than a twenty-five-year-old person.
- The eighty-year-old eye needs three times as much light to see as clearly as it did at age twenty.

Creating greater contrast in your surroundings will optimize your vision. Contrast can be increased either by using dark and light color combinations or by special attention to lighting:

Define the boundaries of the wall and the floor by using different color values. This can be an important source of orientation in a room.

Use contrasting backgrounds to make objects easier to see. A piece of white paper is easier to write on when it is lying on a dark blotter; a piece of candy is easier to pick up when it's on a contrasting plate.

Use contrasting paint to improve visibility. Doorframes (painted a darker shade than the wall), light switch plates, stair railings, doorknobs, drawer handles, dinnerware all can be more visible against contrasting backgrounds.

Consider walls and carpeting as background, and use contrasting shades on furniture. This will make items easier to locate and less likely to be tripped over.

In creating contrast, bear in mind that it is easiest to see the warmer colors — yellow, red, orange. Darker colors — blue, black, and brown — tend to be difficult to distinguish from one another, and after age seventy the green/blue/violet range of colors is hard to tell apart.

Fluorescent light diffuses evenly, throwing less shadow and diminishing contrast, and some people are disturbed by a persistent flicker fluorescent bulbs produce that can cause eye fatigue, tearing, and headaches. A bulb cover may lessen the effect of the flicker. An incandescent bulb creates more shadow and contrast, delineating the objects in a room; it's a good light source for close work. A combination of fluorescent and incandescent lighting could supply general room light and highlight a number of specific areas.

Walls painted a light color reflect additional light into a room. Of course, a higher-wattage bulb also produces more light, but you can only go as high as the maximum wattage allowed in a fixture.

Watt Facts

A twenty-year-old person needs 100 watts to see close work easily.
A forty-year-old person needs 145 watts.
A sixty-year-old person needs 230 watts.
An eighty-year-old person needs 415 watts.

On the other hand, brighter light is not always better for everyone. In some cases too much light can create glare that may make it harder to see. Each person must experiment with the lighting sources in his or her home to arrive at a practical balance. A large picture window through which a bright afternoon sun shines on polished furniture or mirrors can be regulated with a combination of shades, blinds, or drapes to control glare. Reflective surfaces tend to increase glare, whereas upholstered furniture and carpeting can reduce glare.

Some people whose vision is cloudy because of cataracts can see better with a medium level of light. Ninety-five percent of people over age sixty-five experience changes in the quality of the lenses of their eyes. A dimmer switch lets you regulate the light level in response to changing sunlight or to balance other lights in the room so that you can achieve a comfortable level of light.

You should be able to turn on your lights easily, and you should place them so that they illuminate your walking path. The small on/off lever on most light switches may be difficult to manipulate and can be replaced with a rocker switch that can be operated with gentle pressure from one finger, the side of a hand, or an elbow. Wall switches with levers that glow in the dark are easier to find in a darkened room. Arrange the lighting, or install a motion- or sound-sensitive device (one that responds when you clap your hands is available) in a lamp, so that you never have to traverse a darkened room to get to a switch. Light switches, electric outlets, keyholes, and doorknobs are easier to locate in the dark if they're marked with phosphorescent tape. A flashlight can help you see into darkened corners and the backs of drawers and closets.

You can derive a double benefit from installing a remote control system that allows you to turn lights on and off without getting out of your chair *and* provides a house with a "lived-in" look to discourage intruders. Most remote control systems can be installed using the existing wiring in your house. A lamp or appliance is plugged into a module that is plugged into a wall outlet and becomes controllable by means of a remote device that you can put anywhere or take outside with you. Though it sounds complicated, all you do is push buttons on a control similar to the one for a TV or set a timer to operate the light or appliance. Remotely controlled lights may be part of a home automation system that includes other electric appliances, protection devices, and other features.

Resources

Products

Light Bulbs, Lamps, Flashlights:
> LS&S Group catalog, (800) 468-4789, or, in Illinois, (708) 498-9777
> Lighthouse Consumer Products catalog, (800) 829-0500
> Real Goods catalog, (800) 762-7325
> Seventh Generation catalog, (800) 456-1177

Safety Marking Tape. Phosphorescent tape for making objects easy to locate at night, marking hallways, doorknobs, light switches. 1- or 2-inch widths. $11 to $20. Independent Living Aids catalog, (800) 537-2118.

Nite-Lite Phosphorescent Security Tape Shapes. Precut shapes. $4. Sense-Sations catalog, (800) 876-5456.

100-Year Nite-Lite. Two seven-watt bulbs draw only four watts of power for a soft glow when plugged in an outlet. $3. Miles Kimball catalog, (414) 231-4886.

Button Night Light. Small button-shaped light for hallways and bathrooms. Four night-lights for $9. Enrichments catalog, (800) 323-5547.

Light Sensitive Timer. Turns lights on at dusk and keeps them lit the length of time you program, from two hours to all night. $18. Solutions catalog, (800) 342-9988.

Seven Day Light Timer. You customize the on and off times for a whole week to accommodate your schedule or to create a lived-in look for your home. $20. Bruce Medical Supply catalog, (800) 225-8446.

Automatic Night Light. Automatically turns on as the room darkens, turns off in daylight. $6. Maxi-Aids. (800) 522-6294.

Mini-Mag Pocket Lite. 4 inches long, adjusts from a spotlight to a floodlight. Includes spare bulb and belt holster. $20. Visual Aids catalog, (212) 889-3141, or in the West call (415) 221-3201.

Solitare Pocket Flashlight. Adjusts from diffused to pinpoint light, stands on its own, carries replacement bulb. 3¼ inches long. $15. Visual Aids catalog, (212) 889-3141, or in the West call (415) 221-3201.

Light Switch Extension Handle. Turn on a toggle switch using an extension handle that extends 17 inches below wall plate. $12. For a distributor near you, contact Maddak, Inc., 6 Industrial Road, Pequannock, NJ 07440, (800) 443-4926.

E-Z Turn Lamp Knob. A larger grip that fits over the tiny knob on some lamps. $9. AfterTherapy catalog, (800) 235-7054.

Digital Timer. Can be programmed to turn lights or appliances on and off with multiple settings. Accessolutions catalog, (800) 445-9968.

LightMakers. A remotely controlled lighting system. Comes with a central control for up to sixteen lights or appliances and a mobile base to plug in as a receiver, $26. Power timer for up to four lights and appliances, $19. Modules for lamps, appliances, wall switches, less than $10 each. For a dealer nearest you contact Stanley Home Automation, 41700 Gardenbrook, Novi, MI 48375, (800) 521-5262.

Cordless Fluorescent Light. Self-adhesive tape for mounting, battery operated. Black or white unit. 12½ inches, $11. 6½ inches, $8. Miles Kimball catalog, (414) 231-4886.

Halogen Gooseneck Floor Lamp. Fifty-watt bulb provides three times the light of an incandescent bulb. Flexible arm allows light to be positioned where you like. Foot switch. $140. LS&S Group catalog, (800) 468-4789.

Galaxy Table Lamp. Two-hundred-watt lamp with white opal glass diffuser that eliminates glare. 20 inches high, brown with beige shade. $90. Lighthouse Consumer Products catalog, (800) 829-0500.

BriteEye Lamp. This adjustable floor lamp is said to increase contrast without glare, making it easier for some to read. Comes with a bulb that produces as much light as five bare hundred-watt lightbulbs with a life of eight thousand hours without heating up the shade. Brass pole and shade. $125. Visual Aids catalog, (212) 889-3141, or in the West call (415) 221-3201.

Light for Sight Lamp. Has a diffuser shade designed to provide better-quality light with reduced glare and eye fatigue. Up to two-hundred-watt bulb. 20 inches high. $65. Visual Aids catalog, (212) 889-3141, or in the West call (415) 221-3201.

Publications

"Aging and Vision: Making the Most of Impaired Vision," AARP and American Foundation for the Blind. Describes various causes of vision loss and suggests ways of adapting the home and other facets of life to accommodate reduced vision. FREE. AFB, 11 Penn Plaza, Suite 300, New York, NY 10001, (800) AF-BLIND (232-5463.)

Bathrooms

It may be one of the smallest rooms in the house, but the bathroom holds more potential danger per square foot than any other room. A bathroom's hard, shiny surfaces create a glare that increases the risk of falling as it interferes with your vision. A dimmer control in the bathroom may allow you to adjust the lights to help your eyes become acclimated when you go from other rooms to the brightly lit glare of the bathroom.

Problems of balance, vision, and strength are exaggerated by bathroom activities, such as getting on and off the toilet, stepping over the rim of the bathtub, and navigating shiny, wet surfaces. The single most helpful item that can make your time in the bathroom safer is a grab bar.

A grab bar combines with the strength in your upper body to help you change positions or give you a sense of security. You need some strength in your hands, wrists, and shoulders to benefit from using a grab bar. Locating the bar properly is vital to maximizing its usefulness.

Grab Bar Basics

- A vertical grab bar can be used to pull yourself up from a seated or lying down position.
- A horizontal grab bar is used to push or pull yourself up, usually from a seated position, and to help maintain your balance.
- An angled grab bar can combine both the above uses.

More Grab Bar Basics

- The bar should be long enough to provide support throughout the process of going from a seated to a standing position and vice versa.
- The bar should be installed at the point of your greatest strength, usually about the center of your body's height.
- Locate the bar on your stronger side.
- Grab on to a visitor's arm to gauge the best place to position the bar.
- Attach the grab bar to wall studs.
- In a tub/shower combination, use one grab bar for security when standing, and install a second one to assist you in sitting on the tub floor or on a bath seat.

While a towel rack is not sturdy enough to be a substitute for a grab bar, a grab bar may be used as a towel rack.

A strategically located vertical pole with handholds at different heights may provide assistance for using more than one fixture in the bathroom, depending on how closely together the handholds are placed. Separate railings or bars can be used in conjunction with the bathtub, toilet, and sink. Tub rails can be placed over the rim of the tub with strong suction cups or a vise grip at a height that provides the most security for getting in and out. A bath or shower seat can be combined with an extension that fits over the edge of the tube and allows you to swivel your legs over the side to get into or out of the tub. A bath seat is most conveniently used with a handheld shower so that you don't have to think about getting on and off the seat.

A warm bath, rather than a shower, may be part of a treatment program for arthritis or other joint or muscle conditions, and you may find that a bath lift will ease your way into and out of a bath. *Not* an electrical or battery-powered gadget, the bath lift is a special chair that uses water from the tub's faucet to gently raise and lower you in the chair from tub rim to tub floor and back again. Some bath lifts have seats that swivel toward the tub edge and then, when you activate a lever, slowly lower you so that you can take your bath.

If you prefer a shower, you can choose from a wide variety of stick-on treads and bathtub mats for secure footing. If your shower is part of your bathtub, you can ease your entry by using bath seats, bars, or railings. Try placing a chair or sturdy stool close to the edge of the tub so that you can swivel your legs one at a time over the rim. A shower stall should have adequate lighting, soap dishes within easy reach, and a curtain or an outward-opening or sliding door, in case someone needs to help you in an emergency. A roll-in shower that can accommodate walkers and wheelchairs is the ultimate for easy entry and use. Often roll-in showers include seats and shelves as part of the design. A grab bar in a shower can give you support if you feel disoriented should you get soap in your eyes or lose your balance. Without a grab bar you might instinctively reach for the water control and inadvertently adjust the water temperature to too hot or too cold.

Difficulties in getting in and out of chairs are worsened in the case of toilets. Because the usual toilet is four inches lower than most chairs, getting up becomes a particularly difficult chore. The seat can be raised with a portable plastic addition or an adjustable attached seat that adds four, five, or six inches. To figure out how many inches you need, stack some thick books on a closed toilet seat until you can easily get on and off. Special armrests that attach to the toilet can be used to boost you up and help you to sit down. Some toilet armrests can be attached to the floor or the wall or are part of the toilet seat itself. A footstool can be a help if your feet dangle above the floor when the seat is at the height you need. Be sure that the toilet paper supply is within convenient reach and not on the same wall as the toilet, requiring you to reach awkwardly to get it.

Other Safety Tips for the Bathroom

- Use a nonslip floor covering, such as wall-to-wall carpeting or vinyl; avoid a loose rug or bath mat.
- Keep a night-light always lit.
- Don't lock the door.
- Use a bath mat and tub mat of contrasting color to the bathroom floor and the tub to enhance visibility.
- Consider keeping a phone extension or cordless phone in the bathroom in case of an emergency.

Physical activity for enhancing your flexibility and strength and techniques for getting in and out of chairs are detailed in Chapter 9, "Achieving the Four Elements of Mobility."

Magnifying mirrors and cosmetics for skin care and hair care are listed in Chapter 4, "Looking Your Best."

Products

Bath Chairs, Grab Bars, and Other Bathroom Items:
Adaptations catalog, (800) 688-1758
AfterTherapy catalog, (800) 235-7054
Ann Morris catalog, (516) 292-9232
Bruce Medical Supply catalog, (800) 225-8446
Comfort House catalog, (800) 359-7701
Enrichments catalog, (800) 323-5547
Lighthouse Consumer Products catalog, (800) 829-0500
Maxi-Aids catalog, (800) 522-6294
Sears Home HealthCare catalog, (800) 326-1750
Smith & Nephew Roylan catalog, (800) 558-8633

Hand-Held Water-Saver Shower Head. Gentle or brisk spray. $24. Bruce Medical Supply catalog, (800) 225-8446.

Slip-X Safety Treads. Rubber with adhesive backing. Eight 18-inch-long treads, $8. For a distributor near you contact Maddak, Inc., 6 Industrial Road, Pequannock, NJ 07440, (800) 443-4926.

Self-Stick Pre-Cut Bathtub Treads. Vinyl, mildew-resistant treads 10 by ¾ inches. Ten, $5. Comfort House catalog, (800) 359-7701.

Tub or Shower Mat. Cushioned, waffled surface. Tub or shower, $17 each. Maxi-Aids catalog, (800) 522-6294.

Slip-X Tub Mattress. Inflatable full-length cushion with suction cups to attach to tub bottom. $11. Enrichments catalog, (800) 323-5547.

Liquid Level Monitor. Alarm goes off when water reaches desired level. Can be used to alert you when filling the bathtub or in the kitchen or near the hot-water heater as a flood alarm. $16. Lighthouse Consumer Products catalog, (800) 829-0500.

Bathtub Grab Bar. Incorporates two handholds: one inside the tub, one over the edge. Clamps onto tub rim. $45. For a distributor near you contact Maddak, Inc., 6 Industrial Road, Pequannock,

NJ 07440 (800) 443-4926.

Colored Safety Support Bar. Comes in shades that either blend with your existing tiles or contrast for better visibility. May be used near toilet, shower, or bathtub or along any wall. Various configurations available; prices range according to diameter and length. 1½-inch-diameter, 4-foot straight bar, $35, or unassembled as a kit, $25. For a dealer near you, contact Safetek International, 2850 Kirby Avenue, NE, Palm Bay, FL 32905, (407) 952-1300.

Tub Guard Bathroom Safety Rail. Rounded design with textured surface. Mounts to tub rim with clamps with rubber pads. Portable. White, blue, or beige. $50. AfterTherapy catalog, (800) 235-7054.

Two-Level Bathtub Safety Bar. A metal bar with handholds at two heights. Clamps to tub rail. $34. Independent Living Aids catalog, (800) 537-2118.

Adjustable Bath and Shower Stool. $40. Sears Home HealthCare catalog, (800) 326-1750.

Hydrocushion. Cushion fills with water and serves as a rim-high seat for entry to the tub. Water is let out of the cushion when you want to be gently lowered to tub bottom. Refill again to exit. $425. Enrichments catalog, (800) 323-5547.

Dignity Bath. A seat lift for use in a bathtub. Chair swivels and descends using water pressure, not electricity. Also may add whirlpool. $4,700 to $5,700. Electric Mobility catalog, (800) 662-4548.

Roll-In Replacement Shower. The drain lines up with a standard bathtub drain to minimize installation problems. A ramp adjusts to your floor level for barrier-free entry. $530. For a dealer near you, contact Swan Corporation, 1 City Centre, St. Louis, MO 63101, (314) 231-8148.

Combination Bath/Shower. Converts from a step-in shower to a bath by inserting a panel. You may add grab bars, water temperature valve to prevent fluctuations, handheld shower spray, seat. Basic model, $600. Ferno Healthcare, 70 Weil Way, Wilmington, OH 45177, (800) 733-7752.

Vitality Shower. Barrier-free, wheelchair-accessible acrylic shower. Folding stainless steel and plastic seat; grab bars; detachable showerhead slides to raise or lower on a 24-inch rail. Two soap dishes and a shelf. $2,400. For dealer near you, call Lasco Bathware, 3255 East Miraloma Avenue, Anaheim, CA 92806, (800) 877-2005.

J-Dream Shower System. Whirlpool shower, sixteen head-to-toe hydrojets, seat, three adjustable showerheads. Electronic control panel programs each function. $10,000. Jacuzzi Whirlpool Bath, P.O. Drawer J, 100 North Wiget Lane, Walnut Creek, CA 94596, (800) 288-4002.

Accessible Shower. Includes built-in seat, support bar, handheld showerhead. Comes unassembled. $1,200. For a dealer near you, contact Safetek International, 2850 Kirby Avenue, NE, Palm Bay, FL 32905, (407) 952-1300.

Soft Bathtub. Tub is made of spongy urethane foam with a fiberglass covering. Footing is more secure because the surface gives under your weight. Foam core also insulates and keeps the water warmer longer. Nonporous and easier to clean than a ceramic surface. Whirlpool available. Six sizes, $1,700 to $4,000. International Cushioned Products, Suite 202, 8360 Bridgeport Road, Richmond, BC V6X 3C7, Canada, (800) 882-7638.

Toilet Handrail. Not attached to the toilet, white vinyl finished steel. $15. Harriet Carter catalog, (215) 361-5151.

Toilet Guard Rail. Adjustable-height armrests, bolts to toilet. Chrome-plated steel. $35. Maxi-Aids catalog, (800) 522-6294.

Toilet Tissue Holder. Hooks onto rim of toilet bowl. $11. For a distributor near you contact Maddak, Inc., 6 Industrial Road, Pequannock, NJ 07440, (800) 443-4926.

Publications

"Grab Bars." Discusses using and buying rails and bars. FREE. Independent Living, Health and Welfare Canada, Ottawa, Ontario K1A 1B5 Canada.

Home Maintenance

A clean home may be among our highest priorities, but housecleaning chores may be among the lowest. No wonder. No arguments. Few people enjoy the process, but most of us enjoy the result. We cannot live safely, avoiding tripping or stumbling, unless we achieve a minimum standard of neatness and cleanliness by doing the laundry, taking out the garbage, and keeping things in order.

Select your housekeeping appliances with design features that make them easy to use — for example, larger knobs and push buttons and larger lettering on the controls.

Suggestions for Minimal Housekeeping

- Clean only one room a day, and spend no more than twenty minutes or half an hour doing so.
- Do only one job a day: dusting, vacuuming, ironing, laundry, and so on.
- Negotiate with a friend or relative to trade the job you hate doing the most for one he or she would rather not do.
- Inviting a friend over can provide an incentive for tidying up.

Resources

Products

Housekeeping

Home Maintenance Products:

Fuller Brush catalog, (800) 522-0499
Home Trends catalog, (716) 254-6520
Real Goods catalog, (800) 762-7325
Seventh generation catalog, (800) 456-1177.

Extension Dust Mop. Handle extends to help you reach the ceiling or other hard-to-reach places. Dust sticks to polyester fibers; shake or launder to clean. $9. Comfort House catalog, (800) 359-7701.

Lambswool Duster. Lanolin attracts dust and shakes clean. $19. Fuller Brush catalog, (800) 522-0499.

No-Bend Dustpan with Broom. The cover opens when you set the long-handled dustpan on the floor to pick up debris. $15. Comfort House catalog, (800) 359-7701.

Miracle Mop. Wrings out without bending; simply twist handle. Hands stay dry. Mop head is machine-washable. $17. Comfort House catalog, (800) 359-7701.

Bissell Floor Sweeper. Light, nonelectric, handy all-surface sweeper. $25. Enrichments catalog, (800) 323-5547.

Vacuum Extension Hose. Extend your vacuum's hose by 12 feet to avoid dragging the machine. $20. Improvements catalog, (800) 642-2112.

Laundry

Cordless Electric Iron. Six heat settings. Beeps when specified temperature is reached and shuts off automatically when not in use. Recharges in base. $150. Community Kitchens catalog, (800) 535-9901.

Rowenta Lightweight Steam Iron. Special surface on soleplate provides nonstick "glideability." $55. Atlanta Thread and Supply Company catalog, (800) 847-1001.

Iron Safety Guard. Two protective bumpers attach to your iron, preventing your free hand from accidentally touching the hot surface. $45. Lighthouse Consumer Products catalog, (800) 829-0500.

Poldar Premium Ironing Board. Large, 15″ × 48″, wire mesh surface, with padding and cover. Two-position iron rest for right- or left-handed use, electrical cord holder, leg leveling system, nonskid feet. Height adjusts up to 37 inches. $70. Atlanta Thread and Supply Company catalog, (800) 847-1001.

Foldaway Ironing Board. Can be mounted on door or on wall without tools. $40. Atlanta Thread and Supply Company catalog, (800) 847-1001.

Ironing Blanket. Can be used to iron on any flat surface instead of an ironing board. $16. Fuller Brush catalog, (800) 522-0499.

Foldaway Clothes Rack. For just-ironed items. $90. Atlanta Thread and Supply Company catalog, (800) 847-1001.

Retractable Clothesline. Five 12-foot cords extend over the bathtub or elsewhere and retract when not in use. $13. Improvements catalog, (800) 642-2112.

HOME ASSISTANCE

Sometimes a small aspect of our lives temporarily eclipses the rest: You can get to the supermarket, but it's too tiring to cook the food; you can dress yourself, but you can't reach down to tie your shoelaces. So you find yourself compromising: Rather than cook a "real" meal, you eat breakfast foods three times a day; you wear the same slip-on loafers regardless of the occasion. It's okay to make occasional accommodations, but when your health or safety is at risk, you may need to arrange for support services to continue to live in your present home.

Sometimes a special device such as a walker or a buttoning hook is sufficient to maintain your independence. Or maybe you need to find someone to help you dress or bathe safely, manage your checkbook, keep your house clean, and the like. You may be fortunate to have family members who offer to shop for you, friends who can drive you to the doctor, or other private sources of assistance. The federal government has agencies that offer these same services, often without charge. Your local agency for aging is mandated to offer services that will help you manage your daily needs at home. Transportation — to doctors' offices, the supermarket, and senior centers — is frequently provided, and the centers offer meals and social opportunities. Housekeeping and help with personal needs are also available, but they are not intended to include medical care. In general, if you don't need medical care, you don't need nursing home care. Some nursing homes even offer home care, visiting nurse services, and other options that may help you stay in your own home even when you are not perfectly well.

Home care agencies provide many services that can enable you to stay at home. The services range from live-in companions to nurses to homemakers. Volunteer agencies provide support services related to chores, shopping, and homemaking. Some communities have phone assurance programs that are comforting daily phone calls if you live alone.

A combination of home adaptations, selected personal assistance, and community programs can prolong your independent lifestyle in your home.

Resources

Sources of cooked meals and shopping services are mentioned in Chapter 8, "Home Cooking."

Supportive groups that can help you help yourself are noted in Chapter 1, "Embracing a Positive Outlook."

Services

Home Health Program. For a home health program near you, contact the National Association for Home Care, 519 C Street, NE, Washington, DC 20002, (202) 547-7424.

Calldoctor. Doctors who examine and treat you at home with a mobile office equipped to perform most services of a doctor's office. Able to do X-rays, electrocardiograms, blood tests. Currently available in Arizona, California, Florida, and Illinois; for one near you contact Calldoctor, 1355 Snell Isle Boulevard, NE, St. Petersburg, FL 33704, (800) CALLDOC (225-5362).

Publications

"A Consumer Guide to Home Health Care," National Consumers League. Describes mainly medical services, how to locate them, and what government insurance covers. $4. NCL, 1701 K Street, NW, Suite 1200, Washington, DC 20006, (202) 835-3323.

Home Care for Older People: A Consumer's Guide by Anne Werner and James Firman. Practical sources of home-based health services that can help you remain at home despite a health problem. 1994. $11. United Seniors Health Cooperative, 1331 H Street, NW, Suite 500, Washington, DC 20005, (202) 393-6222.

"Making Wise Decisions for Long-Term Care," American Association of Retired Persons. A comprehensive description of long-term care services, financial options, and a consumer checklist. FREE. AARP Publications, 601 E Street, NW, Washington, DC 20049.

BEST BUY. "Staying at Home: A Guide to Long-Term Care and Housing," American Association of Retired Persons. Description of services that can help you remain at home, where to find them, and books and organizations that refer you to them. FREE. AARP Publications, 601 E Street, NW, Washington, DC 20049.

"Community Services," American Association of Homes for the Aging. A brief description of more than a dozen services that can help you in your home. Resources for further information. FREE with SSE. AAHA, 901 E Street, NW, Suite 500, Washington, DC 20004.

Chapter 13

Choosing New Housing

If you decide that it is impossible to adapt your present home to make it safer, or if you have other reasons for moving, there are various housing alternatives that can allow you to preserve your independence in a secure environment. You want a safe place to live where you will feel secure from crime or intrusion from the outside, as well as have ready access to help in an emergency.

The most independent situation is one that offers a place to live where you provide your own services and maintenance and no one monitors your daily routine but yourself. The least independent living arrangement, and the most protected, is a nursing home where your activities are directed and monitored by others. In between these two extremes has grown a remarkable assortment of housing alternatives offering a range of services, supports, assistance, and monitoring. These housing choices are referred to as supportive or assisted living. Some estimates indicate that as many as 50 percent of nursing home residents could live in assisted living homes. In many cases a range of these housing styles is available within a single community. Assisted living allows you to retain your independence by conceding a small part of it. One eighty-five-year-old resident of a group home described it this way: "You have to give away some of your independence, knowing you're doing so for your own development. There are always things that are very small and very private, where you have to moderate your disposition in order to make the fit."

270

The term "assisted living" has been defined inconsistently as various communities mingle in the marketplace. Some services may be offered for an extra fee or may not be available at all. There are no uniformly adopted standards, so you must ascertain *exactly* what services are being provided by the community you are considering.

Most assisted living facilities fall within one of the following broad categories:

Retirement communities. These are either apartment buildings or one-family houses where one family member must be fifty-five or older. The services usually include landscaping, social activities, and athletics and often include security guards. No personal or health services are provided.

Accessory units. These are apartments created in single-family houses. The tenant may agree to provide some home maintenance as part of the rental agreement. The tenant may also serve as reassurance for the homeowner in an emergency.

Elder Cottage Housing Opportunity (ECHO). This is a prefabricated unit temporarily located on the property of a relative. This arrangement permits privacy to coexist with opportunities for supervision and companionship.

Shared housing. In this arrangement each individual has a private bedroom, but other living areas are shared by one or more persons. Benefits include privacy and independence without living alone.

Congregate housing. This option involves separate apartments with meals, housekeeping, and social activities provided. It may include medical monitoring and transportation services.

Board and care homes. Formerly called rest homes, board and care homes offer a variety of arrangements with a range of care. "Group homes," "foster homes," "adult homes," "personal care," and "domiciliary homes" are some of the terms used to describe housing for groups of people who need help with some of their personal needs but require no medical care. (These are not to be confused with room-and-board or boarding homes, where no care is provided.)

Residential care, continuing care, and life care communities. These usually include several levels of supported housing so that when a resident requires nursing care, accommodations are available within the community itself. These may be retirement/congregate/nursing home communities.

Some of these types of housing are limited by local zoning regulations and building codes, but there are indications that these restrictions are changing slowly as the need and demand for assisted living dwellings grow. ECHO housing is now permitted in 40 percent of all communities, and there are four hundred shared housing programs in forty-two states. Two major hotel chains, Hyatt and Marriott, have launched assisted care communities, adding a twenty-four-hour nursing staff and other support services to the usual hotel amenities. Estimates in 1993 had as many as forty thousand assisted living residences in America, with as many as one million residents.

As housing options expand, some communities designed for only a single style of living, such as retirement homes, have begun to diversify in order to compete. At first residents were required to make substantial nonrefundable capital investments to participate in such housing arrangements. Now there is a variety of financial options: Some are rentals; some are cooperatives; some can be purchased with a provision for the community to repurchase your unit if you want to sell in the future.

There are waiting lists for most of these housing categories, an indication not only of their popularity but of the careful advance planning that deciding on a housing change requires. One three-hundred-resident apartment facility and nursing home complex with a pool and community center, including in its entry fee a comprehensive health insurance policy and all nursing home charges, had a waiting list of six hundred people before breaking ground.

Resources

Information about full-time recreational vehicle living is available from sources listed in Chapter 18, "Continuing to Learn."

Financial aspects of housing decisions, including reverse mortgages, are considered in Chapter 20, "Managing Your Finances."

Services

Shared Housing. Provides referrals to the shared housing program in your area and answers to your queries. A self-help guide for homeowners and renters is available. National Shared Housing Resource Center, 321 East 25th Street, Baltimore, MD 21218, (410) 235-4454.

Publications

"A Consumer's Guide to Homesharing," American Association of Retired Persons and National Shared Housing Resource Center. Your answers to a series of self-questionnaires can help you decide if you would like shared housing and how you can achieve an arrangement that suits you. Also includes a model home-sharing lease. FREE. AARP Publications, 601 E Street, NW, Washington, DC 20049.

"The Continuing Care Retirement Community," American Association of Homes for the Aging. Description of services offered at continuing care retirement communities and information that can help you determine if such a community would suit your needs. FREE with SSE. AAHA, 901 E Street, NW, Suite 500, Washington, DC 20004.

List of Continuing Care Retirement Communities. Includes only those communities accredited by the Continuing Care Accreditation Commission, a voluntary evaluation. FREE with SSE. CCAC, 901 E Street, NW, Suite 500, Washington, DC 20004, (202) 783-2242.

"Assisted Living," American Association of Homes for the Aging. A brief description of services, costs, and accommodations in assisted living facilities. FREE with SSE. AAHA, 901 E Street, NW, Suite 500, Washington, DC 20004.

"Assisted Living Checklist," Assisted Living Facilities Association of America. More than fifty items to consider when selecting an assisted living residence. FREE with SSE. ALFAA, 9411 Lee Highway, Suite J, Fairfax, VA 22031, (703) 691-8100.

"Your Home, Your Choice: A Workbook for Older People and Their Families," American Association of Retired Persons and the Federal Trade Commission. A self-administered checklist of considerations that can help you determine which type of housing you should choose. The checklist stimulates thinking about your needs over the short and long terms, your priorities, your financial concerns, and whether you have considered all the important factors. Also describes services you might need if you stay at home. FREE. AARP Publications, 601 E Street, NW, Washington, DC 20049.

"Selecting Retirement Housing," American Association of Retired Persons. An overview of housing options and work sheets to help you decide on a housing situation that suits your needs. FREE. AARP Publications, 601 E Street, NW, Washington, DC 20049.

"Guide to Choosing a Nursing Home," Health Care Financing Administration, Department of Health and Human Services. Raises issues and provides resources for advance planning for entering a nursing home. Suggests how to go about selecting and visiting a nursing home. Includes a checklist to use when comparing two nursing homes. FREE. HCFA, 7500 Security Boulevard, Baltimore, MD 21244, (410) 786-3000.

Chapter 14

Preparing for Emergencies

Certain safety precautions can be as valuable for the reassurance they offer as for the actual protection they provide. Even though we don't really think there will be a fire, we buy fire insurance and smoke alarms. We lock the doors against the chance that an intruder will choose our home and try to enter by turning the door-knob.

We need to be alert to dangers we can control, such as hot-water temperature or a home that is uncomfortably cold or hot. Although our medications are intended to provide relief, we must monitor their use carefully to avoid harm caused by misusing them.

In an emergency we rely on the telephone as our lifeline to help; a remote control button can activate the phone to initiate calls for assistance when needed. Another source of personal security comes from carrying information about your medical history and your doctor's name, address, and phone number in case of a medical emergency. A first aid kit also provides a certain security for when you need immediate medical attention.

ALARMS AND ALERTS

"I just like to feel safe in my own home. Imagine how I would feel to lose all these photos and mem-orabilia of a lifetime. Sure, I worry. But even if I'm fooling myself, I double lock the doors and feel better."

"You need the peace of mind that tells you you're home and things are safe. The worst thought is that a stranger would be rummaging through my drawers."

No one likes to think about intruders in his or her home, but prevention is the key to taking control.

The Burglary Story

- Homes without electronic alarm systems are six times more likely to be burglarized.
- Burglary is the most frequent crime, usually occurring when people are away from home.
- Burglary is the most preventable crime.
- In 1990 more than three million houses and apartments were broken into.

We can make our houses look lived-in by trimming the bushes so they can't be used as "cover" and by using timers to turn on the lights every evening. We can secure the windows and doors and keep the shades drawn to keep valuables from view. When someone is at the door, you should know who it is before you open the door. Windows located near the door can help you observe callers and can be especially useful if it's difficult to hear people identify themselves through the closed door. Motion or sound detectors can activate alarms, either to alert you or to frighten strangers away.

Your electric company may offer lights that illuminate at night from the utility pole, a safety measure especially useful in rural areas.

More than 75 percent of all burglaries involve a door. Doors that have a hollow echo when you knock on them can be easily kicked in. They should be replaced with stronger solid wood or metal doors. On sliding doors, locks that are drilled into the runner are more secure than slip-on locks. For good measure, slip a metal rod or broomstick into the runner to block the sliding door from being opened.

Alarms that sound when windows or doors are opened may be

good deterrents. Another option is a loud, ferocious, angry-sounding barking dog — either real or electronic.

The most sophisticated and expensive security system triggers a call to a central monitoring service that begins a process of alerting police and neighbors that a break-in has occurred. A security system may be one element of a home automation system that allows you to program aspects of your home's environment — lighting, energy use, appliances, and virtually all electric and electronic devices — so that they can be centrally controlled.

A personal alert system is meant for people who may not hear alarms or other sounds that indicate an intruder is near. It can be configured to notify you of everyday sounds, such as the ring of the telephone, an alarm clock, or the doorbell, as well as to sound emergency alarms. These sounds can be communicated to you by a flashing light or by a pocket device that vibrates gently to get your attention when a noise or motion that you have programmed the system to detect is triggered.

Resources

Confronting hearing loss and considering strategies for enhancing communication, including telephone conversations, are discussed in Chapter 3, "Keeping in Touch."

Products

Home Security and Home Automation Systems

AT&T Security Systems. A wireless system that can incorporate protections against burglary, fire, gas leaks, floods, low heat, and carbon monoxide, as well as activation during a medical emergency. May be linked to a central monitoring service or used only with the alarm. Also controls lights inside and outside the house and has intercom and telephone capabilities. A portable remote control device can turn system on and off from a distance. $1,500 to $3,500. Monitoring service, $20 to $30 per month. For a dealer near you, contact AT&T, P.O. Box 850, Freeport, NY 11520, (800) 222-5111.

Butler-in-a-Box. A voice-activated home environmental control system. Operate the telephone — for example, a call to 911 — by voice command alone; no need to lift the receiver. Use the unit to change TV channels, control air conditioning and heating units, and operate any appliance. The system can function automatically, according to programmed instructions, or manually. Thirty-two separate timers can be set individually for up to a year or for each day. When the system detects intruders, it will ask them to identify themselves, dial an emergency number, if necessary, and turn on the lights. It can interface with an existing home security system. Includes an audiocassette and instruction manual to help you get the most benefit from the system. Basic system, $1,800. Without voice option, $1,200. Mastervoice Home Automation, c/o AVSI, 17059 El Cajon Avenue, Yorba Linda, CA 92686, (800) 628-5837.

Motion Detectors

Motion Detector. Receives notice of movement from up to 300 feet away and sounds a low beep. $60. Ann Morris Enterprises catalog, (516) 292-9232.

Wireless Driveway Sensor. Alerts you to anyone approaching the house: expected guests, mail carrier, delivery person, intruders. Motion and heat sensor is silent outside in driveway or entryway, while receiver indoors beeps. $180. Northern catalog, (800) 533-5545.

Motion-Sensing Indoor/Outdoor Lights. When motion is detected outside the house, both interior and exterior lights are lit to alert you that someone is within a 4,000-square-foot area, up to 70 feet away in a 110-degree arc. $50. Northern catalog, (800) 533-5545.

Doors

Wireless Chime. Mount ringer near front door and the chime is heard in any room where the unit is plugged in. $40. Extra receivers available for use in more than one room. $25 each. Accessolutions catalog, (800) 445-9968.

Cordless Electronic Door Chimes. Mount the button unit on the front door, and plug a chime box into an outlet in any room of the house. When the button is pressed, the chime box rings wherever it is located. Any number of extra chime boxes can be plugged in to sound the doorbell in other rooms. Button unit and one chime box, $10. Additional chime boxes, $7 each. Carol Wright Gifts catalog, (402) 474-2161.

Wide Angle Peephole. Provides a 130-degree-angle view of visitors even when you stand up to 4 feet away from the door. $25. Improvements catalog, (800) 642-2112.

Keyless Dead Bolt Lock. Dead bolt operates with a pushbutton combination you choose. $100. Safety Zone catalog, (800) 999-3030.

Portabolt. A strong, portable door bolt that gives the security of a dead bolt without permanent installation. $20. Safety Zone catalog, (800) 999-3030.

Door Jammer. Steel bar prevents a sliding or regular door from opening. Adjustable and portable. $19. Comfort House catalog, (800) 359-7701.

Sliding Door Security Bar. Electronic bar fits in the track of a sliding door and sounds an alarm when an attempt is made to open it. $14. Hanover House catalog, (717) 633-3366.

Entry Alert. No wiring required for 100-decibel alarm that sounds when the door is opened unless you shut it off with a secret code. May also be set to chime. Emergency panic button. $35. Safety Zone catalog, (800) 999-3030.

Door Chain Alarm. Alarm rings if door is opened when the chain is in place. $6. Hanover House catalog, (717) 633-3366.

Sound Sensor Door Light. Portable alarm lights when it senses the vibrations of a knock on the door or the doorknob turning. Can be adapted to light in response to the sound of a telephone or an alarm clock. $30. Maxi-Aids catalog, (800) 522-6294.

Watchdog Security Alarm. Hangs on doorknob and sets off a piercing alarm if the door is touched. $15. Enrichments catalog, (800) 323-5547.

Door Stop Security Alarm. With this doorstop in place, it is impossible to open the door. Also emits a piercing alarm to scare intruders and awaken you. May be installed permanently or used when traveling. Needs no wiring, and it flips up when it is not in use. $5. Carol Wright Gifts catalog, (402) 474-2161.

Windows

Alarm Screens. An imperceptible security circuit woven into a window screen activates an alarm if the screen is cut or removed. Available with a solar weave that allows you to see out but prevents others from seeing in. Custom-fitted on aluminum or stainless steel frames, in colors. Can be added to an existing alarm system. Average price, $80 per screen if added to an existing system; $165 if installed with a new alarm system. For dealer nearest you, contact Imperial Screen Company, 12816 South Normandy Avenue, Gardena, CA

90249, (800) 422-1957.

Wireless Window Alarm. An 85-decibel siren indicates when sliding windows or doors are being used. Three for $30. Northern catalog, (800) 533-5545.

"Dogs"

Electronic Guard Dog. Sound-activated device makes a loud, threatening, realistic barking noise to frighten away intruders. Detects sound from up to 60 feet away. Barking lasts forty-five seconds and resets automatically. Volume and sensitivity to sound can be adjusted. Plugs into a wall outlet. $25. Carol Wright Gifts catalog, (402) 474-5174.

Radar Watchdog. This unit detects moving objects through doors, walls, and glass up to 16 feet away. When someone approaches, the unit emits a loud, angry barking that gets louder and longer as the person comes closer. Sensitivity and volume are adjustable. $130. Safety Zone catalog, (800) 999-3030.

Alerting Systems

Door Knock Light. Flashes a bright light when there is knocking at the door. Attaches with Velcro to the inside of bathroom, bedroom, or hotel door. Portable. $30. Accessolutions catalog, (800) 445-9968.

Knock Sensor. Light flashes when device senses a knock at the door and shuts off after five seconds until it is activated again. $35. Silent Call Corporation, P.O. Box 868, Clarkston, MI 48347, (800) 572-5227.

Doorbell/Telephone Transmitters and Receivers. Alerting devices that activate a lamp or pocket vibrator to notify you if doorbell or telephone bell rings. Transmitter, $100. Receiver, $50. Nationwide Flashing Signal Systems, 8120 Fenton Street, Silver Spring, MD 20910, (301) 589-6671.

Silent Page II. Wrist receiver vibrates when a sound is perceived within a 100-foot range by a transmitter. $440. Additional transmitters, $160. Accessolutions catalog, (800) 445-9968.

Personal Alert System. A vibrating receiver alerts you when the doorbell, telephone, smoke detector, or any sound activates it. You wear or carry a device like a pager. Receiver, $200. Transmitters, $60 to $100. Silent Call Corporation, P.O. Box 868, Clarkston, MI 48347, (800) 572-5227.

Alertmaster. Notifies you of telephone, doorbell, or other sounds by flashing a light or vibrating your bed. Can accommodate second receivers that can be used in other rooms. Basic system, $170. Harris Communications catalog, (800) 825-6758.

Sonic Alert. A three-part personal alert system: control unit, sensor, and receiver. Sound sensors transmit signals to the control unit, which activates receivers that operate through lights, horns, or vibrators. Plug-in components are sold separately to accommodate your needs. Control unit, $330. Signalers, about $80. Receivers, about $45. Maxi-Aids catalog, (800) 522-6294, or for dealer near you, contact Sonic Alert, 1750 West Hamlin Road, Rochester Hills, MI 48309, (313) 656-3110.

Watchman Signaling System. Will alert you with a flashing lamp to doorbell, telephone, other sounds, and in-house pager. $250. Harris Communications catalog, (800) 825-6758.

Publications

"Signaling and Assistive Listening Devices for Hearing-Impaired People" by Diane Castle. Information and resources on alerting and warning devices. FREE. Alexander Graham Bell Association for the Deaf, 3417 Volta Place, NW, Washington, DC 20007, (202) 337-5220.

"Devices for Deaf and Hard of Hearing People," National Information Center on Deafness. A list of manufacturers of products that alert people who have hearing problems. NICD, Gallaudet University, 800 Florida Avenue, NE, Washington, DC 20002, (202) 651-5051.

"How to Protect Your Home," American Association of Retired Persons. A brief summary of methods of securing doors and windows. FREE. AARP Publications, 601 E Street, NW, Washington, DC 20049.

"How to Conduct a Security Survey," American Association of Retired Persons. About twenty questions that can help you discover what you need to do to make your home more secure. FREE. AARP, Criminal Justice Services, Program Department, 601 E Street, NW, Washington, DC 20049.

"Bless This House," Aetna Life and Casualty Company. A review of precautions you can take to protect against burglary of your home. FREE. Aetna, 151 Farmington Avenue, RWAC, Hartford, CT 06156, (203) 273-2843.

PROTECTING AGAINST FIRES AND OTHER HAZARDS

Eighty percent of elderly people who die in fires either have no working smoke detectors or none at all. Early warning from a smoke alarm can allow you a few extra minutes to get out of the building. To ensure that you always have a functioning alarm, change smoke alarm batteries on your birthday.

People between sixty-five and eighty years old may have a reduced ability to smell smoke, and 50 percent of those over age eighty do. People who move slowly or with walkers will benefit in an emergency from as much extra warning as possible. Smoke alarms should be in hallways with at least one on each level of a house. If it's hard to hear your alarm or its low-battery indicator, look for an alarm that has a different sound level or frequency or one that alerts you by means of a flashing light or bed vibrator.

Rules for Smoking in the House

- The main cause of fires is smoking.
- Smoking should be restricted to a designated area, preferably outside the home. If inside the home, the area should have a functioning smoke detector and not be a room where smokers would be likely to fall asleep, such as while watching TV or reading.
- Smoking hours should be restricted to a time when you are least likely to be sleepy. DO NOT SMOKE IN BED.
- Use large, stable, standing ashtrays.
- Use a lighter rather than matches, which might remain ignited inadvertently.
- Smokers should not be under the influence of either alcohol or medications.

Many fires begin in the kitchen, and a surprising number occur when a sleeve is ignited as someone reaches across a burner. Pot-holders, aprons, or dish towels also are often the kindling for kitchen fires. Special smoke detectors are available for use in the kitchen that allow for a moderate amount of smoke from cooking before they are activated.

Avoiding Kitchen Fires

- Wear clothing with sleeves that won't accidentally be ignited by a heating element. Bathrobes and nightgowns often have loose-fitting sleeves.
- Resist using a dish towel in place of a potholder.
- Monitor food frequently during the cooking process.
- Clean the stove regularly to prevent accumulating grease that might add fuel to a fire.
- Keep all combustible items far from the heating element.

Firefighters suggest that every room have two avenues of escape in case of fire, and this is particularly important in the kitchen. Buy and learn how to use a fire extinguisher, and keep a large pot lid or a cookie sheet handy to smother a fire. Baking soda and salt can also do the job, but do not use the exhaust fan, and do not use water on fires fueled by grease or electricity. You may decide to designate a window as one fire exit from your bedroom or kitchen to account for a situation in which the door is blocked by flames or smoke. A portable ladder can be hung over the windowsill and dropped down to the ground.

Special precautions may be required when you use the following:

- Portable heaters. Kerosene heaters should use only 1-K kerosene, not gasoline or any other fuel. Electric heaters should be placed three feet from wall coverings, drapes, or bedding.
- Fireplaces. Charcoal gives off invisible, odorless, and lethal carbon monoxide gas when burned in a fireplace. No fire should be unattended, and the damper must be open when hot ashes remain.
- Electric cords. Cords can become frayed and start fires if they run under carpets or dangle from overloaded outlets.
- Electric blankets. Heat builds up in a folded or rolled blanket or heating pad, causing a short or igniting bedding. Electric blankets should not be tucked in or covered.

Smoke detectors can be linked into home alarm systems to trigger automatically a call to the police or fire department. Sprinklers that function when a certain temperature is reached are designed to limit a fire to the room where it begins. About seven hundred communities now require sprinkler systems for new homes. A further protection is to purchase nonflammable or flame-retardant items, particularly nightwear, bedding, fabrics, etc. Wallpaper made of material that triggers a smoke alarm at lower than usual temperatures is available to give you more time to get out.

Preventing Scalds

It's alarming to discover that your hot-water heater is capable of producing water that can give you first-degree burns in just *one second*. Several states have passed laws prohibiting water heater settings above certain temperatures, and in order to avoid national regulation, manufacturers may decide to limit the maximums to 125 degrees or 130 degrees F.

In many homes turning on the cold water in the kitchen can suddenly siphon off the cold water in the shower, leaving the hot water on alone for a few seconds. Slower reaction time, reduced agility, and the very confinement and vulnerability normally experienced in a shower or bath make one particularly defenseless to a jet of scalding hot water. You can determine the temperature of your water by letting it run for one or two minutes and holding under the faucet a thermometer, such as a meat thermometer or any one that reaches 150 degrees F. If necessary, adjust the setting on your water heater to warm or medium. For added safety, begin a shower by letting only the hot water run for a minute or two until it reaches maximum temperature and then adding the amount of cold water you need for comfort. A protective valve can be installed to prevent water above a certain temperature from coming out of the faucet or showerhead. Confusion between the hot and cold faucets may be avoided by using two different handle designs. Indicate the direction to turn the water on or off by drawing an arrow above the faucet, using nail polish, waterproof marker, or some other easily visible sign.

Miscellaneous Alarms

If you want to be alerted to other potentially serious situations in your home, install devices that detect hazards in the air or water leaks.

Gas detectors. Place the device near the ceiling for natural gas, near the floor for propane and gasoline.

Leak detectors. These can be installed under sinks and refrigerators, near bathtubs and washing machines.

Carbon monoxide detectors. The indicator changes color or sets off an alarm in the presence of carbon monoxide gas.

Resources

Ideas for organizing your kitchen to improve accessibility of stored items are discussed in Chapter 8, "Home Cooking."

Programs that train animals to assist people with mobility or hearing problems are mentioned in Chapter 3, "Keeping in Touch."

Products

Smoke Detectors and Fire Alarms

Light Socket Smoke Detector. Device is screwed into an overhead light socket underneath the bulb and uses household current with a backup battery. It has a 95-decibel pulsating alarm, test button, and low-battery signal. $25. Independent Living Aids catalog, (800) 537-2118.

Fire Alarm. Operates without wiring or batteries; you wind it like a clock. A shrill alarm is activated at 125 degrees. When not functional (because it needs winding or was tampered with), a flag is displayed. Reusable. White or flame red. $8. Boston Firewarning, Box 73G, Cochituate, MA 01778.

Smoke Alarm. Portable, with 85-decibel horn. $10. Maxi-Aids catalog, (800) 522-6294.

Christmas Tree Fire Detectors. They look like tree ornaments but actually contain a 110-decibel alarm that sounds if the temperature rises above 113 degrees. Test alarm by placing it in the heat of a hair dryer or candle. Battery-operated. $13. Safety Zone catalog, (800) 999-3030.

Firex Smoke Alarm. Flashing safety light and 85-decibel alarm. $40. Hear-More catalog, (800) 881-HEAR (4327).

Smoke Detector with Strobe and Horn. A portable unit that can be plugged in anywhere. When smoke is detected, a high-intensity strobe light flashes and a 90-decibel horn sounds. $150. Potomac Technology catalog, (800) 433-2838.

Vibrator Smoke Alert. Mounted next to a smoke alarm, it transmits to a pillow or bed vibrator or to flash a lamp. $55. Maxi-Aids catalog, (800) 522-6294.

Portable Visual Smoke Alarm. High-intensity flashing strobe light plugs into wall outlet. $237. Hear-More catalog, (800) 881-HEAR (4327).

Portable Shake-Up Smoke Detector. Vibrator wakes you up when the smoke alarm is activated. $220. Silent Call, P.O. Box 868, Clarkston, MI 48347, (800) 572-5227.

Ladders and Other Products

Res-Q-Ladder. Hooks over windowsill and hangs down with chain sides. Two-, three-, and five-story sizes, $42, $55, $135. Miles Kimball catalog, (414) 231-4886.

Redi-Exit Escape System. A permanently attached aluminum fire escape that looks like a downspout. A release lever outside the window unfolds the device into a rigid, sturdy aluminum ladder. Available in different lengths. 18-foot ladder for a two-story house, $700 plus installation. For a dealer near you, contact Karsulyn Company, 542 Industrial Drive, Lewisberry, PA 17339, (717) 938-0256.

Automatic Range Top Fire Extinguisher. Sprays extinguishing material from beneath the range hood and turns off the power to the range when it detects flames. $500 to $600, installed, for electric or gas stoves. For nearest dealer, contact 21st Century International Fire Equipment and Services Corporation, 3249 West Story Road, Irving, TX 75038, (800) 786-2178.

Kitchen Fire Extinguisher. Dry chemical snuffs out fires. For grease and electrical fires. $13. Lighthouse Consumer Products catalog, (800) 829-0500.

All-Purpose Fire Extinguisher. Dry chemical for fires fueled by flammable liquid and wood, paper and cloth; also electrical fires. $20. Safety Zone catalog, (800) 999-3030.

Kitchen Fire Extinguisher. Designed like an aerosol can, it sprays nontoxic material to extinguish a fire. For grease, gasoline, combustibles. Not for electrical fires. $20. Improvements catalog, (800) 642-2112.

Antiscald Devices

Scaldsafe. Stops water flow when temperature reaches 114 degrees, restarts at push of a button. Faucet aerator, $7. Shower attachment,

$15. Tub spout, $25. Accent on Living catalog, (800) 787-8444.

Shower Gard. Antiscald safety valve shuts water flow to a trickle when water temperature is between 110 degrees and 120 degrees F. $23. Maxi-Aids catalog, (800) 522-6294.

Thermometer/Bath Alert. Water temperature shows in digital display and alarm lets you know when tub is filled. $18. LS&S Group catalog, (800) 468-4789.

Bath Thermometer. Registers up to 150 degrees F. In a hardwood housing. $17. For a dealer near you, contact Apothecary Products, 11531 Rupp Drive, Burnsville, MN 55337, (800) 328-2742.

Temperature Tub Mat. Nonslip tub mat with adhesive backing, incorporating a temperature indicator to guard against scalding. $15. Dr. Leonard's Health Care Products catalog, (800) 785-0880.

Miscellaneous Alarms

Water Alarm. A 70-decibel alarm sounds for up to three days when sensor detects water. Use for potential leak or to alert you when sink overflows. $15. Improvements catalog, (800) 642-2112.

Leak Detector. Battery-operated sensor on floor sets off 85-decibel alarm and warning light when it detects a small amount of water. $20. Safety Zone catalog, (800) 999-3030.

Gas Alarm. An 85-decibel alarm is activated when unit detects methane or propane gas. Plugs into outlet. $80. Safety Zone catalog, (800) 999-3030.

Carbon Monoxide Alarm. Sensor detects presence of carbon monoxide and sounds an 85-decibel alarm until gas level drops. $80. Safety Zone catalog, (800) 999-3030.

Publications

"Stopping Fires Cold! A Safety Program for Older Adults," National Safety Council. Summary of various prevention methods and what to do in case a fire should occur. $1. NSC, P.O. Box 558, Itasca, IL 60643, (800) 621-7619.

CLIMATE CONTROL

If you feel heat and cold more than you used to and you always keep an extra sweater handy, your body temperature may not be regulating itself efficiently. The old 98.6-degree F. standard for a healthy body temperature has been discarded after a new study discovered that body temperature normally fluctuates throughout the day in healthy people. Whatever your temperature is under normal conditions, if it goes below 95 degrees F. or rises as high as 105 degrees F., it is life-threatening.

The Cold

In winter, house temperature should be set at seventy degrees or higher. To save money on your heating bills, contact your heating company for ways of keeping the heat inside, but the thermometer should read between sixty-five and seventy degrees. If you can arrange it, keep one or two rooms at seventy, and stay in those rooms.

Lowering your thermostat in order to economize may put you at risk for hypothermia, a severe drop in body temperature. Hypothermia can occur in temperatures that are not extreme, between fifty and sixty-five degrees — nowhere near freezing. The temperature may even seem relatively mild to most people, especially if they are moving around. According to the National Institute on Aging, accidental hypothermia kills approximately twenty-five thousand Americans a year, almost all of them older adults. Signs of hypothermia are hard to notice in oneself since mental confusion is a principal symptom. Other symptoms include poor coordination, pale and cold skin, apathy, forgetfulness, difficulty in speaking, shallow breathing, slow heartbeat, stiff muscles, sleepiness, puffy face, trembling, and shivering. If you live alone, it's especially important to guarantee yourself proper temperatures by setting the thermostat at about seventy. If you live with others, be sure they are aware that you need their help to maintain the temperature indoors at seventy. Let your housemates read this section so that they will recognize hypothermia symptoms and know what to do. For symptoms of hypothermia, the remedy is not a hot shower. Shock can result from a too-rapid rise in temperature, so body temperature should be raised at the rate of about one degree per hour. A doctor should be consulted for appropriate treatment.

Factors That Contribute to Hypothermia

- Prescription medications that adversely affect the body's ability to generate heat
- Inability to participate in activities that would raise the body temperature
- Alcohol, which dilates the blood vessels, impairing the body's ability to conserve heat
- Poor nutrition
- Inadequate winter clothing
- Poorly insulated homes

In a cold climate choose wool clothing or synthetics, rather than cotton, for warmth. Warm, dry gloves, socks, and a good head covering are important since the cold is felt first in fingers, toes, and ears. When the temperature outside is twenty degrees Fahrenheit, more than 40 percent of the body heat you lose escapes from the head. Ski hats do a good job of covering the ears and can be pulled down to cover the neck and face. A ski mask — a knitted hood that covers the entire head with openings for eyes, nose, and mouth — can keep the head warm efficiently.

Another item of clothing borrowed from skiers and other winter sports enthusiasts is underwear made of polypropylene, a very lightweight material worn next to the skin that wicks away sweat and keeps you dry and warm. Mittens insulated with down are lightweight and keep you warm under the same principle as that of a down comforter: by trapping heat generated by your own body. If your hands or feet feel cold, soak them in warm water and wear socks to bed.

If you can't get warm at night, use extra blankets, a down quilt, or an electric blanket, or sleep in a sweater, sweatpants, or other warm clothes. Your bedroom will feel warmer if you raise the humidity with a pan of water near the radiator.

In winter, eating and drinking well, especially hot meals and warm drinks, is important. In addition, check with your doctor about whether your medications make you more susceptible to the cold.

If finances are your motivation for keeping home temperatures low, some heating companies offer discounts and special consideration for customers over age sixty.

When heat builds in the body faster than it can be cooled either by air conditioning or perspiration, hyperthermia can occur. If such a condition persists, heat exhaustion — weakness, dizziness, mild confusion, but no real change in body temperature — results. This can lead to heat stroke, a medical emergency in which the body temperature climbs to over 104 degrees and the person exhibits disoriented behavior and has a rapid pulse. Perspiration usually provides a cooling effect as it evaporates on the skin, but when the humidity is high or if the sweating mechanism doesn't work effectively, heat can build in the body. If the body's temperature reaches about 105 degrees, the enzymes that regulate metabolism stop working normally.

How to Keep Cool If You Don't Have Air Conditioning

- Drink at least one *gallon* of liquid a day, unless of course a physician does not permit you to do so. Avoid alcoholic drinks, which act as a diuretic.
- Use a fan, either electric or paper, to move the air around.
- Take frequent cool baths or showers.
- Wear a hat and lightweight, light-colored, loose clothing.
- Drink cool water, which works more effectively than ice water to keep your temperature down.
- Between noon and 4:00 P.M., the hottest part of the day, avoid activity and spend as much time in air-conditioned places as possible.
- Do a minimum of cooking, and don't eat hot, heavy, spicy foods.

Resources

Products

Oversize Non-Compression Socks. These all-cotton, nonallergenic socks are sized to accommodate swollen feet. White. Small, medium, large, $6. Maxi-Aids catalog, (800) 522-6294.

Lava Buns. A cushion that keeps your seat warm (or cool) for up to eight hours. Intended originally for use in the bleachers at sports events. Microwave for five minutes just before leaving home, or cool in the refrigerator during hot weather. $30. Sharper Image catalog, (800) 344-4444.

Footwarmer. An electric heat mat that radiates heat from the floor up to keep feet and legs warm. Heavy-duty rubber. $45. Carpeted version also available, $60. Indus-Tool, 300 North Elizabeth Street, Chicago, IL 60607, (800) 662-5021.

Kool Kollar. A terry cloth collar with a built-in ice compartment for use around your neck. Not only does it keep the neck cool, but it lowers body temperature by cooling the blood as it travels to and from the brain. For use during activity or just to keep cool. $10. Aerobics and Fitness Association of America, 15250 Ventura Boulevard, Suite 200, Sherman Oaks, CA 91403, (800) 446-AFAA (2322).

Insulated Socks. These socks have a polyester lining in a quilted acetate shell and can be used as socks, boot liners, and slippers or to sleep in. Small, medium, or large. $4. Carol Wright Gifts catalog, (402) 474-4465.

Ear Pops. Fleece earmuffs without a connecting band. Sized to fit small, medium, or large ears. One pair, $8. Solutions catalog, (800) 342-9988.

Cool Bandanna. Soak in cool water and scarf will retain coolness to assist in lowering body temperature. Tie around joints for a cold pack. $8. Bruce Medical Supply catalog, (800) 225-8446.

Publications

"Hyperthermia: A Hot Weather Hazard for Older People," National Institute on Aging. Describes the danger signs of heat stroke, how to avoid it, and what to do if someone you know gets heat stroke. FREE. NIA Information Center, P.O. Box 8057, Gaithersburg, MD 20898, (800) 222-2225.

"Accidental Hypothermia: The Cold Can Be Trouble for Older People," National Institute on Aging. Cautions regarding hypothermia. FREE. NIA Information Center, P.O. Box 8057, Gaithersburg, MD 20898, (800) 222-2225.

USING MEDICATIONS PROPERLY

Although medications prescribed for you by a doctor are intended to make you feel better, they sometimes cause unpleasant side effects. They may, for example, lead to mental confusion, physical weakness, or other serious consequences, especially if you are taking more than one. It's important to monitor your medications to avoid taking too much (an overdose) or using drugs that cause adverse reactions when taken together or with alcohol.

To be sure you avoid mistakes, be scrupulously organized about fulfilling your medication schedule, especially if you must keep track of several dosages and requirements. A daily chart or medication memo can be a useful reminder.

Devices such as small alarm clocks or timers attached to pill bottle caps or incorporated into pillboxes also may serve as reminders. These will alert you when it's time to take your next dose. One device gives you a message on a small computer screen, naming the medication you need and how much to take, as well as keeps a record of doses you take or miss. Some medicine labels come with a series of scratch-off dots to indicate how many doses you have taken. A bedside clock, pillbox, and alarm combination includes a printer for keeping a record of the time and date of doses taken or missed. You can select from a large assortment of plastic, compartmentalized pill holders for a daily or weekly supply. The depressions in an egg carton can be adapted for a twelve-hour or weekly allotment of pills.

Some container reminder systems are not efficient if the medications are liquid or must be kept under refrigeration. An assortment of pills of different colors and sizes all collected in one daily box may create confusion even if an alarm alerts you to take a pill. If you find it easier, keep your medications in their original containers with the original labels and maintain a daily written diary of your pills.

When prescribing medications, a doctor may rattle off the dosage information and any precautions quickly while scribbling the prescription. Though a pharmacist often gives more explicit information when he or she gives you the medication, your doctor is responsible for answering the following questions for you, as recommended by the National Council on Patient Information and Education.

Some pharmacists maintain computer databases to monitor your medications so that they can alert you to problems that can occur if you combine certain medications, but drug interactions are an issue best raised with your doctor. When you visit the doctor, bring a medication memo — a list of all medications you presently take and their dosages — so that he or she can see what medications another physician may have prescribed for you and assess their interactions with new medications.

Be sure to ask your doctor under what circumstances you should contact him or her and when you should stop taking the medicine. People over age sixty-five are considerably disadvantaged by the lack of research on the effects of medicines on that age-group. Despite the fact that the over-sixty-five segment of the population consumes more than 30 percent of prescription medicines and 40 percent of nonprescription medicines, it is excluded from premarket testing. Slower metabolic rates may cause a medication to build up to toxic levels within the body of a person over sixty-five. The liver may be slower to break down medications, intestines less effective in absorbing, and kidneys up to 50 percent less efficient in excreting chemicals. Doses that suit younger people may cause adverse reactions in people over sixty-five.

Side effects from medications may assert themselves slowly so that it may be difficult to draw a connection between increasing sleepiness, for example, and a new medication that you began taking a week or so earlier. Many side effects are symptoms you may not associate with a medication at all: memory loss, confusion, and behavior or personality changes.

Ask Your Doctor About Your Medications

- What is the name of the medication and what is it expected to do?
- How often, how much, and when should it be taken, and for how long?
- What food, activity, or other medication should be avoided while taking it?
- Are there any side effects?
- Is there any written information about the medication?

Many over-the-counter medicines also can cause problems when used without a doctor's supervision, especially if they are added to an assortment of other medications already prescribed by your doctor.

Paying for medications is the largest out-of-pocket expense for three quarters of Americans age sixty-five and older. Sixty percent have no insurance to cover these costs. Some states may have special programs to subsidize medications for people over sixty-five, and some pharmacies offer special discounts to attract the over-sixty-five market. Your doctor may be able to recommend a less expensive generic substitute for your medication and tell you how it may differ from the name-brand version. Because generics are not identical to brand-name medicines, do not switch to generic brands without checking with your doctor. Medicare currently doesn't cover medicines.

When you go for an annual medical checkup, take a moment to empty your medicine chest of old or unused medicines. Flush old medications down the toilet. Check the expiration dates — using a magnifying glass if you need one — and bring with you to your doctor the ones you decide to keep so that you will be sure exactly which medications you should continue to take and which might cause problems when taken together.

Discard Medications If . . .

. . . you haven't used them in more than a year.

. . . you don't remember what they are for.

. . . the expiration date has passed.

. . . you are cured of the condition for which the medication was prescribed.

. . . the color or smell of the medication has changed.

. . . labels or package instructions are missing.

The bathroom is not the ideal place for storage of medicine since it frequently is hot and steamy, conditions that may cause some medications to deteriorate. A dry, cool place, even if it seems less convenient, is usually best for retaining the efficacy of most medications. As a compromise, consider keeping only a week's supply in the bathroom medicine cabinet and the rest in a linen closet or other storage until needed. Always ask your pharmacist to put an expiration date on the label, and be particularly alert to it if you plan to purchase a several months' supply.

New Developments

* The Food and Drug Administration is evaluating a plastic device, similar to a watch, that can propel medicine through the skin according to a preset schedule and dosage.
* Some medications are available now in patch form, a Band-Aid-like device that provides medication directly through the skin.
* For those who have trouble swallowing pills, one researcher is working on a pill that turns to liquid after three or four seconds in the mouth.
* An effort is being made to require that labels on all medications be in print that is easy for everyone to read.
* Some pharmacies are providing lids for prescription medicines that incorporate a window that displays the day of the week and the number of doses taken so far that day.
* A triple-function gadget may be soon available to use to pry open bottles with match-up-the-arrows-style caps, break the protective inner seal, and pull out the cotton.

Resources

A choice of timers you can use as medication reminders is available in Chapter 8, "Home Cooking."

Some issues relating to medical care costs and medical insurance are discussed in Chapter 21, "Planning Your Health Care."

Products

Drink-A-Pill Cup. The pill rests on a shelf in the cup and flows into the mouth as you drink the liquid. $1. Lighthouse Consumer Products catalog, (800) 829-0500.

Pill Bottle Opener. Unscrews, pries, and flips open even childproof caps. $2. Comfort House catalog, (800) 359-7701.

Timers/Reminders/Organizers

Medi-Dot. Labels to attach to pill containers with dots that can be rubbed off to keep track of each dose as it is taken. This may help you avoid missed doses or mistaken overdoses. $2. For a dealer near you, contact Apothecary Products, 11531 Rupp Drive, Burnsville, MN 55337, (800) 328-2742.

Pill Reminder. Alarm alert indicator for four pill times a day, plus a pill storage compartment. $45. Maxi-Aids catalog, (800) 522-6294.

Pill-Alert. Alarm beeps to remind you to take pill. $10. LS&S Group catalog, (800) 468-4789.

Medicine Reminder. Alarm can be set for thirty-one different times. Small enough to fit in a pocket. $15. Maxi-Aids catalog, (800) 522-6294.

Seven-Day Pill Reminder. Divided into seven compartments, each with a transparent door. Choose from three sizes depending on the size of your pills and how many you need each day. Three small for $3. Two medium for $5. One large for $3. Miles Kimball catalog, (414) 231-4886.

Weekly Pill Organizer. Seven compartments in one 5½-inch-long container. $1. Independent Living Aids catalog, (800) 537-2118.

Pillbox and Timer. Buzzing alarm lasts for about one minute. Press reset button for next time interval. Holds pills too. $11. Independent Living Aids catalog, (800) 537-2118.

Reminder Pillbox. Round box with alarm. $8. Lighthouse Consumer Products catalog, (800) 829-0500.

Medicine Chest Reminder. A tray holds seven removable four-compartment pill holders labeled "morn, noon, eve, bed." $7. Miles Kimball catalog, (414) 231-4886.

Programmable Pill Reminder. Beeps ten and five minutes before next dose alarm, resets automatically. Two compartments for pill storage. $10. Sears Home HealthCare catalog, (800) 326-1750.

Medication Reminder System. A pocket-size container houses a digital timepiece that keeps track of your medication schedules. It beeps when you are due for medication $15. Bruce Medical Supply catalog, (800) 225-8446.

Automated Medication Dispenser. One week of medication and vitamins organized and dispensed according to your schedule. When the pills are dispensed into a removable drawer, a buzzer sounds until they are removed and the drawer is replaced. $800. CompuMed, 1 Pitchfork Road, Meeteetse, WY 82433, (800) 722-4417.

Medicine Memos

Personal Health Planner. A booklet that provides a central place for recording medications, appointments, medical history, allergies, etc. $5. Harvard Medical School Health Publications Group, 164 Longwood Avenue, Boston, MA 02115, (617) 432-3939.

Health Journal. A record-keeping booklet for medications, with space for insurance numbers, blood type, etc. FREE. Pennsylvania Department of Aging, 231 State Street, Harrisburg, PA 17101.

Medication Passport. A passport-size booklet in a plastic envelope for recording your medical information. Includes space to list your medications, allergies, blood pressure, doctor's name, etc. $5. Informative Amenities, P.O. Box 1280, Santa Monica, CA 90406, (800) 553-3886, or in California call (310) 394-6992.

Personal Health Journal. Medical history, medications, allergies, vaccinations, and more can be listed in this pocket-size booklet. $5. Bruce Medical Supply catalog, (800) 225-8446.

Don't Forget Your Medicines When You Travel. Wallet card to record your medications. FREE. Council on Family Health, 225 Park Avenue South, Suite 1700, New York, NY 10003, (212) 598-3617.

Personal Medication Record. Space for listing medications, medical conditions, doctors' names. Convenient for pocket, purse, or first aid kit. FREE with SSE. Elder-Health, University of Maryland, School of Pharmacy, 20 North Pine Street, Baltimore, MD 21201.

Mail-Order Pharmacies

AARP Pharmacy Service. House brands and name brands of drugstore items and prescriptions filled by mail. 500 Montgomery Street, Alexandria, VA 22314, (800) 456-2277.

America's Pharmacy. Call for prices for prescription medications. P.O. Box 10490, Des Moines, IA 50306, (800) 247-1003.

Action Mail Order Drug Company. Prescriptions, especially generics, and vitamins and health care products. P.O. Box 787, Waterville, ME 04903, (800) 452-1976.

Genovese Home Delivery. Order prescriptions or other drugstore items by phone. Catalog available. (800) 544-4554.

Non-Prescription Health Care Items. Generic vitamins and minerals. Health care products and cosmetics also. Star Professional Pharmaceuticals, 1500 New Horizons Boulevard, Amityville, NY 11701, (800) 274-6400.

List of Discount Pharmacies. Most of these offer mail-order service. FREE with SSE. Parkinson Disease Foundation, 650 West 168th Street, New York, NY 10032, (800) 457-6676.

Services

Ask the Pharmacist. A registered pharmacist provides information about medications around the clock. $1.95 per minute. (900) 4200-ASK (420-0275).

National Council on Alcoholism and Drug Dependence. A referral service in case you are concerned about alcoholism or other drug addiction. NCADD, 12 West 21st Street, New York, NY 10010, (800) NCA-CALL (622-2255).

Publications

"Safe Use of Medicines by Older People," National Institute on Aging. Advice on taking medications safely. FREE. Age Page, NIA Information Center, P.O. Box 8057, Gaithersburg, MD 20898, (800) 222-2225.

"What's Really Inside Those Pills, and Why It May Make a Difference!," Elder-Health. A brochure discussing tablets and capsules and what to do if you have trouble swallowing them. FREE with SSE. Elder-Health, University of Maryland, School of Pharmacy, 20 North Pine Street, Baltimore, MD 21201.

"Consumers Guide to Prescription Medicines," Pharmaceutical Manufacturers Association. General information regarding medication storage, communicating with your doctor, and other issues. FREE. PMA, 110 15th Street, NW, Washington, DC 20005, (202) 835-3450.

"Food and Drug Interactions," National Consumers League. Describes classes of drugs and common brand names and how they may interact with certain foods. $1. NCL, 1701 K Street, NW, Suite 1200, Washington, DC 20006, (202) 835-3323.

"Health Alert: Over-the-Counter Drugs," National Center for Health Promotion and Aging. A fact sheet and self-test about storing and using medication safely. FREE. National Council on the Aging, 409 3rd Street, SW, Washington, DC 20024, (202) 479-1200.

BEST BUY. "Using Your Medicines Wisely: A Guide for the Elderly," National Institute on Drug Abuse. Suggestions for maintaining a medication schedule. Includes a pocket-size "Passport to Good

298

Health Care," in which you can record your medical condition and which medications you take in case of emergency. FREE. National Clearinghouse for Alcohol and Drug Information, P.O. Box 2345, Rockville, MD 20847, (800) 729-6686.

"Alcohol, Drugs, and Seniors: What You Should Know." A chart that describes the consequences of mixing alcohol and specific medications. Bergen County Council on Alcoholism and Drug Abuse, P.O. Box 626, Paramus, NJ 07653, (201) 261-2183.

"Medicines and You: A Guide for Older Americans," Council on Family Health. Tips on medicine-related concerns. Chart is provided for you to list your medications. FREE. CFH, 225 Park Avenue South, Suite 1700, New York, NY 10003, (212) 598-3617.

Prescription Drug Handbook, AARP Pharmacy Service. A guide to medicines most frequently prescribed for persons age fifty and older. One thousand entries describing side effects, combinations of medications that may be harmful, a chart with illustrations to help you identify drugs. $18. AARP Pharmacy Service, 500 Montgomery Street, Alexandria, VA 22314, (800) 456-2277.

BEST BUY. *Worst Pills Best Pills: The Older Adult's Guide to Avoiding Drug-Induced Death or Illness* by Sidney M. Wolfe, M.D., and Rose-Ellen Hope, R.Ph. Discusses medications most frequently prescribed for older adults and their side effects, also alternative medications. Explicit descriptions of medications, what they are usually prescribed for, and what the dangers are. Includes 119 drugs the authors consider too dangerous to take and others that can serve as substitutes. $12. Public Citizen Health Research Group, 2000 P Street, NW, Suite 700, Washington, DC 20036.

OBTAINING EMERGENCY HELP

"Without a phone I feel like I'm stranded on a desert island in a snowstorm. I might as well be too. If I can't call or be called, I might as well not exist."

The telephone is remarkable for the reassurance it provides, even if it just sits silently on a table. Of course, you must hear its rings and hear the caller. Phone companies offer an expanding number of services that make the telephone a more valuable and potentially lifesaving instrument. Some communities have monitoring programs that verify your safety with a daily call. A computer may call you and be programmed to send help if you don't respond by pressing a certain phone button; other programs are more personal and take the time to chat. There are some that include regular visits from people who can help you do things at home or go shopping with you.

Some telephones have memories so that you can dial the police or your neighbors by pressing a single button. A speakerphone allows you to have a conversation without holding the receiver. The idea of calling for help just by pressing a button stowed in your pocket or suspended around your neck is reassuring, especially if you think you might fall or feel ill and not be able to get to the phone. Other telephone models can be activated by remote pendant buttons to play prerecorded messages, so that assistance can be sent to you. A monitoring center can receive your emergency call, activated with a remote button, and notify a neighbor or the police to send help. Some personal emergency response systems can be programmed to call the police directly or 911, without connection to a monitoring center. These can also be part of a home security system that activates the telephone to dial the police.

For the reassurance of always being in contact with a family member, you can rent a pager that beeps or vibrates when you are being called.

New technology is available to modify the telephone so that it:

- Can be made smaller, pocket size
- May be operated by touching a screen with a stylus or your finger
- May be operated by voice alone
- May permit you to call another extension in your home

Telephone companies plan to offer voice dialing as an option to permit a caller to speak a name and have the number dialed automatically. Several phone companies are developing a national wireless phone network that would permit callers to communicate from virtually anywhere, like Dick Tracy and his wrist radio.

When an emergency occurs, it is the rare individual who is calm enough to remember vital information that a police officer or emergency assistance personnel may need: your doctor's name and phone number, medications you are taking and those you're allergic to, or other medical conditions. For those situations, wallet-size cards or a special bracelet or necklace containing such information are available. Some medical identification services provide stickers for you to affix to your refrigerator that direct emergency personnel to a medical ID card in your wallet or medicine chest.

As a first line of defense in an emergency, be sure that your medicine chest contains the minimum ingredients for first aid should you need it. Of course, first aid is only a temporary measure and does not replace a visit to a doctor.

A Basic First Aid Kit

- Large Band-Aids, 4″ × 4″ and 2″ × 2″ gauze pads, and adhesive tape
- Burn ointment, antiseptic ointment, and petroleum jelly
- An instant ice pack or a freezer bag of frozen peas or corn
- Large safety pins, stretch bandage, small scissors
- Q-Tips, premoistened towelettes
- A small towel

Resources

Equipment that facilitates using the telephone, including text telephones and telecommunications relay services, is listed in Chapter 3, "Keeping in Touch."

Products

Telephone Dialing
Telephone Dialer Stick. A plastic pointer with a fat handle to use with rotary phones. $14. For a distributor near you contact Maddak, Inc., 6 Industrial Road, Pequannock, NJ 07440, (800) 443-4926.

Voice-Activated Phone. Phone automatically dials fifty numbers by voice, speed-dials an additional hundred. Hearing aid-compatible. Includes alarm clock, hold key, and more features. $200. Lighthouse Consumer Products catalog, (800) 829-0500.

Phone Home. This device permits you to use a public phone without money to dial a collect call. Held against the mouthpiece of a telephone, it automatically dials the number you program, up to a sixteen-digit number, when button marked "Home" is pressed. Batteries included. $20. Nimrod International Sales, Inc., P.O. Box 565, Clarksburg, NJ 08510, (609) 259-3754.

Personal Emergency Response Systems

CareLine. Connects to the phone like an answering machine. When a portable button activates the system, it dials up to five numbers you have preselected. It keeps dialing until someone answers and then plays a message you have recorded. A speakerphone permits two-way conversations within voice range, and when it is activated in an emergency, phone calls are answered automatically. Can also be used as a silent alarm for a security emergency. Desk- or wall-mounted with voice-assisted setup. $330. Sears Home HealthCare catalog, (800) 326-1750, or for your nearest dealer, contact Personal Communication Systems, 2596D Reynolda Road, Winston-Salem, NC 27106, (800) 691-9222.

Personal Emergency Phone. When the alert button is pressed, the phone automatically dials each of four emergency numbers until it reaches someone. It may be programmed to call emergency numbers if the phone is not used for a specified period. The keypad flashes as the phone rings. $400. Accessolutions catalog, (800) 445-9968.

MedicAlert Response Service. Monitoring service with remote activator button. Price is $50 to start, plus $40 per month for leasing and monitoring. To purchase, $600, plus $20 per month for monitoring. MARS, (800) 642-0045, extension 500.

Lifeline Systems. A monitored emergency response system activated with a small button. The central service tries to communicate with you by speaker when the device is activated and contacts whomever you have designated. $20 to $90, installation. $25 to $40 a month. For nearest dealer, contact Lifeline, 1 Arsenal Marketplace, Watertown, MA 02172, (800) LIFELINE (543-3546).

Medical Identifications

"Get the Answers." A wallet card with spaces for listing medications, blood type, allergies, medical condition, and doctor and emergency numbers. FREE with SSE. National Council on Patient

Information and Education, 666 11th Street, NW, Suite 810, Washington, DC 20001, (202) 347-6711.

Medical Identification Data Corporation. A crimson plastic ID card with medical information on both sides and stickers to alert people that you carry a medical ID. MIDC, 1119 Springfield Road, Union, NJ 07083.

Bracelets, Necklaces, or Tags. Imprinted with information to alert medical personnel to specific problems. Under $10. Imp-Prints, P.O. Box 3, Okauchee, WI 53069, (414) 569-9234, or in southeastern Wisconsin (800) 585-9234.

Medical Alert. Bracelet and card with medical conditions engraved on the back. Bracelet, $5. Card, $2.50. Maxi-Aids catalog, (800) 522-6294.

Medic Alert. Bracelet or pendant with personalized engraving detailing your medical condition and emergency number. Includes wallet card and twenty-four-hour telephone number that provides information from computerized medical records. Stainless, sterling, gold-filled, $35 to $75. $15 annual fee, including updates. Medic Alert Foundation International, 2323 Colorado Avenue, Turlock, CA 95382, (800) ID-ALERT (432-5378).

Jewelry-style Medical ID. Medical conditions engraved in three lines on reverse. Pendant or bracelet, silver or gold. Petite pendant, silver, $60, or gold, $139. Bruce Medical Supply catalog, (800) 225-8446. Medic IDs, Inc., 18730 Oxnard Street, Unit 210, Tarzana, CA 91356, (800) 92-MEDIC (63342).

Sav-ur-life. Emergency identification system. Provides emergency personnel with accurate, easy-to-read information to allow them to give you proper treatment until you get to a hospital emergency room. Identifies previous conditions, blood type, medications, allergies, etc.; also provides names of your doctor and people to contact in an emergency. Includes stickers to alert emergency personnel to look for card in your wallet. Four microfilm slides are embedded into the card, two containing information sheets you provide and two containing information from your doctor, EKG, charts, or other information. $20. Medi-Quik Info Services, P.O. Box 582, Glen Rock, NJ 07452.

Lifedata Card. A condensed summary of your medical history in a legible form for immediate use in case of emergency. It is actually a folded form that fits in a credit card-size plastic holder. $8. For dealer nearest you, contact Lifedata America, 1 Alin Plaza,

2107 Dwight Way, Suite 100, Berkeley, CA 94704, (510) 644-3366.

BEST BUY. Heart Chart. A wallet-size laminated card containing basic information, doctor's name, whom to call in an emergency, medical history, and allergies. On the reverse is a miniaturization of your most recent electrocardiogram to provide a baseline ECG that emergency personnel can use for comparison. It doesn't need to be read by a microfilm reader. $18. P.O. Box 221, New Rochelle, NY 10804, (914) 833-0667.

Vial of Life. A magnet on the refrigerator door alerts medical emergency personnel to look inside for vital health information. Your health details, medications, doctor's name, and other information are placed in a special plastic container. FREE. Call for nearest CVS Pharmacy, (800) 444-1140.

Computer Medical Record Keeper. Helps you maintain medical records on your home computer and generates a wallet-size summary. Also helps you create advance directives such as a living will. Program assesses interactions of various medications for your safety. $70. Pixel Perfect, 10460 South Tropical Trail, Merritt Island, FL 32952, (800) 788-2099.

First Aid

"Emergency Care Guide: What to Do Until Help Arrives." A slide guide to get you through the early stages of sixteen emergencies, such as stomach pain, electric shock, burns. FREE. Our Lady of Mercy Medical Center, Office of Marketing, 600 East 233rd Street, Bronx, NY 10466, (718) 920-9251.

All-Purpose First Aid Kit. Bandages, tape, wipes, cream, cold pack, Tylenol, scissors, tweezers, guide, and gloves. $40. Safety Zone catalog, (800) 999-3030.

First Aid Kit. Metal box with bandages, antiseptic, burn ointment. $20. Northern catalog, (800) 533-5545.

First Aid Kits. Either filled or empty, three sizes: basic, compact, and standard, $10, $17, $20 empty, or $22, $35, $50 stocked. Also mini kit stocked, $9. Campmor catalog, (800) CAMPMOR (226-7667).

Dental Emergency Kit. Includes temporary filling, temporary cement, wax, repair liquid, repair powder, toothache drops, cotton, tweezers, and more. $15. Campmor catalog, (800) CAMPMOR (226-7667).

Comprehensive Adventure Medical Kit. Includes manual, splints, scissors, iodine tablets, basic medications, etc. $130. Campmor catalog, (800) CAMPMOR (226-7667).

Emergency Burn Kit. Burn dressings, burn wrap, sterile burn sheet, tape, gauze, sterile water, scissors, and gloves, instructions. $80. Safety Zone catalog, (800) 999-3030.

Computer Programs

Computer Medical Advice. Dr. Schueler's Home Medical Advisor. A computer program that can answer your questions until you can reach a doctor. Analyzes symptoms and suggests diagnosis, care; poison information; medications and side effects; nutrition information. $88. Pixel Perfect, 10460 South Tropical Trail, Merritt Island, FL 32952, (800) 788-2099.

Publications

"PERS (Personal Emergency Response System) Product Report," American Association of Retired Persons. Explains and compares emergency response systems. Describes features and prices of twenty models. FREE. AARP Publications, 601 E Street, NW, Washington, DC 20049.

"First Aid for Eye Emergencies." A list of instructions in cases of chemical burns to the eye, specks in the eye, blows to the eye, or cuts on eye or eyelid. Can be applied to the inside of a medicine cabinet or first aid kit. FREE. Prevent Blindness America, 500 East Remington Road, Schaumburg, IL 60173, (800) 331-2020.

Chapter 15

Feeling Safe on the Road

"People thought I was so virtuous when I told them I tore up my driver's license. What I didn't tell them was about the accident I almost had because I misjudged how fast a car was coming as I made a turn. I will never forget that sound of screeching brakes — the other car's, not mine — and just in the nick of time."

When you leave the comfort of home, you want to feel safe driving your car or walking, whether you are out for pleasure or running errands. Often a few simple changes or devices can help you be a safe driver or pedestrian.

DRIVING SAFELY

The closer your birth date is to the beginning of this century, the less likely it is that you had formal driving lessons or took a driving test before getting your license. There may be some new traffic rules you should be aware of, as well as some power features on newer cars you could learn to use. You may feel quite comfortable driving in your neighborhood, but unfamiliar streets or superhighways may seem confusing and make you feel less secure. Drivers also can be affected by changes in vision, hearing, physical abilities, or mental alertness.

If you find that pedestrians, other cars, or objects appear "out of nowhere" as you drive, your vision may be putting you at risk. Poor vision, loss of peripheral vision, sensitivity to sun glare or the glare of lights at night, and slowed rate of focusing all can affect the way you drive. Sunglasses may help even out the light values of the sun, but driving at dawn or dusk may still present special problems.

Allow your eyes to adjust to the darkness before you begin driving at night. If you feel blinded by oncoming headlights, use the median line or the opposite edge of the road as a guideline.

Experiment to determine if you drive better with or without your hearing aid and whether or not you should keep a window open to get cues from background sounds. Test to determine if you can hear a warning horn or a railroad crossing bell. You may find that listening to the radio while driving is too much of a distraction. If interior car noises overwhelm those from the outside, ask passengers to whisper when they talk among themselves, so that you can concentrate on the sounds outside.

A Driver's Warm-up

Before you get in the car and about once an hour on long drives, do the following routine:

- Arch your back.
- Turn your head from side to side.
- Raise yourself up on your toes.
- March in place, raising your knees as high as you can.
- Walk around the car a few times.
- When you get back into the car, concentrate on relaxing your shoulders and body.
- As you drive, try to keep relaxed, change your hand position on the steering wheel frequently, and learn to use cruise control if you have it on your car, so that you can flex your legs.

Driving safely requires you to maintain your basic fitness. You should be able to turn your head to either side well enough to check oncoming traffic before making a lane change. Your legs should be strong enough and agile enough to find the gas pedal and distinguish it from the brake pedal.

One sure sign that you feel tentative about driving is that you avoid making left turns on two-way streets. Rather than drive dangerously, detour by using successive right turns to circle to the street you need. Buy a street map, and figure out a "long, scenic route" with which you feel comfortable.

Learn to use all the power equipment in your car: how to adjust the side view mirrors, the driver's seat, the defogger, and so on. The easier maneuvering afforded by power brakes and power steering can compensate for some loss of reaction time. Get used to using your safety belt; if it feels too tight, take it to your car dealer to have it adjusted.

Signs of Unsafe Driving

- Driving consistently *below* the speed limit
- Not staying within the lane markings
- Switching lanes frequently, especially without signaling
- Not understanding the meaning of some road signs
- Not coming to a full stop at a stop sign

The youngest drivers (between ages sixteen and nineteen) cause fatalities at a higher rate than the oldest drivers, but the latter are more likely to have accidents when measured by the number of miles driven. Thirty-two states and the District of Columbia offer an automobile insurance discount to older drivers who attend a defensive driving course. Other states are introducing more frequent testing for license renewals. For example, in Illinois, a seventy-five-year-old driver must take driving and vision tests before renewing a license; after age eighty, a driver must renew again after two rather than four years, and after age eighty-five renewal is every year. Illinois offers a driver refresher course, and other states have instituted similar age restrictions.

If you are considering purchasing a new car, check for the ease of operating the air conditioning, heater, headlights, and radio controls without needing to look at them. Legible numbers on the speedometer, an easy-to-read gas gauge, and an audible beep that reminds you to turn off headlights or put on your seat belt are other important features that can add to the safe operation of a car.

A car's operation can be modified for easier use, by altering the shift, the accelerator, or the brake mechanism. For example, right-hand shifts can be switched to left-handed use; foot brakes can be adapted for operation by hand. These alterations may be done by private mechanics. Some manufacturers offer rebates for the cost of installing adaptive equipment in a new car.

A Driver's Emergency Equipment

The following items should be a permanent part of your car's accessories. Fit under the front seat as many of these items as possible, especially those in italics. In this way you avoid having to exit the car in bad weather or bad neighborhoods to get access to the car's trunk compartment.

- A *battery-operated radio, plus extra batteries*
- A *flashlight, plus extra batteries*
- A *blanket*
- Booster cables (be sure to get a lesson in their use)
- A fire extinguisher (be sure to get a lesson in its use)
- *A small first aid kit in a coffee can,* with a quarter taped to the plastic lid for an emergency phone call
- Flares and *a large sign that says CALL POLICE*
- A shovel and a tool kit
- *Bottled water and raisins*
- *Maps*
- *A car phone*

Resources

Suggestions for improving your strength and flexibility through physical activity are offered in Chapter 9, "Achieving the Four Elements of Mobility."

Products

Electro Flares. Alternative to one-time-use flares. When the tripod legs are unfolded, a signal light flashes once a second and stops when the legs are folded again. Reusable. Battery-operated. Two for $15. Hanover House catalog, (717) 633-3377.

Four-bladed Windshield Wipers. Easy to install. Four blades are incorporated into one to sweep, clear, clean, and protect. Guaranteed for as long as you own your car. Two front blades for $20. Safety Zone catalog, (800) 999-3030.

Electric Windshield Scraper. Plugs into the cigarette lighter socket and heats up in two minutes for melting ice and snow. Reaches all the windows on your car, and stores in the glove compartment. $13. Safety Zone catalog, (800) 999-3030.

Car Door Opener. Use this plastic device to open either push-button or lift-up car door handles. $20. AfterTherapy catalog, (800) 634-4351.

Panoramic Rear View Mirror. Enlarges the viewing area threefold, eliminating blind spots. 13-inch, $28. 17-inch, $30. Comfort House catalog, (800) 359-7701.

Blind Spot Mirrors. Convex mirror attaches with self-adhesive backing to side view mirrors to avoid blind spots. Adjustable. $6. Brookstone catalog, (800) 926-7000.

LaneChanger. An extra large rearview mirror that includes the areas to the side and rear of car. $29. Safety Zone catalog, (800) 999-3030.

Visor Extender. Adds 9 inches to right or left side of the visor and additional sunscreen to combat glare. $8. Vermont Country Store catalog, (802) 362-2400.

Foam Seat Booster. Either to add 3 inches to car's seat or for use as a backrest. $9. Hanover House catalog, (717) 633-3366.

Foam Wedge Cushion. Keeps you from sinking too far into the car's seat and improves your view of the road. $6. Carol Wright Gifts catalog, (402) 474-4465.

Back Cushion. Adjusts to nine different positions to fit the curve of the lower spine. $40. Solutions catalog, (800) 432-9988.

Shoulder Belt Cushion. Washable, cotton twill covered ½-inch-thick cushion. Three colors available. $10. Bruce Medical Supply catalog, (800) 225-8446.

Home and Auto Back Massager. Plugs into cigarette lighter or may be used at home with a converter. $50. Sears Home HealthCare catalog, (800) 326-1750.

Acu-cushion. Washable cotton and polyester cushion with a bumpy surface resembling large bubble wrap. Large back and seat portions held in place with a strap around the seat back. $30. Northern catalog, (800) 533-5545.

Swivel Seat Cushion. Allows you to turn and get in or out of car with less effort. $15. Comfort House catalog, (800) 359-7701.

Driving Controls and Driving Aids. Either motorcycle-type throttle or right-angle operation. $275 to $400, plus installation. Wells-Engberg Company, P.O. Box 6388, Rockford, IL 61125, (800) 642-3628.

Automatic Clutch Operating System. With this installed in a manual-shift car, as the driver begins to shift, the clutch operates automatically. A dashboard switch allows return to normal clutch function. About $2,500. Access Unlimited, 570 Hauce Road, Binghamton, NY 13903, (607) 729-7530.

Parking Alert. Battery-powered green, yellow, red traffic light helps you determine your car's position. For use in garage, tight driveway, or other driving situations. Activates when car's head- or taillights are on. $50. Parkrite. Solar Wide, P.O. Box 7600, Wilton, CT 06897, (800) 765-5090.

Blinker Buddy. An electronic turn signal reminder. Sounds a tone and flashes a light when the turn signal is on. The longer the turn signal is on, the louder the tone gets. $80. Accessolutions catalog, (800) 445-9968.

Parking Guide. When you hit the rubber wheel stop, you will know you're in proper position in the garage. Movable. $24. Home Trends catalog, (716) 254-6520.

Flashing Emergency Strobe Alert. A bright light, which stays magnetically attached to the roof of the car, flashes every second. Stay in the car, and wait for help. $20. Northern catalog, (800) 533-5545.

Car Phone. Free 911 emergency calls and free American Automobile Association calls with preprogrammed buttons. Uses cigarette lighter power. Specially designed for members of the AAA. Three-year warranty. $200 to $300. About $15 to $30 a month service fee from your local cellular phone company. AAA/Auto Club Cellular Corporation, Attn. Laura Reed, 6 Penns Trail, Suite 105, Newtown Pavilion, Newtown, PA 18940, (800) 942-2220, extension 128.

Tire Check. A tire valve cap that changes color when your tires lose air. Four for $10. Safety Zone catalog, (800) 999-3030.

Emergency Car Kit. Includes jumper cables, gas siphon hose, fire extinguisher, flares, "Help" flag, hammer, pliers, screwdriver, emergency tape and Fix-a-Flat, first aid kit, and towelettes. $65. Safety Zone catalog, (800) 999-3030.

Refresher Driving Courses

Safe Driving for Mature Operators. Guidance for traffic accident prevention and risk management for drivers age fifty-five and older. Special attention is given to suggestions for compensating for physical changes, such as diminished vision and hearing. Sponsored by local American Automobile Association (AAA) clubs and taught by certified instructors. Price varies according to location and may even be FREE. For a location near you, contact AAA, Driver Safety Services, 1000 AAA Drive, Heathrow, FL 32746, (407) 444-7961.

"55 Alive." Driver-retraining classes by the American Association of Retired Persons volunteers. Six-session, eight-hour refresher course. Focuses on age-related physical changes, declining perceptual skills, rules of the road, local driving problems, license renewal issues. Some states require a rebate in insurance premium for drivers who take it. Must be over age fifty. $10. For a course near you, contact AARP Traffic and Driver Safety Program, 601 E Street, NW, Washington, DC 20049, (202) 434-6014.

Coaching the Mature Driver. A defensive driving course for drivers over fifty-five. Explains how to compensate for changes caused by aging. $45. National Safety Council, P.O. Box 558, Itasca, IL 60143, (800) 621-7619.

Services

GM Mobility Program. General Motors offers up to $1,000 off the cost of installing adaptive equipment on a newly purchased or leased vehicle. Financing is available on both the car and the equipment at the time of purchase. A list of driver assessment facilities, adaptive equipment installers, and other mobility conversion funding sources is available. GM Mobility Assistance Center, P.O. Box 9011, Detroit, MI 48202, (800) 323-9935.

Chrysler Corporation's Automobility Program. A cash incentive for expenses of up to $1,000 to install adaptive equipment for driver or passenger for up to two new vehicles. Resource information. Chrysler's Automobility Resource Center, P.O. Box 3124, Bloomfield Hills, MI 48302, (800) 255-9877.

Ford Mobility Motoring Program. Purchasing or leasing a new Ford car, truck, or van, you receive up to a $750 rebate when you install adaptive driving or passenger equipment, a complimentary cellular telephone, and one-year membership in Ford Auto Club for emergency road service. Assistance locating and selecting appropriate equipment, dealers, installers in your area. FREE. P.O. Box 529, Bloomfield Hills, MI 48303, (800) 952-2248.

Publications

"The Older Persons' Guide to Safe Driving" by Myron Brenton. Pamphlet highlights some situations that may present driving problems and how to confront them. $1. Public Affairs Committee, 381 Park Avenue South, New York, NY 10016.

"Good Vision . . . Vital to Good Driving," American Automobile Association. How to compensate when you drive if you have declining vision. FREE with SSE. AAA, Corporate Communications, 1000 AAA Drive, Heathrow, FL 32746, (407) 444-8000.

"A Flexibility Fitness Training Package for Improving Older Driver Performance," AAA Foundation for Traffic Safety. Exercises that can improve flexibility and an explanation of how they can help you be a better, safer driver. FREE with SSE. AAA Foundation for Traffic Safety, 1440 New York Avenue, NW, Suite 201, Washington, DC 20005, (202) 638-5944.

PEDESTRIAN SAFETY

"I keep hearing about how good walking is for me, but I'm much more nervous about getting hit by a car or bicycle or mugged than I am about being out of shape."

Naturally you want to feel safe while you walk outdoors. You may wonder if you can jump out of the way of a speeding car or bicycle, and you may not always be sure of your footing. Problems with vision, hearing, or balance can make you feel less secure on the street; just walking in an urban area can heighten worries about personal security. You think about traffic, other pedestrians, and crime. A study found what most women know from experience: You don't walk as fast or as securely in high heels as in flat shoes. And if you are hampered in your stride or balance in any way, you must start across an intersection with enough time before the light changes. Yet a study of pedestrians at a Los Angeles intersection found that 27 percent of older people needed a longer time to reach the opposite curb than the traffic lights allowed; many pedestrians were as much as an entire traffic lane short of the curb when the light changed.

Tips for Safe Walking

- Check and double-check the traffic before crossing the street, and don't assume that drivers will see you.
- Wear light-colored clothing.
- Don't jaywalk.
- Always assume drivers will turn right on red.

Although it is true that people over sixty-five are more likely to be victims of a purse snatcher or pickpocket, this age bracket has the lowest rate of incidence for other types of crime. Unfortunately there is greater fear of violent crime among those over age sixty-five than is justified by actual figures. Using old-fashioned common sense can allow you the freedom to be out during the day, preferably with a companion and with only a small amount of cash in your pocket. To avoid a purse snatching or pickpocketing, women can use waist packs rather than purses, and men should carry their wallets in front pants pockets or in inside jacket pockets.

If it makes you feel more secure, carry a portable alarm or one of the defensive pepper sprays to use in case you feel threatened. (Use of defensive sprays may not be legal in certain states; check with your local police for information about your area.) Walking with a dog may give you a good sense of safety and may even deter some criminals.

A walking program is suggested in Chapter 10, "On the Move."
Programs that provide dogs trained specifically to alert you to sounds you need to hear are noted in Chapter 3, "Keeping in Touch."

Products

Clip-On Flasher. Battery-operated flashing red light to make you visible on the road from a distance of up to 2,000 feet. $9. Jogalite, Box 125, High Street, Silver Lake, NH 03875, (800) 258-8974, or in New Hampshire call (603) 367-4741.

Strobe Light. A 2-inch flashing light visible from 2,000 feet. Wear on wrist or ankle or belt. $13. Ann Morris catalog, (516) 292-9232.

Reflective Stripes. 3½- by ½-inch stripes attach to your clothing back and front so that you are visible to others at night. $4. Ann Morris catalog, (516) 292-9232.

Safety Vest. Mesh vest with reflective stripes. Fluorescent orange, white, or lime. $16. Jogalite, Box 125, High Street, Silver Lake NH 03875, (800) 258-8974, or in New Hampshire call (603) 367-4741.

Reflective Wrist Wallet. To carry "mad" money and keys while on the road. $6. Jogalite, Box 125, High Street, Silver Lake NH 03875, (800) 258-8974, or in New Hampshire call (603) 367-4741.

Personal Alarms

Personal Attack Alarm. When the pin is pulled, a 104-decibel piercing screech is emitted. The size of a beeper, the alarm can be clipped to a pocketbook with the strap on your wrist. If the purse is taken, the pin will be pulled, setting off the alarm, which lasts up to two hours and can be turned off only by replacing the pin. Battery-operated. Original, $25. Alarm incorporating a flashlight, $30. For a distributor near you, contact Quorum International, 1550 West Deer Valley Road, Phoenix, AZ 85027, (602) 780-5500.

Snap-on Portable Alarm. Attaches to a cane, walker, or umbrella. Emits a loud alarm when the button is pressed until the button is pressed again. $42. For a distributor near you, contact Maddak, Inc., 6 Industrial Road, Pequannock, NJ 07440, (800) 443-4926.

Keychain Alarm. When ring is pulled, a 105-decibel alarm goes off. May be used as a door or window alarm. Includes a heat fuse for a fire alarm. $16. Safety Zone catalog, (800) 999-3030.

Flashlight Alarm. Flashlight and key chain and a 100-decibel alarm in response to the slightest motion, if panic button is pushed, or if strap is detached. $15. Improvements catalog, (800) 642-2112.

SoundMate. The 120-decibel siren activated with one squeeze on the cylinder continues, even if you drop it, until you deactivate it with a code. $30. Safety Zone catalog, (800) 999-3030.

HelpAlarm. Signals for help when it is knocked loose, worn like a beeper. $20. Lighthouse Consumer Products catalog, (800) 829-0500.

Self-Defense Sprays

NOTE: Use of defensive sprays may not be legal in certain states; check with your local police for information about your area.

Sprays. Tear gas and pepper spray, $16. Pepperfoam, $20. Safety Zone catalog, (800) 999-3030.

Mace. Compact with belt clip and key chain. $13. Campmor catalog, (800) CAMPMOR (226-7667).

Services

Security Guard Dogs. Borrow a trained, defensive dog to join you for a walk, a jog, or any outdoor activity. Trained to match an assailant's aggression by growling, barking, and baring their teeth, the dogs are not attack dogs. They are intended as deterrents. FREE for people over age sixty. For a location near you, contact Project SafeRun, P.O. Box 22234, Eugene, OR 97402, (503) 345-8086, a twenty-four-hour answering service.

Publications

"Peace of Mind, Senior Citizen Self Protection" by Linda Kenoyer and Py Bateman. A pamphlet enumerating ways of preparing yourself to confront threatening situations by maximizing your defenses. $4. Alternatives to Fear, 2811 East Madison, Suite 208, Seattle, WA 98112, (206) 328-5347.

"Directory of Animal Support Programs for People Who Have Disabilities." A list of programs that supply service animals. FREE. Information Center for Individuals with Disabilities, Fort Point Place, 27-43 Wormwood Street, Boston, MA 02210, (617) 727-5540.

Organizations

Handi-Dogs. Provides dogs for people with various needs. Newsletter. P.O. Box 12563, Tucson, AZ 85732, (602) 326-3412.

Canine Companions for Independence. Four regional centers provide service dogs. P.O. Box 446, Santa Rosa, CA 95402, (800) 572-BARK (2275).

Part Five

An Alert Mind

Chapter 16

Enhancing Your Memory and Vision

Your own innate curiosity and interest in what goes on around you can go far toward helping you keep an alert mind. We stimulate our minds when we pursue interests that engage us, challenge us, inspire us to commit our time and concentration. Of course, a good memory is essential to learning new things. Thankfully there is no truth to the idea — generally accepted until the 1960s even by researchers — that after a certain age learning isn't possible.

A basic tool for continued mental stimulation is reading: for pleasure and to activate our imagination, for information and to keep up with current events, or for education. Even if your eyesight is poor, there are things you can do to enable you to continue reading.

A NIMBLE MEMORY

The most cheering message of recent decades indicates that loss of brain function is *not* an inevitable condition of aging. Scientists find that mental capacity can be enhanced by using your mind for learning, traveling, being with stimulating people, and continuing to grow, improve, and enjoy life. Far from waiting for an inevitable mental decline, we are told that we have the power to maintain agile minds.

Amazingly your intelligence doesn't decline when your brain loses nerve cells, a process that begins after age thirty or forty and progresses until 60 percent is lost by age ninety. You need never experience an interruption in your everyday activities. You may take more time to learn something new or you may learn it in a different way from the way you used to, but your judgment and general fund of knowledge remain constant.

Core memory — the accumulation of experiences, feelings, and learning unique to us — usually remains the same throughout life. This is what allows us to tie our shoes, call someone by name, discuss a past event, use information we once learned, and react to and understand life. *Semantic memory,* which involves knowledge and factual information, and *implicit memory,* which refers to automatic skills, such as buttoning, are more or less stable regardless of age. *Episodic memory* refers to the commonplace items most people over age forty-five have trouble with — remembering where they put items, remembering names — but these signs of forgetting are not omens of irreversible enfeeblement. The brain cells involved in short-term memory — what you had for lunch or a new fact — are the first to die. The fact is, your lunch menu may never register in the brain at all; therefore, it can't be retrieved later.

Remaining mentally active, at work, through community involvement, or with hobbies will keep your memory keen and your brain's ability to function at a high level.

Confusion and forgetfulness may result from a specific and treatable condition, so you shouldn't assume they are either a normal consequence of aging or signs of brain disease.

Of course, all changes in the way your body — or mind — functions should be reported to a physician.

So how can we avoid the annoyance of misplacing our keys, eyeglasses, or wallet or forgetting what we ate for lunch? We can learn tricks to help us remember, most of which are designed to focus our attention. When you think of the items you never lose, you may discern a helpful truism: When things are always in the same place, you know where they are. Probably you don't forget where your telephone is located, unless it is portable. That is one clue to remembering. We "lose" something when our attention is distracted and we don't notice where we put it. One cure for forgetfulness lies in always putting items in the same place or having

Some Causes of Confusion or Forgetfulness

- Lack of alertness can be a side effect of medication or the interaction of several medications. Consult your physician if you suspect this is a problem for you.
- Dehydration diminishes blood volume and thus may reduce the oxygen supply to the brain.
- Lack of certain nutritional elements — particularly sodium and potassium — may affect the brain's functioning.
- Infections, such as urinary tract infections, pneumonia, or other treatable medical problems, may cause disorientation.
- Hearing or vision problems may affect what you learn and remember.
- Depression or withdrawal resulting from emotional trauma may cause uninterest or inattention.
- Retirement or a less structured day may make your recollection of the day and its date less significant or may reduce your chances for social interchange. If you don't know what "everyone else" knows — the names of current movie stars, political figures — you may feel "out of it."

multiple sets of keys, eyeglasses, pens in the several places where you usually look for them. With items that are frequently hard to find, try to develop a convenient habit: keys always on a hook near the door, reading glasses on a cord around your neck, a pen attached to the phone, appointments on *one* calendar, things to do on *one* list.

A daily routine, such as creating a schedule and list at breakfast time, allows you to ponder the events of the day to come and put them in order by location (first the post office, then the cleaner) or by time (a twelve-thirty lunch, a two-thirty appointment), including a notation of things to bring or pick up, coupons to take to the supermarket, and so forth.

Beware of holding yourself to an unreasonably high standard. We all forget things; it's human nature to do so. That's what lists are for. Forgetting to mail a letter or leaving the grocery list at home is not a sign of "old age"; it's a function of a busy life: When you are trying to remember to take your gloves, you leave behind the grocery list.

If you worry about forgetting something, do something about it now if you can. Put what you need by the door when you think of it. Find some memory trick that fits your routine: If you need your keys before you leave the house, put other items you must take near your keys or put your keys near your coat or hat.

To keep a limber brain, exercise it with card games, chess, puzzles, and other mental challenges. Try a mind test or two: Count backward from one hundred by sevens or sixteens, or have a friend read a random entry from the phone book and try to recall it after ten minutes of conversation about other matters.

Learning is a complicated process that relies on complex interactions between brain cells. You may learn by repetition, by association, verbally, visually, or a combination of these. You may learn or retain information better before or after a meal or in the morning or evening, depending on conditions under which you are most alert.

Resources

A choice of timers to use as reminders is available in Chapter 8, "Home Cooking."

Suggestions of products to use to record family histories are offered in Chapter 2, "Nourishing Relationships."

Products

Parking Timer. An alarm sounds ten minutes and five minutes before the alarm time. Key chain attached, pocket size. $5. Charles Allyn International, 315 West 9th Street, Suite 323, Los Angeles, CA 90015, (213) 624-0112.

Four Task Timer. Multifunction timer that keeps track of four chores at once. Also functions as a clock and stopwatch. Stands on countertop, clips to belt, or adheres magnetically to refrigerator. $25. Home Trends catalog, (716) 254-6520.

Talking Memo. A credit card-size recorder will let you remind yourself of chores, directions, and so forth. Sixty-word capacity. $16. Easier Ways catalog, (410) 659-0232.

Publications

"Now Where Did I Put My Keys?," American Association of Retired Persons. A brief overview of factors that affect your memory and how to improve it. FREE. AARP Publications, 601 E Street, NW, Washington, DC 20049.

Our Remarkable Memory: Understanding It, Improving It, Losing It? by Edith Nalle Schafer. A succinct, but comprehensive, discussion of what is known about memory functions. Tips for improving memory. 1992. Starrhill Press, P.O. Box 32342, Washington, DC 20007.

"10 Simple Ways to Improve Your Memory." Suggestions for remembering names, phone numbers, and other frequently forgotten items. FREE with SSE. Memory Assessment Clinics, 8311 Wisconsin Avenue, Bethesda, MD 20814, (800) FIT-MIND (348-6463).

"What's on Your Mind? A Quiz on Aging and the Brain," National Institute on Aging. Information in question-and-answer form to clarify new understanding of the "normal" aging of the brain and mental functions. FREE. NIA, National Institutes of Health, HPIZ, P.O. Box 8057, Gaithersburg, MD 20898, (800) 222-2225.

RELYING ON YOUR VISION

You depend on your visual ability for many stimulating activities that will keep your mind alert. Reading (for pleasure, to keep up with world events, or for learning); watching television, a computer screen, movies, or other cultural events; and enjoying the beauty of nature and art are just a few vision-dependent activities that keep you alert and engaged.

Visual acuity is said to peak at age eighteen and then decline gradually until it stabilizes at age fifty-five. After age thirty, less light enters the eye and more must be provided artificially as the size of the pupil decreases. By age seventy it takes three times longer for your eyes to adjust to the dark than when you were twenty-five years old, and you need more illumination in a room or when you do detailed tasks. After age eighty you will need three times more light to see clearly than when you were a twenty-year-old.

Around age forty the eye's lens, located in the center of the pupil, starts to lost its flexibility. This lessens the ability to focus, particularly on close objects, a condition called presbyopia. Although the eye's muscles may move properly, the lens cannot respond to permit clear focusing. This can be corrected with bifocal eyeglasses.

Changes in Your Vision

- Difficulty changing focus (from distant to near or vice versa), blurring of near vision (presbyopia)
- Needing more light to see properly
- Sensitivity to the glare from a car's headlights or the sun
- Narrowed peripheral vision
- Problems distinguishing among colors
- Reduced night vision
- More frequent episodes of seeing spots, floaters, or patterns

You may notice vision changes indirectly. For example:

- You tire more easily than usual.
- You sit closer to the television set.
- You expend more effort to do routine tasks.
- You lose things more frequently.
- You can't locate items easily in the supermarket.
- You need to be at the corner to read street signs.
- You don't recognize people on the street.
- You don't notice housekeeping lapses.
- Your balance is sometimes unsteady.

Damage from some eye diseases can be limited if they are caught at early stages. For example, people with diabetes are at high risk for diabetic retinopathy, which can be detected by an ophthalmologist. Similarly, glaucoma, a disease that can cause total loss of vision, can be controlled with treatment if detected early. Deterioration of the macula, the central portion of the retina, causes distortion in the central portion of vision. The remainder of vision is not affected in macular degeneration, and with prompt treatment some improvement may be possible. Any change in your vision should be reported to an ophthalmologist.

Some warning signs of potentially serious problems:

- Hazy or blurred vision
- Recurrent pain in eye area
- Double vision
- Seeing flashes of light or halos around lights
- Change in color of pupil

326

- Sensitivity to light and glare
- Darkness or visual distortions in center of vision

By age sixty 50 percent of us will begin to develop cataracts — clouding of the eye's lens. This clouding is attributed to damage from exposure to the sun's ultraviolet rays, some medical conditions like diabetes, or a natural deterioration. Damage from ultraviolet rays of the sun may be delayed by wearing sunglasses that block between 60 and 92 percent of visible light.

Sunglass manufacturers have agreed to provide labels that specify the amount of protection from ultraviolet radiation and visible light you can expect from the lenses you buy.

Sunglass Labels Explained		
Category	**Protection**	**Purpose**
Cosmetic	Blocks 70%UVB, 20% UVA, and 60% visible light	While shopping or doing chores
General purpose	Blocks 95% UVB, 60% UVA, and 60–90% visible light	Hiking, driving
Special purpose	Blocks 99% UVB, 60% UVA, and 97% visible light	At the beach, skiing, and other bright locations

Recent research indicates that some cataracts may be forestalled with sufficient dietary intake of antioxidants, including vitamins E and C, and beta-carotenes.

Cataracts sometimes cause only minimal visual loss without interfering at all with daily activities. On the other hand, you may find it difficult to see small details and impossible to do certain activities, such as needlepoint, reading normal print, or driving a car. In some cases a cataract stabilizes and doesn't worsen, and it may take ten years or longer for it to develop to the point where it prevents you from carrying out your normal routine. Some people with cataracts are able to enhance their vision with better lighting, by reducing glare, or by using magnifying glasses for reading and close work. When these methods are not sufficient for maintaining your activities, surgical removal and replacement of the clouded lens are a commonplace treatment. In 1992 Medicare paid for 1.4 million cataract extraction/lens implant procedures, the single most common surgery for beneficiaries. Cataract surgery, generally done with a local anesthetic on an outpatient basis, usually takes under an hour and permits a speedy recovery and return to normal activities. Generally the new lens is adjusted for far vision, and you will need glasses for close vision.

New Developments

* The Food and Drug Administration has under review lenses with bifocal, or multifocal, capability that could be implanted after cataract removal. Approval of these lenses might avoid the need for wearing glasses for near vision.
* Drug companies are developing substances that may prevent or treat cataracts by preventing the formation of the clouding.
* The FDA plans to require that *all* sunglasses permit less than 1 percent of UVB and less than 5 percent of UVA radiation to reach the eye. The new requirements will include standards for impact resistance, require use of nonflammable materials, and regulation of health claims.

Resources

Solutions to lighting problems in your home are offered in Chapter 12, "Adapting the Old Homestead."

Techniques for enhancing your vision when driving an automobile are mentioned in Chapter 15, "Feeling Safe on the Road."

NOTE: The organizations and services in this "Resources" listing, even those whose name specifies "blind," also provide advice and assistance for people with low or poor vision.

Products

Plastic Simulator. A card with four special areas, each representing a different eye condition. When you look through each area you can understand how people experience impaired vision. 55 cents. Lighthouse National Center for Vision and Aging, 111 East 59th

Street, New York, NY 10022, (800) 334-5497.

Home Vision Tests

"Adult Home Eye Screening." Kit to measure vision and to help you detect cataracts, macular degeneration, or eyeglass prescription errors. $3. Sight & Hearing Association, 674 Transfer Road, St. Paul, MN 55114, (800) 992-0424.

BEST BUY. "How's Your Vision? Family Home Eye Test," Prevent Blindness America. Materials you can use to test for distance and near vision, glaucoma, and macular degeneration. FREE. PBA, 500 East Remington Road, Schaumburg, IL 60173, (800) 331-2020.

Services

Mission Cataract, U.S.A. Ophthalmologists provide eye screening and surgery FREE to people who can't afford it and have no insurance. For a participating doctor near you, contact Mission Cataract, U.S.A., c/o Info-Media, 6716 North Cedar Avenue, Suite 212, Fresno, CA 93710, (800) 343-7265.

National Eye Care Project. Volunteer ophthalmologists offer care to those age sixty-five and older who do not have ophthalmologists. Patients receive comprehensive medical exams and treatment for eye diseases (not for eyeglasses). Information on prevention and treatment of eye problems. National Eye Care Project, P.O. Box 429098, San Francisco, CA 94142, (800) 222-EYES (3937).

Publications

BEST BUY. "Low Vision Information," Lighthouse. Includes a photographic essay on partial sight, illustrating various ways a person with low vision might be seeing. FREE. Lighthouse National Center for Vision and Aging, 111 East 59th Street, New York, NY 10022, (800) 334-5497.

"Cataract in Adults: A Patient's Guide," Agency for Health Care Policy and Research. FREE. AHCPR Publications Clearinghouse, P.O. Box 8547, Silver Spring, MD 20907, (800) 358-9295.

"Your Guide to Cataract Surgery," Prevent Blindness America. General discussion of cataracts, how they form, and what you may expect if you need surgery. FREE. PBA, 500 East Remington Road, Schaumburg, IL 60173, (800) 331-2020.

"About Cataract Surgery in Adults," American College of Surgeons. A description of surgery to remove cataracts and what a patient should anticipate. FREE. American College of Surgeons, 55 East Erie Street, Chicago, IL 60611, (312) 664-4050.

"The Eyes Have It!," American Association of Retired Persons. Description of eye care and some common disorders. AARP Publications, 601 E Street, NW, Washington, DC 20049.

Cataracts by Julius Shulman, M.D. A survey of the condition, ranging from what causes cataracts to how they can be treated. A guide to types of cataract surgery and lens implants. Easily legible print. 1993. St. Martin's Press.

"Living More Comfortably with Glaucoma," Prevent Blindness America. An explanation of the disease, its detection, and treatment options. FREE. PBA, 500 East Remington Road, Schaumburg, IL 60173, (800) 331-2020.

Organizations

Foundation Fighting Blindness. Information on diseases of the retina. The organization maintains a national registry of patients with retinal degeneration. Coordinates a retina donor program for research. FFB, 1401 Mount Royal Avenue, 4th Floor, Baltimore, MD 21217, (800) 683-5555.

Prevent Blindness America. Publications on vision and eye health — for example, age-related macular degeneration, floaters, and dry eye. Information about free glaucoma testing. Referral to low-vision centers. PBA, 500 East Remington Road, Schaumburg, IL 60173, (800) 331-2020.

Magnifying or Speaking the Words

We often need to read the fine print — for example, on a medication label or the ingredients list of a food. Of course, we need to see the controls on our appliances to use them properly. Reading correspondence, newspapers, and books is a necessary part of life's enjoyment and routine. When these items are magnified or if you can listen to the text, low vision isn't an obstacle to full engagement in daily activities.

Range of Visual Acuity

- 20/20: You and others with normal vision are able to recognize an object from a distance of twenty feet.
- 20/40: You can recognize an object from twenty feet that people with normal vision can see from forty feet. (At this level you can read a newspaper, and in some states this is the minimum to qualify for a driver license.)
- 20/70: This level indicates the loss of 40 percent of your vision.
- 20/200: With this level of vision, or a field of vision less than twenty degrees, you are legally blind. (Total blindness is the absence of useful vision or light perception.)

Visual acuity describes how near an object you need to be to recognize it and is usually represented in terms of your ability to see what a person with average eyesight would see.

An eye care specialist can advise you about whether your vision problems can be alleviated with prescription eyeglasses. Eye doctors in some areas provide their services at no charge for seniors who cannot pay.

Today's eyeglasses are light in weight and have thin lenses, and you may economize by reusing the frames and replacing only the lenses when your prescription is changed. Over-the-counter glasses, sold at drug and department stores without prescriptions, called readers, cost about one tenth of made-to-order frames and lenses and may be suitable for you. Unfortunately readers are not appropriate for people who need to wear glasses all the time or have an astigmatism (an irregular lens) or different viewing abilities in each eye.

Take other measures to improve your vision. Experiment until you find the right combination of lighting, positioning, magnification, or contrast. Vision rehabilitation is a process that combines several strategies to enhance residual vision, allowing people with low vision to perform their daily activities. Trained specialists at low-vision clinics can help you devise new ways of approaching your activities and suggest some devices to enable you to see better. When you have low vision, you may see light, color, movement, dimension, shape, and size even though objects appear blurred, faded, or distorted and it may be difficult to differentiate slight shadings of colors or intensities of light.

Don't worry about further damaging your vision by holding objects too close to your eyes, overusing your vision, or sitting too close to the TV. A magnifier can enlarge print or objects. You can choose something as basic as a handheld magnifier or something as elaborate as a closed-circuit monitor. You will find a method that suits you by experimenting: a portable magnifier to use at the supermarket or to read a menu and a desktop model for home use.

Position a magnifier by starting with it close to the print, slowly raising it toward your eyes until you can read clearly. Illumination should fall between the print and the magnifier. The closer you can hold the magnifier to your eyes, the less interference you will experience from glare or reflected light. Hand magnifiers are intended for use by both eyes, so you usually place them closer to the text or object.

Magnifiers are not only for enlarging print. Standing models allow you to do crafts or other tasks that require close viewing while leaving your hands free to fill out a check, write a letter, or thread a needle.

You can view text — from a book, magazine, or newspaper, package labels, instructions, and so forth — on a closed-circuit television (CCTV) or computer monitor linked to an electronic scanner. The scanner — similar to the devices that read bar codes in the supermarket — projects the material onto the monitor as much as sixty times larger than the original. CCTVs can also be used for grooming fingernails, viewing crafts or fine detail, labels, and more.

Copy machines can enlarge originals as much as 200 percent and may be an alternative means of magnifying material you refer to often, such as knitting instructions, a special recipe, directions, or

---

Magnifying Terminology

- Power: the strength of a lens. For example, "3×" means the lens multiplies an image three times.
- Field of view: the area that you see through a magnifier.
- Focal length: the distance between the lens and the object at which the image is sharply defined.

The stronger the lens, the longer the focal length and the larger the field of view.

map information. Large-print books are available from your library, from bookstores, or through mail-order catalogs. Usually the text is in fourteen-point type — this size.

The display on a computer monitor can be enlarged either through a software program or with a magnifier mounted on the screen. You can use a computer for correspondence and balancing your checkbook, as well as for services like shopping or reading news stories through a computer network link.

Chores the Computer Can Help You Accomplish

- Store and dial telephone numbers
- Issue checks, balance a checkbook, keep your budget, and other accounting tasks
- Remind you of appointments
- Shop and make hotel and transportation arrangements
- Read newspapers and other periodicals

A computer is smarter than a typewriter, does more things better, and is just as easy to use. The print on a computer screen can be more legible if it appears black on a white background. Simple stick-on overlays can enlarge the keyboard letters, and special tactile locators can be applied for correct finger placement on keys. Many printers operate with large type. Using a scanner, you can store text in the computer and display it on the monitor in larger type or print it out in large type to read later.

Another option for access to printed material is to listen to the words, rather than reading them. For people who have trouble reading type, the National Library Service makes available special tapes and disks that must be played on special machines. Tapes, disks, and the players are provided FREE and are sent through the mail at no charge to you. Spoken books are becoming increasingly commonplace, and a large selection of current and classical titles is available at most bookstores and through some mail-order companies.

Local radio services broadcast local news and read newspapers and periodicals on a dedicated frequency, or closed channel, that can be heard through a special receiver, provided to you FREE. Selected magazines and newspapers are available by subscription on National Library Service's special audiotape or on regular audiotape.

Contact the service to determine if you are eligible for its FREE benefits (see Resources, page 336).

With the use of an optical character reader and a scanner, text can be translated into synthesized speech. "Talking" capability may facilitate use of a computer by speaking the letters and punctuation to you as you type them or reading aloud a word, line, or page as you go along. This feature can be used with headphones.

Products that magnify or speak the text must accommodate individual differences in vision and other conditions; therefore, be sure to try before you buy. Check catalogs for an idea of the range of products and prices, but contact an eye care professional or a low-vision clinic for assistance in selecting what is best for you.

Resources

Computers as networking or communication tools and a source of news and information are discussed in Chapter 1, "Embracing a Positive Outlook."

Products

Wide Selection of Magnifiers:
Bossert Specialties catalog, (800) 776-5885
Independent Living Aids catalog, (800) 537-2118
Just for You catalog, (800) 541-7903
Lighthouse Consumer Products catalog, (800) 829-0500
Maxi-Aids catalog, (800) 522-6294
Science Products Magnilog catalog, (800) 888-7400
Sense-Sations catalog, (800) 876-5456
TASH ADL catalog, (416) 686-4129
Visual Aids catalog, (212) 889-3141 in eastern United States;
    (415) 221-3201 in western United States

"Talking" Products — Clocks, Watches, and Other Items with Synthesized Speech:
Ann Morris Enterprises catalog, (516) 292-9232
Just for You catalog, (800) 541-7903
Lighthouse Consumer Products catalog, (800) 829-0500
Maxi-Aids catalog, (800) 522-6294
Technology for Independence catalog, (800) 331-8255

Luxo Combo Lamp. Twenty-two-watt fluorescent tube and sixty-watt incandescent bulb with adjustable arm and 9½-inch-diameter shade. Clamp to table or weighted base. $215. Visual Aids catalog, (212) 889-3141 in eastern United States; (415) 221-3201 in western United States.

Big Eye Lamp. High-intensity magnifying lamp. A combination of illumination and magnification. 2× magnifier. Table, $45. Floor, $75. Visual Aids catalog, (212) 889-3141 in eastern United States; (415) 221-3201 in western United States.

Credit-Card Sized Magnifier. Carry it in your wallet in case you need to read menus, maps, package labels, and so forth. Comes with carrying case. $2. Magellan's catalog, (800) 962-4943.

BriteEye. Hundred-watt spotlight reflector bulb with its power reduced electronically to only fifty-three watts, changing its beam of intense white light to a very bright but soft yellowish light, "like a ray of setting sun." Affords high visibility without eye strain. Floor lamp, $100. Visual Aids catalog, (212) 889-3141 in eastern United States; (415) 221-3201 in western United States.

Talkman VI. Plays both four-track (National Library Service) and two-track (standard) tapes. Records with built-in microphone or directly from built-in radio. Includes variable speed control, headphones, and carrying case. $200. Technology for Independence catalog, (800) 331-8255.

Large Print Overlay. Makes the letters on a computer keyboard easier to see. More than 101 keys, blue on ivory. $25 a set. Data-Cal Corporation, 531 East Elliot Road, Suite 145, Chandler, AZ 85225, (800) 223-0123.

Closed Circuit Television (CCTV). Objects placed under camera lens are magnified up to 60 times on 20-inch monitor. Switches from black on white to white on black. Various models from about $3,000. Technolog catalog, (800) 522-6294.

Eye Relief. A large-type word processor that can enlarge the on-screen type to five times normal size. $300. SkiSoft Publishing Corporation, 1644 Massachusetts Avenue, Suite 79, Lexington, MA 02173, (800) 662-3622.

Readers. Four lens strengths and five frames to choose from, using eye chart in the catalog. $10. Bruce Medical Supply catalog, (800) 225-8446.

Language Master Special Edition. A portable "speaking" computer reference incorporating a dictionary, thesaurus, grammar guide, and ten educational games. Typewriter-style keyboard, ¼-inch characters on display screen, headphones. $500. Franklin Electronic Publishers, 122 Burrs Road, Mount Holly, NJ 08060, (800) 762-5382.

Large-Print Books and Periodicals

"Directory of Sources for Books in Large Type, on Audiotape, or Braille," National Library Service. NLS, 1291 Taylor Street, NW, Washington, DC 20542, (800) 424-8567.

Large Print Loan Library. More than three thousand titles circulate by mail, postage FREE. National Association for Visually Handicapped, 22 West 21st Street, 6th Floor, New York, NY 10010, (212) 889-3141.

Large Type Publications. Mainly textbooks and some general interest titles. Catalog. American Printing House for the Blind catalog, (800) 223-1839.

Large Print Books by Mail. Catalog lists a wide variety of best-sellers, mysteries, and cookbooks in hardback and paperback. Books are printed on nonglare paper. Thorndike Press & G.K. Hall Large Print, 200 Old Tappan Road, Old Tappan, NJ 07675-9808, (800) 223-2336.

Large Print Books. Hardcover and paperback editions of popular and classical books by mail. Catalog available. FREE shipping. Ulverscroft Large Print Books, Helen D. Boyle, 279 Boston Street, Guilford, CT 06437, (800) 955-9659.

Isis Large Print Books. Classic and contemporary literature, self-help books, reference works. Catalog available. Transaction Publishers, Rutgers University, New Brunswick, NJ 08903, (908) 932-2280.

Doubleday Large Print Home Library. Fiction and nonfiction. Catalog available. 6550 East 30th Street, P.O. Box 6325, Indianapolis, IN 46206, (800) 688-4442.

Random House. Publications printed in sixteen-point type. Catalog available. 400 Hahn Road, P.O. Box 100, Westminster, MD 21157, (800) 733-3000.

New York Times Large-Type Weekly. Sampling of the week's news and features, crossword puzzle. One year's subscription, $70. NYT, P.O. Box 9564, Uniondale, NY 11555, (800) 631-2580.

World at Large. Tabloid-size biweekly large-type (twenty-point) newsmagazine with stories selected from *U.S. News & World Report,*

Time, and other magazines. News, politics, and large version of Los Angeles *Times* Sunday crossword puzzle. One year's subscription, $40. Sample issue FREE with SSE with $1.47 postage on 9″ × 12″ envelope. World at Large, P.O. Box 190330, Brooklyn, NY 11219, (800) AT-LARGE (285-2743).

Reader's Digest Large-Type Edition. Monthly selection of articles. $9. Reader's Digest Fund for the Blind, P.O. Box 241, Mount Morris, IL 61054, (815) 734-6963.

Books and Periodicals on Audiotape

Reader's Digest and *Newsweek* magazine. Available on four-track cassette. FREE. Requires cassette player, which is available FREE from the National Library Service. American Printing House for the Blind, P.O. Box 6389, Louisville, KY 40206, (800) 223-1839.

"*Newsweek* on Air." Weekly 54-minute audiotape of a radio program that is based on five major stories from the magazine. Ten-week subscription, $30. MARK56 Records, P.O. Box 1, Anaheim, CA 92815, (800) 227-7388.

Audio Magazine Anthology. Articles, fiction, and poetry selections from over one hundred magazines and newspapers. Bimonthly subscription, 8 hours on four-track cassette tapes. FREE. To be used with four-track tape player, provided FREE from the National Library Service. Choice Magazine Listening, P.O. Box 10, Port Washington, NY 11050, (516) 883-8280.

Magazines in Special Media. Lists magazines available FREE in large print, four-track audiotape and disk. FREE. National Library Service, 1291 Taylor Street, NW, Washington, DC 20542, (800) 424-8567.

Audiobooks. Unabridged recorded books to rent for thirty days and return in mailer provided. Classics and current best-sellers. For example, *The Firm* by John Grisham, ten cassettes, 14¾ hours, $17.50; *Crime and Punishment* by Fyodor Dostoyevski, eighteen cassettes, 25½ hours, $23.50. Recorded Books, 270 Skipjack Road, Prince Frederick, MD 20678, (800) 638-1304.

Books on Tape. Unabridged best-sellers in a catalog of more than twenty-five hundred selections for thirty-day rental, postage paid. From five to fifteen cassettes, each with a running time of from 5 to 22 hours, $9 to $20. P.O. Box 7900, Newport Beach, CA 92658, (800) 626-3333.

Services

National Library Service for the Blind and Physically Handicapped. FREE loan of recorded books and magazines for people who cannot see well enough to read print or cannot handle printed material. Special equipment loaned FREE to play recorded material, including headphones or an amplifier. About seventy magazines available with FREE subscriptions. For the participating library nearest you and an application, contact NLS, 1291 Taylor Street, NW, Washington, DC 20542, (800) 424-9100.

National Institute for Rehabilitation Engineering. Help in selecting a computer and a large-screen display that suits your needs. Advice by telephone, personal consultation (for a fee), or referral to a local source. NIRE, P.O. Drawer T, Hewitt, NJ 07421, (800) 736-2216.

Apple Computer Disability Solutions Store. A listing of devices that will help you use a Macintosh computer — for example, a keyboard with a layout that facilitates touch typing with one hand. Includes a list of resources for further information, database of adaptive devices, software programs, publications, and networks. FREE. Apple, P.O. Box 898, Lakewood, NJ 08701, (800) 600-7808.

Computer Access Advice. Technical assistance with computer technology for people with visual problems. Sensory Access Foundation, 385 Sherman Avenue, Suite 2, Palo Alto, CA 94306, (415) 329-0430.

American Printing House for the Blind. Large-type books and magazines, recorded publications, or textbooks on computer disk. Catalog of instructional aids, tools, and supplies. APH, 1839 Frankfort Avenue, P.O. Box 6085, Louisville, KY 40206, (800) 223-1839.

Low Vision Clinics. For information and referral to a clinic near you. American Council of the Blind, 1155 15th Street, NW, Suite 720, Washington, DC 20005, (800) 424-8666.

Support Groups. For a group near you geared specifically for people your age with vision problems, contact National Center for Vision and Aging, 111 East 59th Street, New York, NY 10022, (800) 334-5497.

Periodicals via Radio and Telephone

In Touch Networks. A twenty-four-hour reading of magazines, periodicals, and newspapers for people who can't read them unaided. Available on closed-circuit radio by means of a special receiver that is provided to you FREE. For an affiliate in your area, contact ITN, 15 West 65th Street, New York, NY 10023, (800) 456-3166.

Telephone Accessible Newspaper. Listen to the news over the phone with Touch-Tone selection of stories you want to hear. May be a toll-free call. FREE or with a small monthly subscription fee, depending on location. Service available in selected areas. For information, contact the National Federation of the Blind, 1800 Johnson Street, Baltimore, MD 21230, (410) 659-9314.

National Association of Radio Reading Services. One hundred forty stations nationwide offer programming specifically for those who can't use newspapers, magazines, and books. Special receivers are provided FREE. To locate stations with this service, contact NARRS, 2100 Wharton Street, Suite 140, Pittsburgh, PA 15203, (412) 488-3944.

Publications

"Products for People with Low Vision." A list of sources for closed-circuit television, magnifiers, and other products. American Foundation for the Blind, National Technology Center, 11 Penn Plaza, Suite 300, New York, NY 10001, (800) AF-BLIND (232-5463).

"Low Vision Resource Guide." List of sources for low-vision products and service providers. Foundation Fighting Blindness, 1401 Mount Royal Avenue, 4th Floor, Baltimore, MD 21217, (800) 683-5555.

Living with Low Vision: A Resource Guide for People with Sight Loss, Resources for Rehabilitation. A large-print directory of services, organizations, products, and publications that can be of help to people who have low vision. $35. Resources for Rehabilitation, 33 Bedford Street, Suite 19A, Lexington, MA 02173, (617) 862-6455.

"Resources for Individuals with Visual Impairment," National Eye Care Project. A list of organizations and sources for reading material and devices, with services and products for a person who has difficulty seeing. FREE. NECP, P.O. Box 429098, San Francisco, CA 94142, (800) 222-EYES (3937).

"Low Vision Questions and Answers: Definitions, Devices, Services," American Foundation for the Blind. Explanations about low vision with photos of how people with certain vision limitations see and suggestions for what can be done to improve low vision. FREE. AFB, 11 Penn Plaza, Suite 300, New York, NY 10001, (800) AF-BLIND (232-5463).

"I Keep Five Pairs of Glasses in a Flower Pot" by Henrietta Levner. Poignant, realistic description of one person's adaptation to vision loss. $2. National Association for Visually Handicapped, 22 West 21st Street, New York, NY 10010, (212) 889-3141.

Organizations

National Eye Institute. Information on current research into eye care and disease. NEI, National Institutes of Health, Building 31, Room 6A-32, 9000 Rockville Pike, Bethesda, MD 20892, (301) 496-5248.

American Foundation for the Blind. Information, referrals, publications. National Technology Center for evaluation and demonstration of computer equipment or reading machines and advice about different models. Also a database of manufacturers. AFB, 11 Penn Plaza, Suite 300, New York, NY 10001, (800) AF-BLIND (232-5463).

National Association for Visually Handicapped. Publications, referral. Discussion groups for seniors and clearinghouse of information about low-vision centers. FREE large-print loan library. Newsletter and catalog of visual aids available. NAVH, 22 West 21st Street, New York, NY 10010, (212) 889-3141, or 3201 Balboa Street, San Francisco, CA 94121, (415) 221-3201.

Lighthouse National Center for Vision and Aging. Information and resources about age-related eye disorders, low-vision clinics and training for independent living, self-help groups. Newsletter, videos, referrals, catalog of low-vision products, vision rehabilitation. NCVA, 111 East 59th Street, New York, NY 10022, (800) 334-5497.

American Council of the Blind. Information about causes and treatment of blindness and visual impairment, referrals to low-vision clinics, local services, and support groups. Publications, including lists of computer resources, self-help guides, and information from other organizations. Newsletter with ads for used equipment. 1155 15th Street, NW, Suite 720, Washington, DC 20005, (800) 424-8666.

Council of Citizens with Low Vision International. Support groups, information, and referrals. Large-print newsletter. CCLVI, 5707 Brockton Drive, Number 302, Indianapolis, IN 46220, (800) 733-2258.

Chapter 17

Getting Enough Sleep

To keep your mind fresh for the day's activities, you need to sleep well at night. When you feel rested during the day and don't need to depend on coffee or other caffeinated drinks to stay awake, you know you are getting enough sleep. "Enough" may range from five to ten hours a night, an amount that isn't affected by your age but is determined by genetic factors.

Research finds that as people grow older, the quality, rather than the quantity, of their sleep changes: Dreaming sleep, short periods of rapid eye movement (REM), shrinks from about a quarter to closer to a fifth of total sleep time. The deeper, quieter sleep (non-REM) also declines by about one half by age sixty-five. Since you are sleeping more lightly, you are liable to be awakened by noises that you used to sleep through: a barking dog, a snoring mate, even an unsettling dream.

People age sixty and over are found to awaken as many as 150 times a night, compared with about 5 times for younger adults. Even if this waking period is only a few seconds and not remembered in the morning, you may feel tired the following day. If disturbed sleep means you must nap in the afternoon, your sleep schedule can be thrown off kilter since naps count toward your daily sleep total. If you do nap, keep to a schedule, preferably midafternoon.

Sleep disruptions also can be due to health conditions, medications, or depression. Some people have a condition called restless legs syndrome that creates an uncomfortable sensation in the legs that is relieved by keeping them in motion, making sleeping impossible. You may wake at night because of snoring or breathing problems, such as the momentary cessation of breathing called apnea. Sleep apnea may interrupt your sleep, leaving you tired the next day if it occurs frequently. Snoring may become progressively louder until it crescendos to a loud gasp or snort that may awaken you briefly. Apnea and snoring are more likely to occur if you are overweight.

Snoring may be hereditary and may become more of a problem as you get older. After age sixty, 60 percent of men and 40 percent of women snore regularly.

To Control Snoring

- Sleep on your side, not your back.
- Sew a tennis ball onto your pajama at the back to discourage you from rolling over.
- Wear an electronic wristband that sounds an alarm to wake you if noise exceeds a certain volume.
- Use either special pillows designed to encourage correct positioning of the head or two pillows.
- Control your weight.
- Maintain a proper exercise routine.
- Avoid alcohol, a stimulant, within three hours of bedtime.

The most common sleep problem, experienced by about twenty million people, is insomnia — insufficiently restful sleep — characterized by frequent waking, taking more than one-half hour to fall asleep, or waking too early without being able to fall back to sleep in less than a half hour.

Whatever the cause, if you don't get enough sleep, your mental ability, physical energy, and attitude are likely to be adversely affected. It can affect your short-term memory, your ability to make decisions or concentrate, and your reaction time. You may be more subject to accidents and somewhat unaware of your surroundings.

Temporary insomnia may result from jet lag, personal problems, or stress. Consult a physician when, despite your own efforts, sleep problems persist for longer than two weeks.

Putting Yourself to Sleep

To relax

- Soak in a warm (body temperature) bath two to four hours before bed.
- Increase exercise in the late afternoon, at least three hours before bed. Physical fatigue helps your body relax.
- Eliminate stress.
- Do deep-breathing exercises before bedtime or in bed.
- Don't smoke; nicotine is a stimulant.
- Having sexual relations helps some people feel sleepy.

To drink

- Milk or herbal tea
- No alcoholic beverages after dinner
- No beverage containing caffeine after 4:00 P.M. (coffee, black tea, soft drinks, hot chocolate)

To eat

- Don't overeat close to bedtime, but don't go to bed hungry. Try carbohydrates and protein for a bedtime snack: crackers, not cookies, and milk.
- Avoid foods that give you digestive problems, particularly those containing the flavor enhancer MSG, as well as fats, spicy foods, and especially garlic.

To prepare for bed:

- Arrange your pillow so that your head is in the same relation to your shoulders and neck as if you were standing. Use a firm pillow if you sleep on your side, medium firm if you sleep on your back, soft if you sleep on your stomach.
- If you don't fall asleep after about fifteen minutes, get out of bed. Do something, and try later.
- Don't approach bedtime with dread because falling asleep is too daunting a challenge for you. Let sleep overtake you; don't wait for it.
- Reserve your bed or bedroom only for sleep and sex.
- Use an electric blanket only for the falling-asleep period; attach a timer to turn it off after one or two hours. Your body temperature rises during the night, and being over heated may awaken you.
- Turn your clock to the wall.
- Determine your bedtime to allow you to wake at the same

time each day. If you are tired too early in the evening, plan an activity, go for a walk, do your supermarket shopping at night, or do the laundry, so that you delay going to sleep until the established time.

- Prepare relaxation thoughts, either visualizations (try numbers), monotonous repetitions, calling up memories, or playing recall games. Avoid thinking about problems you need to solve.
- Go to sleep only when you feel sleepy and don't use an alarm clock to wake up.

Treatment for episodes of stubborn insomnia may include *short-term* use of sleeping pills (long-term use may cause persistent drowsiness during the day and other dangerous side effects, including addiction).

To establish your bedtime and wake-up times, determine how much total sleep you need to feel rested, decide on a convenient time for you to wake up, and figure your bedtime from that. Then always keep your wake-up time constant, making adjustments only to your bedtime. Restrict your time in bed to the total sleep time you need. Then get up even if you haven't slept the full amount. The next time you may. Don't stay in bed too long. If you have a disturbed night, keep to the original timetable, and try to avoid taking an afternoon nap. Think of insomnia as a bad habit that you can change by adjusting your behavior.

If you want to change a bedtime-wake-up pattern, gradually adjust your bedtime every few days by an hour or two until you're back to a desirable schedule.

Resources

Sources for pillows and other products for bed comfort and suggested sleeping positions to alleviate back pain are enumerated in Chapter 11, "Overcoming Obstacles to Being Active."

Products

No-Snore Pillow. Incorporates a roll of foam that fits under the neck, tilting the chin enough to keep breathing passages open. $18. Pillows for Ease catalog, (800) 347-1486.

Neck-Preserving Pillow. Maintains spinal alignment for sleeping on back or side. Supports head, neck, and shoulders. Firm or soft. Standard, $45. Traveler size, $38. Pillows for Ease catalog, (800) 347-1486.

Digital Sound Conditioner. "White noise" machine with seven different sounds from which to choose, among them surf, babbling brook, waterfalls, and rain. Customize for rate and intensity. Allows you to add other digitally recorded sound effects. $150. Signals catalog, (800) 699-9696.

Services

Accredited Sleep Centers. Centers that provide diagnosis and treatment of sleep-related disorders and are accredited by the American Sleep Disorders Association. For centers near you, contact National Sleep Foundation, 1367 Connecticut Avenue, NW, Suite 200, Washington, DC 20036.

Publications

"The Good Night Guide," Better Sleep Council. Summary of sleep needs, falling-asleep techniques, and bedding. FREE. BSC, P.O. Box 19534, Alexandria, VA 22320, (703) 683-8371.

Sleep Right in Five Nights: A Clear and Effective Guide for Conquering Insomnia by James Perl, Ph.D. Techniques for more restful sleep and a self-diagnosis questionnaire to help you pinpoint causes. Suggestions include utilizing your wakeful time and waking every day at the same time. 1993. Quill/William Morrow.

"The Nature of Sleep," National Sleep Foundation. A review of various sleep disorders and their symptoms. FREE. NSF, 1367 Connecticut Avenue, NW, Suite 200, Washington, DC 20036.

"Sleep as We Grow Older," American Sleep Disorders Association. A description of age-related changes in sleep patterns some people experience. National Sleep Foundation, 1367 Connecticut Avenue, NW, Suite 200, Washington, DC 20036.

Sleep: Problems and Solutions by Quentin Regestein, M.D., and David Richie. A discussion of sleep, including an explanation of your "sleep clock," stages of sleep, and such disturbances as sleepwalking and some treatment options. 1990. Consumers Union.

"Breathing Disorders During Sleep," National Center on Sleep Disorders Research. A review of breathing disorders that affect sleep, including sleep apnea. FREE. NCSDR, National Heart, Lung, and Blood Institute Information Center, P.O. Box 30105, Bethesda, MD 20824, (301) 251-1222.

Organizations

National Sleep Foundation. Education and the dissemination of information about sleep disorders. NSF, 1367 Connecticut Avenue, NW, Suite 200, Washington, DC 20036.

National Center on Sleep Disorders Research. Supports and conducts research, and provides education about sleep disorders. NCSDR, National Heart, Lung, and Blood Institute, P.O. Box 30105, Bethesda, MD 20824, (301) 251-1222.

Restless Legs Syndrome Foundation. Information and current research on the syndrome. FREE with SSE. RLS Foundation, P.O. Box 314, 514 Daniels Street, Raleigh, NC 27605.

Chapter 18

Continuing to Learn

Healthy minds, like healthy bodies, perform at their best when they're active. Your mind retains its sharpness when you are interested in the world, learning new things, and involved in events around you. Travel is inherently educational and stimulating and can be enhanced when combined with formal study. Courses in many subjects are available at local cultural institutions or for home study, and television is a source of information about current events, history, and general cultural topics.

TRAVELING

Seeing new places can be exciting and stimulating, as well as a source of wonderful memories. Travel is a learning experience that you can absorb on the spot and appreciate again at home, as you look through your photographs and remember what you saw. There are so many ways to travel; you won't have trouble finding a mode that suits your style. You can choose a guided tour or go solo, relax or plan a strenuous activity, stay in one place or tour, go first-class or budget, or combine some of these options.

There are travel agencies that specialize in senior travel. Some even match single individuals who want companionship or to economize by using double-room rates. If you book your own accommodations, remember to ask for discounts, usually available for travelers over age fifty, even on foreign airlines and hotels. Discounts often are available for members of certain clubs or organizations

348

(AAA, AARP), so don't be shy about asking.

When you make hotel reservations, find out if there are grab bars in the bathrooms should you need them and if there is a long flight of stairs or other inconveniences to negotiate. Adaptation of hotels and sight-seeing destinations has made these more easily accessible for wheelchairs, and enhancements for travelers with hearing or vision problems are more common. For example, in Washington, D.C., the subway system is wheelchair-accessible, and the view from the top of the Washington Monument can be seen with a periscope. The National Park System has braille trail symbols, barrier-free facilities for wheelchair users, and closed-captioned films at its facilities. In larger American cities, such as New York City, theaters and concert halls are being altered to attract wider audiences, including people with hearing or vision problems, to cultural events; some restaurants are installing wheelchair ramps; and other such adaptations are being made.

You may enjoy renting a recreation vehicle (RV), combining hotel and transportation in one. Staying in an RV campground is an opportunity for social interchange, and the RV life gives you the freedom to set your own pace rather than keep up with a tour. Besides economy, RV living eliminates the need for frequent packing (and unpacking) and dealing with variably convenient hotels.

Travelers should take special precautions to protect their health while away from home.

Medical Reminders for Travelers

- Take an extra pair of eyeglasses and a copy of your most recent prescription.
- Prepare a concise medical history, particularly with reference to any conditions you currently have and the treatment that has been prescribed for you. List previous surgeries, major illnesses, and your current physicians' names and phone numbers.
- List medications you are taking, their strengths, and dosages. Note the chemical names too.
- List a family member or close friend as an emergency contact should you fall ill. A good place for this name and phone number is next to your own identification — either your passport or driver's license.

Medical issues are less urgent when you travel in America; Medicare or your private insurance will cover your medical expenses in the United States and, in some instances, in Mexico and Canada. If you travel abroad, you may wish to consider travel health insurance. This shouldn't be confused with insurance against trip cancellation or for airline travel. The health coverage you are offered should include hospital and physician expenses and even medical evacuation by helicopter, which may help you get access to medical care in a major foreign city or even the United States. This insurance may cost between $3 and $6 a day.

As you plan your foreign travel, especially to places where you don't know the language, find out how to ask for help. You may need or write down some phrases so that you can point to one. For example, "I need a doctor [cardiologist, allergist]." "Where is the nearest pharmacy [emergency room, optometrist]?"

The U.S. State Department offers the following travel tips:

- Sign your passport, and be sure it doesn't expire before your return. Photocopy and keep separate the identification page to facilitate replacement.
- Before leaving home, follow current events at your destination, and find out about any official travel advisories.
- Follow local customs and laws.
- Contact the U.S. consul in an emergency.

U.S. consulates are a source of help and advice in foreign countries, but in a medical emergency their assistance is limited to the names of doctors and instructions for wiring funds from your home bank. If you travel with specialized equipment, even something as mundane as an electric wheelchair, it's best to alert an airline or hotel in case there are special restrictions or assistance it needs to provide to you.

Resources

Booklets for recording your personal medical information, pill containers, and medical identification bracelets are listed in Chapter 14, "Preparing for Emergencies."

Products

Swiss Army Traveler Set. A Swiss Army knife with its tiny tools, packaged in a compact leather case with a flashlight, magnifying glass, compass, and thermometer. $70. Magellan's catalog, (800) 962-4943.

Traveling Hearing Gear. A suitcase containing a telecaption decoder, telephone display, telephone alert flasher, strobe light smoke detector, bed-vibrating alarm clock, and door-knock alert. $800. HITEC Group International catalog, (800) 288-8303.

Personal Health Kit. Equipment for bandaging, cleaning wounds. $40. TravelSmith catalog, (800) 950-1600.

Easy-Care, Lightweight Travel Clothes. Packable clothes for every climate. Some are made of no-iron fabrics that can be folded or rolled to save space. TravelSmith catalog, (800) 950-1600.

International Travel Medical Kit. Familiar products to deal with health needs in foreign countries. Includes a variety of bandages and over-the-counter medications for common conditions. $50. Magellan's catalog, (800) 962-4943.

Survival Tool. A stainless steel rectangle, 3⅛ by 2 inches, with tools carved along the edges. Includes a screwdriver, saw, ruler, can opener, and more. Carrying case and instructions. $10. Magellan's catalog, (800) 962-4943.

Discount Travel Opportunities

Travel Clubs. Members are eligible for special discounts, including travel, hotels, insurance, and other benefits. Age limits vary.

American Express, P.O. Box 31562, Salt Lake City, UT 84131, (800) 423-6444

Amtrak, (800) USA-RAIL (872-7245)

Days Inn September Days Club, P.O. Box 4001, Harlan, IA 51593, (800) 241-5050

Howard Johnson Travel Saver Plus Club, P.O. Box 5115, Harlan, IA 51593, (800) 257-2298

Sears Mature Outlook, 6001 North Clark Street, Chicago, IL 60660, (800) 336-6330

TraveLodge, 1973 Friendship Drive, El Cajon, CA 92020, (800) 545-6343

TWA Senior Travel Coupons, P.O. Box 733, Plymouth Meeting, PA 19462, (800) 221-2000

Worldwide Discount Travel Club, 1674 Meridian Avenue, P.O. Box 855, Miami Beach, FL 33139, (305) 534-2082

Golden Age Passport. Americans age sixty-two and older may enter all national parks, some state parks, recreation areas, and monuments FREE for a lifetime. Purchase in person at National Park Service locations that charge a fee. $10. More information from NPS, Office of Public Inquiries, P.O. Box 37127, Washington, DC 20013, (202) 208-4747.

Services

Penfriends and Partnership. Personal ads for travel partners. Saga Holidays, 222 Berkeley Street, Boston, MA 02116, (800) 343-0273.

Travel Companion Exchange. Helps you find a same-sex or opposite-sex traveling partner. Six-month introductory rate for same-sex listings, $36. Sample copy available FREE. TCE, P.O. Box 833, Amityville, NY 11701, (516) 454-0880.

Golden Companions. Travel network for people who seek companions age forty-five and over. Membership includes newsletter, mail forwarding, and access to voice mail exchange. P.O. Box 5249, Reno, NV 89513, (702) 324-2227.

Theater Access Project. Offers of preferential seating to theater, dance, and music performances for people with visual, hearing, or physical impairments. Theater Development Fund, 1501 Broadway, New York, NY 10036, (212) 221-0013.

Travel Information Service. Information and advice for travelers with physical or medical requirements. FREE. TIS, MossRehab Hospital, 1200 West Tabor Road, Philadelphia, PA 19141, (215) 456-9600.

International Association for Medical Assistance to Travellers. FREE membership that includes a directory of qualified English-speaking physicians worldwide who adhere to a fixed fee schedule (office visit, $45). Publications available regarding malaria, climate conditions, immunizations. IAMAT, 417 Center Street, Lewiston, NY 14092, (716) 754-4883.

Traveling Nurses' Network. RNs available to meet your health care needs while you travel. Arrangements for medical equipment and other special needs. TNN, P.O. Box 129, Vancouver, WA 98666, (206) 694-2462.

International Traveler's Hot Line. Information about which immunizations are needed for your destination, as well as medical cautions and alerts about outbreaks of diseases and other health data. Centers for Disease Control and Prevention, (404) 332-4559.

U.S. Consular Information Sheets and Travel Warnings. These describe conditions for each country's entry or currency regulations, existing political disturbances, areas of instability, and other information to help you plan your trip. Warnings are issued in cases where travel is discouraged. FREE. Available from: (1) *passport agencies.* Washington Passport Agency, 1425 K Street, NW, Washington, DC 20524, (202) 647-0518, or one of the other twelve offices; (2) *hot line.* Twenty-four hours a day with Touch-Tone phone, (202) 647-5225; (3) *by computer.* Consular Affairs Bulletin Board, (202) 647-9225, with software set to N-8-1; (4) *airlines' ticket agents.*

Senior Tours

Close Up Foundation. Weeklong trip to Washington, DC, including discussion of national and international issues and meetings and seminars with legislators and policy makers. For travelers age fifty and over. Accommodations and all meals, $981. 44 Canal Center Plaza, Alexandria, VA 22314, (800) 232-2000.

Outdoor Vacations for Women over 40. Hiking, biking, camping, skiing vacations for women over age forty and some multigenerational trips including women over age eighteen. For example: a three-night Windjammer cruise on a schooner, $525; biking and barging in Amsterdam, Holland, ten nights, $2,600. P.O. Box 200, Groton, MA 01450, (508) 448-3331.

Hostelling International-American Youth Hostels Discovery Tours. "Youth" includes all ages! Special groups for participants age fifty and over, though most tours are mainly skill-rated rather than age-restricted. You are responsible for transportation to and from the beginning and end points of the tour. For example, three weeks of van travel and hiking in Alaska parks, average four to seven miles per day over moderately hilly terrain, age fifty and over, $1,525. Tours also available in Europe. Membership includes access to low-cost, simple accommodations in hostels. HI/AYH, 733

15th Street, NW, Washington, DC 20005, (202) 783-6161.

Walking the World. Outdoor trips to appreciate natural aspects of an area for active adventurers age fifty and over. United States and abroad. For example, eleven-day walking tour of Scotland, seven to ten miles a day, mainly moderate, $2,000. P.O. Box 1186, Fort Collins, CO 80522, (800) 340-9255.

Country Walkers. Travel vacations for adults. Walks and hikes in various parts of the world. Between four and twelve miles of easy-to-moderate terrain a day, walking from three to five hours, led by local residents experienced in the natural and historical details of the area. For example, seven days in Nova Scotia, easy-to-moderate terrain, $1,360. P.O. Box 180, Waterbury, VT 05676, (802) 244-1387.

Senior Escorted Tours. No age requirements for trips to such places as the Catskills, Orlando, or Australia. For example, eighteen-day national park trip, most breakfasts and dinners, including airfare, $2,600. P.O. Box 400, Cape May Court House, NJ 08210, (800) 222-1254.

Seniors Abroad International Homestay. Host a visitor in your home or be hosted on your travels in the United States or abroad. For example, three weeks in Scandinavia; two days each week in a hotel, five days with hosts in Denmark, Sweden, and Norway, $2,500. 12533 Pacato Circle North, San Diego, CA 92128.

Evergreen Club. If you can host one or two people in your home, you will get a directory so that you can take advantage of the $10 or $15 a night rate. SSE for information. P.O. Box 44094, Washington, DC 20026, (703) 237-9777.

Saga Holidays. For mature travelers, a variety of tours and cruises, educational programs, garden tours. Includes medical insurance and cancellation protection. For example, twelve nights in Poland and the Czech Republic, $2,300. You can also join Saga Club, a membership arrangement that provides special discounts, a newsletter, and correspondence exchange. 222 Berkeley Street, Boston, MA 02116, (800) 343-0273.

Grand Circle Travel. Extended vacations, escorted tours, cruises, and "soft" adventures. Accommodations selected without steps, not on hills, and with good elevator service. For example, two weeks in an apartment in London, including airfare, $1,200. 347 Congress Street, Boston, MA 02210, (800) 859-0852.

AARP Travel Experience from American Express. Escorted,

"soft" adventures, loosely structured trips. 400 Pinnacle Way, Suite 450, Norcross, GA 30071, (800) 927-0111.

Flying Wheels Travel. Group or individualized tours and cruises and arrangements for people who use wheelchairs. Tours outside the United States are all escorted. For example, fifteen days in China and other countries in the Orient, $3,600. 143 West Bridge Street, P.O. Box 382, Owatonna, MN 55060, (800) 535-6790.

50 Plus Club. Two-week tours at first-class hotels. Some examples: Spa Tour of Italy with side trips, $2,100; seventeen days in Israel, $2,500. A.J.S. 50 Plus Club, 177 Beach 116th Street, Rockaway Park, NY 11694, (800) 221-5002, or in New York call (718) 945-5900.

Go-Ahead Vacations. Tours for active mature travelers to all parts of the world. For example, a week home stay with a family in London, including airfare and two meals a day, $765; Russia and the Baltics, seventeen days, $2,500. 1 Memorial Drive, Cambridge, MA 02142, (800) 242-4686.

Audiotapes and Videotapes

Tours on Tape. Audiotapes and videotapes as a travel preview or to accompany you as a walking or auto tour guide of U.S. and foreign destinations. For example, 90-minute audiotape tour of northern and southern New Mexico, $14. Catalog. Tours, P.O. Box 227, 2 Elbrook Drive, Allendale, NJ 07401, (201) 236-1666.

Publications

Travel Books. Catalog of guidebooks and maps available. The Complete Traveller Bookstore, 199 Madison Avenue, New York, NY 10016, (212) 685-9007.

"Directory of Physicians Who Specialize in Travelers' Health and Tropical Medicine" by Dr. Leonard C. Marcus. Doctors listed are located mostly in the United States and Canada. FREE with SSE, 8½" × 11" envelope with $1.01 postage. Travelers' Health and Immunization Services, 148 Highland Avenue, Newton, MA 02165.

InterContinental Medical Directory. A list of hospitals and physicians for the countries on your itinerary. Names of specialists available in case you want to contact them in advance. $29 for three countries, $3 for each additional country. InterContinental Medical Ltd., 2720 Enterprise Parkway, Suite 106, Richmond, VA 23294, (800) 426-8828.

"Directory of English-Speaking Physicians," International Association for Medical Assistance to Travellers. Doctors included have agreed to a set payment schedule for members. Membership FREE. IAMAT, 417 Center Street, Lewiston, NY 14092.

"World Immunization Chart," International Association for Medical Assistance to Travellers. Lists required and recommended immunizations and routine immunizations that may need boosters. FREE. IAMAT, 417 Center Street, Lewiston, NY 14092.

The Diabetic Traveler. A quarterly newsletter designed to assist people who have diabetes plan safe travel. $20 a year. Diabetic Traveler, P.O. Box 8223 RW, Stamford, CT 06905, (203) 327-5832.

"Insulin Adjustment During Jet Travel Across Multiple Time Zones." A credit card-size guide specifying adjustments for both eastbound and westbound travel. FREE with SSE. Diabetic Traveler, P.O. Box 8223 RW, Stamford, CT 06905, (203) 327-5832.

"Management of Diabetes During Intercontinental Travel" by Edward A. Benson, M.D. A brief guide to what to bring with you, how to adjust your dosage, and how to find medical assistance. FREE with SSE. Diabetic Traveler, P.O. Box 8223 RW, Stamford, CT 06905, (203) 327-5832.

"Travel Tips for Older Americans," Bureau of Consular Affairs, U.S. Department of State. Health, safety, and travel information. $1. Superintendent of Documents, U.S. Government Printing Office, Washington, DC 20402, (202) 783-3238.

"World Climate Charts," International Association for Medical Assistance to Travelers. A set of twenty-four charts detailing climate, clothing suggestions, sanitary conditions, water and food purity worldwide, and specifics for 1,440 cities. Donation requested. IAMAT, 417 Center Street, Lewiston, NY 14092.

"Going Abroad, 101 Tips for Mature Travelers," Grand Circle Travel. Good travel advice and reminders. FREE. Grand Circle, 347 Congress Street, Boston, MA 02210, (800) 221-2610.

The 50+ Traveler's Guidebook by Anita Williams and Merrimac Dillon. A broad selection of accommodations, health-oriented vacations, hotel resorts with special programs, guided tours, and a good assortment of ideas and resources. 1991. St. Martin's Press.

Get Up and Go! A Guide for the Mature Traveler by Gene and Adele Malott. Nuts-and-bolts information for senior travelers, lists of resources, tips on currency exchange, and other practical matters. 1989. Gateway Books.

Mature Traveler. A monthly newsletter featuring special issues on airfare, hotel, and other travel discounts for those age fifty and over. $30 subscription. P.O. Box 50400, Reno, NV 89513, (702) 786-7419.

"Information Sources: Camping and the RV Lifestyle," Recreation Vehicle Industry Association. Contacts for renting RVs, locating campgrounds, publications, and RV clubs. FREE. RVIA, P.O. Box 2999, Reston, VA 22090, (703) 620-6003.

"Go Camping America Camping Vacation Planner," Recreation Vehicle Industry Association. Resources for locating campgrounds near your destination, a guide to different types of RVs, and sources for further information. FREE. RVIA, P.O. Box 2999, Reston, VA 22090, (800) 47-SUNNY (477-8669).

Travel Smart. Monthly newsletter of travel bargains and deals. One year, $37. 40 Beechdale Road, Dobbs Ferry, NY 10522, (800) FARE-OFF (327-3633).

Access for All: A Guide for People with Disabilities to New York City Cultural Institutions, Hospital Audiences, Inc., and WCBS News-radio 88. Includes physical accessibility information for two hundred restaurants, theaters, and cultural institutions in New York City and services for people with hearing or vision problems. Includes location of rest rooms, water fountains, parking facilities. Updates available. $5. HAI, 220 West 42nd Street, 13th Floor, New York, NY 10036, (212) 575-7663.

Travel Insurance

Medical Insurance and Travelers Assistance. A central assistance office coordinates payments, monitors treatment, and provides advice. $100,000 of comprehensive medical insurance for travelers under age seventy-six or $50,000 between ages seventy-six and eighty-four. $3 per day, $100 deductible. Wallach & Company, 107 West Federal Street, P.O. Box 480, Middleburg, VA 22117, (800) 237-6615.

Companies That Offer Travel Insurance:
Access America, (800) 284-8300
Health Care Abroad, (800) 237-6615
International Legal Defense, (215) 977-9982

Mutual of Omaha Travel Assure, (800) 228-9792
Travelers' Travel Insurance Pak, (800) 243-3174
US Assist, (800) 756-5900

International SOS Assistance. If you become ill while traveling, the company directs you to an English-speaking physician. If necessary, FREE emergency evacuation to the United States is arranged, and emergency message transmission to relatives, access to a lawyer, and other services are provided. $40 per person for a fourteen-day trip. P.O. Box 11568, Philadelphia, PA 19116, (800) 523-8930.

Organizations

Society for the Advancement of Travel for the Handicapped. Referrals and information about traveling when you have special access requirements. SATH, 347 5th Avenue, Suite 610, New York, NY 10016, (212) 447-7284.

Recreational Vehicle Industry Association. Information and publications about recreational vehicles and the RV lifestyle. RVIA, P.O. Box 2999, Reston, VA 22090, (703) 620-6003.

Good Sam Club. An emergency service for recreational vehicles. Also offers discounts and other membership benefits. 64 Inverness Drive East, Englewood, CO 80155, (800) 234-3450.

Loners on Wheels (LOWS). A group of single people who like camping and have recreational vehicles. 2940 Lane Drive, Concord, CA 94518.

Worldwide Discount Travel Club. Members receive notice of last-minute spaces available on cruises, airlines, and tours at a discount of up to 50 percent. Travel Club, 1674 Meridian Avenue, P.O. Box 855, Miami Beach, FL 33139, (305) 534-2082.

Education and Travel

If travel is a learning experience in itself, imagine what happens when it's linked with an educational component! You learn the backgrounds of places you visit, the histories and cultures of the people you meet. Sometimes a course or two is simply combined with a lovely setting or takes place at an academic institution. These opportunities are becoming more numerous and make a week's vacation a multifaceted stay.

Services

Interhostel. International study-travel program for those age fifty and over, led by local educators who explain local culture and historical and cultural sites. For example, ten nights in Jerusalem, two nights in a kibbutz guesthouse, and one night in Tel Aviv, $2,700. Accommodations are frequently on campuses and include three meals a day. Participants should be in good health. C/o University of New Hampshire, 6 Garrison Avenue, Durham, NH 03824, (800) 733-9753.

Smithsonian Odyssey Tours. Lectures and excursions accompanied by both a study leader and a tour manager for combination learning and travel. For example, sixteen-night multicity tour of Greece, $3,200. C/o Saga International Holidays, 222 Berkeley Street, Boston, MA 02116, (800) 258-5885.

Elderhostel. An education adventure offering stimulating activities with others age sixty and over. Also offers short-term academic programs by educational institutions around the world and low-cost, weeklong academic programs. Experience culture and traditions of the location. Abroad or United States and Canada. For example, a weeklong residential study program in liberal arts at a college or university, about $300. No homework, tests, or grades. International programs last two to four weeks, each week at a different site. Meals usually are the indigenous food of the country; no special diets accommodated. For regular sight-seeing, stay longer. 75 Federal Street, Boston, MA 02110, (617) 426-8056.

Road Scholar Program. International learning programs for travelers fifty-five years of age and over. Guided tours "off the beaten tourist paths" with an educational component related to the country you're visiting. For example, university program: three-week study of cathedrals: Bristol, London, Reims. $2,700; sixteen-night "Chinese Civilization: Past and Present": Shanghai, Beijing, and other cities. $3,800. Saga Holidays, 222 Berkeley Street, Boston, MA 02116, (800) 621-2151.

Chautauqua Institution. A 358-acre bucolic resort with cultural and educational offerings. Summer packages include accommodations and entry to some events such as symphony performances, lectures, popular concerts. Theme weeks are offered with daily lectures on a topic, and opera and theater performances available. For example, three nights at lakeside hotel with meals, $334. Chautauqua Institution, P.O. Box 28, Chautauqua, NY 14722, (800) 836-ARTS (2787).

Archaeological Excavations. A week assisting exploration of Pueblo culture and history by working with artifacts in the lab and excavating in the field. $800. Cultural art workshops and tours of historical sites available. Crow Canyon Archaeological Center, 23390 County Road K, Cortez, CO 81321, (800) 422-8975.

Folkways Institute. Educational adventures for travelers age fifty-five and over. Some examples: three-week Sherpa cultural trek in the Himalayas with tent accommodations and porters carrying the gear, $3,800, one week walking and hiking in the Swiss Alps, $2,650. Folkways Institute, 14600 SE Aldridge Road, Portland, OR 97236, (800) 225-4666.

Publications

Learning Vacations by Gerson G. Eisenberg. Five hundred education travel programs, worldwide, organized by subject matter (such as music, gastronomy, the outdoors) and other special categories. Not just a listing but a summary of the courses, costs, and comments. 1989. Peterson's Guides.

TAKING COURSES

To keep your mind alert, you may decide to take a class or read books on your own. Public libraries often offer "mobile" services that bring books to your home, or you can order from mail-order catalogs, sometimes at discount prices. If you have deferred your education, you can decide to reenter college, perhaps just for a few courses or perhaps to complete requirements for a degree.

Colleges find that older students learn as well as younger ones; flexible entrance requirements often allow credit for life experience. Courses on a wide variety of subjects can be taken in a number of ways, depending on the facilities available in your community.

- Enroll in a college or university as a resident or nonresident.
- Audit courses that interest you. You may attend classes

and follow assignments, but there are no papers, no exams, no credit. Inquire about availability at the institution.

- Take a course at the local community college. Usually there are no prerequisites and you get no credit.
- Courses of a practical nature are often offered to adults in evening schools.
- Courses may be taught by your peers, organized by a local learning institution.
- Museums, botanical gardens, or other cultural institutions may offer courses related to their specialties.
- Look into home study or correspondence courses, computer-linked courses, phone-linked courses.
- Check on courses on audiotape, videotape, or television.

Returning students often fear they have forgotten how to study, or don't have the skills needed to succeed in an academic setting, or will be intimidated by the other (younger) students. To allay these worries, you might start in private with a home study course and build on that experience in a school setting. After time out of school it is easy to underestimate skills you have accumulated in your work environment or as a homemaker that are useful for learning. Returning students may be more organized, have broader general knowledge, and understand aspects of human nature and life events with more clarity than a student just out of high school. A study of older learners at a community college found improvements in depression, social satisfaction, and health problems, but the good effects disappeared six weeks after the programs ended.

If you need help holding a book or turning pages, you can use a book stand and a battery-operated page turner or a lap desk.

Resources

Products

Pagemate. Book holder keeps pages flat. $25. Touch Turner, 443 View Ridge Drive, Everett, WA 98203, (206) 252-1541.

Easi-Reader Bookstand. Holds all reading material open without hands. Lightweight chrome-plated steel, folds flat. $6. Available in office supply or book stores or directly from the manufacturer: Hoyle

Products, P.O. Box 606, Fillmore, CA 93016, (800) 345-1950 or, in California call (805) 524-1211.

Wooden Desk Top Reading Stand. Tilts to five positions, has page holder, and 18- by 23¾-inch surface will accommodate large-print books. $83. American Printing House for the Blind catalog, (800) 223-1839.

Lightweight Folding Book Stand. Wire book holder. $6. Visual Aids catalog, (212) 889-3141 in eastern United States; (415) 221-3201 in western United States.

Mydesc. A tilt-top acrylic desktop attached to a frame that is stabilized by a sofa pillow, bed mattress, or chair cushion. $320. Also available for scooters and wheelchairs. Mydesc, 476 Ellis Street, Mountain View, CA 94043, (800) 4-MYDESC (469-3372).

Book Butler. Spring-loaded posts hold pages open and allow easy turning. $16. AfterTherapy catalog, (800) 235-7054.

Touch Turner. Page-turning device. Uses flashlight batteries or adapter. Available with various types of switches. For hardcover books or magazines, $520. With bidirectional turning, $655. 443 View Ridge Drive, Everett, WA 98203, (206) 252-1541.

Mail-Order Books

Current, Rare, and Secondhand Books. Catalog available. Strand Book Store, 828 Broadway, New York, NY 10003, (800) 366-3664.

New Hard-Cover Publishers' Overstocks, Closeouts, Remainders. Catalog available. Edward R. Hamilton, bookseller, Falls Village, CT 06031.

Remainders. Catalog available. Daedalus Books, P.O. Box 9132, Hyattsville, MD 20781, (800) 395-2665.

Discount Books. All categories of books at discount prices; also audiotapes and videotapes. Catalog available. Barnes & Noble, 126 5th Avenue, New York, NY 10011, (800) 242-6657.

Correspondence Courses

University of Wisconsin Independent Study. More than six hundred courses available in every university department, and some on a high school level, to complete at your own pace. Written assignments are graded, corrected, and returned by mail. Certificates of completion awarded, and credit, if desired. Catalog available. University of Wisconsin — Extension, 209 Extension Building, 432 North Lake Street, Madison, WI 53706, (800) 442-6460.

Courses on Audiotape, Videotape

Self-Instruction Language Programs. Offers 264 courses in ninety-one languages on audiotape. Some related material, such as travel information, on videotape. For example, Modern Russian I, 28½ hours on twenty-four cassettes, plus a 480-page text and manual, $235. Also, films with subtitles on videotape and audiotape of some Russian literature. Audio-Forum, 96 Broad Street, Guilford, CT 06437, (800) 243-1234.

Learn a Language. Speedy system for learning conversational words and phrases for about twenty different languages. Each system: two ½-hour cassettes plus phrase dictionary. Good for travelers. $17. Signals catalog, (800) 669-9696.

The Teaching Company. Audiotape and videotape recordings provide a condensed version of a one-semester course given by a respected professor. Eight 45-minute lectures: audiotape, $90; videotape, $150. Option for rental and discounts for multiple purchases. For example, "Comedy, Tragedy, History: The Live Drama and Vital Truth of William Shakespeare," taught by Peter Saccio, Ph.D., professor, Dartmouth College. 7405 Alban Station Court, Suite A-107, Springfield, VA 22150, (800) 832-2421.

Services

Great Books Foundation. Provides the texts (which you purchase), a guide to following the "shared inquiry" method of reading and discussion, and questions to stimulate discussion on the selections. For help starting a Great Books group or to find one near you, contact the foundation, 35 East Wacker Drive, Suite 2300, Chicago, IL 60601, (800) 222-5870.

Federal Student Aid Information Center. Information regarding your eligibility for a federal student loan, how financial aid awards are determined, and how to find out if a school participates in federal aid programs. Federal Student Aid Information Center, P.O. Box 84, Washington, DC 20044, (800) 4-FED-AID (433-3243).

Publications

"The Student Guide: Financial Aid from the U.S. Department of Education." Information about federal student financial aid assistance. Federal Student Aid Information Center, P.O. Box 84, Washington, DC 20044, (800) 4-FED-AID (433-3243).

"Directory of Accredited Home Study Schools," National Home Study Council. Includes a list of subjects offered. Educational institution provides lesson materials prepared in a sequential and logical order for study by students on their own. Assigned work is submitted and graded and corrected and returned by qualified instructor. Courses include vocational subjects, brush-up business courses, hobbies. About ninety institutions listed. Completion times vary from a few weeks to several years. FREE. NHSC, 1601 18th Street, NW, Washington, DC 20009, (202) 234-5100.

"Directory of Learning Opportunities for Older Persons," American Association of Retired Persons. A list of 334 educational programs specifically designed for older students. Also describes various settings and opportunities for education. AARP Publications, 601 E Street, NW, Washington, DC 20049.

"The Back-to-School Money Book: A Financial Aid Guide for Midlife and Older Women Seeking Education and Training," American Association of Retired Persons. Scholarships and other ways of financing your education. FREE. AARP Publications, 601 E Street, NW, Washington, DC 20049.

ENJOYING TELEVISION

Television is an excellent link to the news of the day and contemporary culture as well as a source of entertainment for all tastes. The sound can be augmented with special devices, but you have to test them on your set to be sure they work well. All television sets sold in the United States since 1993 are caption-ready, meaning that anyone can view captions for programs that offer them. The captions are subtitles that let you know what has been spoken as well as the sound effects of actions that occur off-screen, which are designated "SFX." The first captions, in 1972, were run along the bottom portion of the screen, and all viewers saw them; they were open captions. Since then closed captions were accessible only with a decoder, which is still needed for older TV sets. Most programs and movies are captioned and are marked in TV listings and on videotape containers with the symbol CC (closed captions).

Resources

Hearing problems and methods of improving communication, especially on the telephone, are discussed in Chapter 3, "Keeping in Touch."

Products

Decoders for Closed Captions. To enable you to read the dialogue of a program or movie on the TV screen. TeleCaption 4000, attaches to your TV set, $190. TeleCaption VR-100, requires a VCR, cable converter, or satellite receiver, $120. Harris Communications catalog, (800) 825-6758, or for a list of retailers in your area, contact National Captioning Institute, 5203 Leesburg Pike, Falls Church, VA 22041, (800) 533-WORD (9673).

Zenith VHS VCR with Closed-Caption Capability. Captions viewed with live-broadcast programs and videotapes. $350. Harris Communications catalog, (800) 825-6758.

AudioLink. For watching TV or in specially equipped theaters or other auditoriums. Headset (1.4 ounces), with tone and volume control tailored to your hearing needs by a hearing health care professional, and transmitter, attached to TV or VCR. $280. Harris Communications catalog, (800) 825-6758, or for a list of retailers in your area, contact National Captioning Institute, 5203 Leesburg Pike, Falls Church, VA 22041, (800) 533-WORD (9673).

Sound Amplifier. Compact headphones and a small microphone to amplify sounds. Can be used for TV, lectures, and theater to enhance your hearing. $25. Potomac Technology catalog. (800) 433-2838.

Beamscope TV Magnifier. Mounts in front of the screen to double its diagonal size. To enlarge 17- to 19-inch picture to 30-inch diagonal, $83. To enlarge 12- to 15-inch picture to 25-inch diagonal, $70. Science Products Magnilog catalog, (800) 888-7400.

Services

Captioned Films/Videos. Educational and theatrical films and videos with subtitles for loan to individuals with hearing loss who cannot attend group showings. ½-inch VHS videotapes include prepaid return postage labels. FREE. Request an application. Modern Talking Picture Service, 5000 Park Street North, St. Petersburg, FL 33709, (800) 237-6213.

Descriptive Video Service (DVS). Narration of public television programs in which the movement of the characters, body language, and the scenes are described during pauses in the sound track. The viewer needs either a stereo TV or VCR that includes a Second Audio Program (SAP) feature or a SAP adapter. FREE. For a list of stations with DVS and a program guide, contact DVS, WGBH, 125 Western Avenue, Boston, MA 02134, (800) 333-1203.

National Institute on Deafness and Other Communication Disorders Information Clearinghouse. Information about captioning and devices for hearing the TV. NIDCD Clearinghouse, 1 Communication Avenue, Bethesda, MD, 20892, (800) 241-1044.

Videotapes

Critics' Choice Video. A catalog is available of more than two thousand movies on videotape, some with closed captions: classics, family subjects, musicals, and more. Most under $20. Critics' Choice Video, P.O. Box 749, Itasca, IL 60143, (800) 367-7765.

Described Movies on Video. Description of settings, actions, and other visual elements of the movie is interjected without interrupting the dialogue. Some public television programs are also available with description on video. No special equipment other than a TV and a VCR is necessary. Call for a catalog and a demonstration. Descriptive Video Service, WGBH, 125 Western Avenue, Boston, MA 02134, (800) 333-1203.

Chapter 19

Creating Your Retirement

Retirement may hold more opportunities for "working" than you may imagine. Today many people who have retired from their jobs are returning to work, either starting their own businesses or adopting more flexible schedules. Sometimes "work" is an unpaid volunteer job or a full-time community commitment. Hobbies may expand to fill a bigger share of your day. Whatever you do, it will be part of a new definition of retirement — more active, more individual.

CHOOSING TO WORK

"I used to think 'work' was a four-letter word! Now I feel 'retirement' is the curse."

"Retirement's not easy. You have to work at it."

Positive aspects of the workaday world become more obvious only when you retire. Regardless of how financially secure you are, a weekly paycheck is income, tangible recognition of your worth in the marketplace. A daily routine, even when it is a source of stress, provides structure and predictability. The workplace is often the main source for your circle of friends. A demanding job may keep your intellectual powers sharp by requiring you to solve problems and organize projects. Work that involves services to others may give you personal gratification. Having a job makes you feel useful and productive. Some people enjoy the work they do. Work often lifts the spirit and raises self-esteem.

You can find many of these benefits in other activities, of course, but it's no wonder that many people prefer to extend their work lives into their retirement years.

According to the Commonwealth Fund, a research foundation, more than five million people over age fifty-five would be willing to work (six million wanted to volunteer — see below). The American Association of Retired Persons found that one third of retired people would like to work, at least part-time. Though a part-time job doesn't offer the same job benefits as a full-time position, the other rewards may be similar, such as providing a sense of purpose and a source of friends and social interactions.

Part-time work comprises arrangements like job sharing, flextime, flexiplace, telecommuting, phased retirement, and home-based work. Other less than full-time commitments include seasonal, temporary, contract, or freelance work. These part-time arrangements facilitate the "new" retirement, which includes travel, leisure, *and* work.

Gradually more companies, particularly small businesses, are finding, as a 1992 study showed, that retired people are reliable, punctual, loyal, and easy to train. Smaller companies often have more tasks that can be accomplished by part-time employees; health care coverage is less of an expense since more than 80 percent of workers over age sixty-five were eligible for Medicare.

Working through a temporary employment agency lets you control your own work schedule, including (unpaid) vacations when you want them, and still offers the benefits of working. Temporary agencies court retired workers by offering brush-up sessions or training in new office equipment, including computers. A temporary position can develop into a full-time permanent job and is frequently used as a trial period by employers and workers seeking new skills or changing careers.

Working less than full-time gives you the opportunity to retire gradually, letting you explore ways of spending your leisure time.

When you've been out of the work force for a number of years, you may feel at a disadvantage as you apply for a job. Skills that prepare you for the current needs of employers are taught by some employment agencies and support groups.

When you apply for a job, your résumé will include two invisible reinforcements: the Federal Age Discrimination in Employment Act, which protects the rights of people over age forty to be hired solely on the basis of their ability, rather than age, and the findings of the Untapped Resource, a study supported by the Commonwealth Fund. This five-year project found that people over age fifty-five do not live up to the popular beliefs held about them: When compared with their younger counterparts, older workers were found to be as quickly trained in new technologies, as flexible about hours and duties, less frequently absent, and less likely to quit, and often better salespeople. So you can approach a job opportunity with confidence since you offer valued qualities. You might ask your future employer about such options as flexible scheduling or the possibility for part-time work, without loss of benefits, and training to allow you to improve your skills.

If you believe you have been turned down because of your age for a job for which you are qualified, you can pursue redress through the Equal Employment Opportunity Commission. In 1994 the AARP

Tips for Finding Jobs

- Find out which companies seek out mature workers. (Examples are hotels: Days Inns, Marriott; banks; travel agencies; hardware stores: Home Depot, Builder's Emporium; companies that have telephone services for taking reservations or phone orders: American Airlines; the Travelers Insurance Company; SupeRx, a drugstore; McDonald's, the fast-food chain.)
- Depend on word of mouth. Ninety percent of job openings are filled without being advertised in the newspaper. Learn how to network.
- For part-time work, look into retail sales. Sears, Roebuck & Company, the nation's leading retailer, is also the largest single employer of part-time help.
- Explore the possibility of government employment.
- Offer to learn a new skill; prospective employers may not realize you would be both willing and able to be trained.

found that more than one quarter of companies that received two résumés, identical except for age (one claimed to be thirty-two, the other fifty-seven) discriminated against the older applicant.

Every state is required to include a specialist at each employment service office to help older people find jobs.

Resources

Services

Forty Plus Club. A cooperative group that helps you conduct an effective job search and provides a base of operations. For one in your area, contact Forty Plus Club, 15 Park Row, New York, NY 10038, (212) 233-6086.

AARP WORKS. A series of job-search workshops to help mature workers prepare for new employment. Teaches job-hunting skills, employment planning, ways of building your self-confidence. For a workshop near you, contact AARP WORKS, Work Force Education, 601 E Street, NW, Washington, DC 20049, (800) 424-3410.

Operation ABLE (Ability Based on Long Experience). A network of ten agencies across the country counsels laborers, skilled workers, and professionals over age forty-five to find jobs. Job training and placement. For the agency nearest you, contact Operation ABLE, 180 North Wabash Avenue, Chicago, IL 60601, (312) 782-7700.

National Employment Lawyers Association. For referrals to attorneys who practice employment law to help you if you feel discriminated against by your employer because of age. NELA, 600 Harrison Street, Suite 535, San Francisco, CA 94107, (415) 227-4655.

List of Federal Employment Information Centers. For information about federal job opportunities and for application forms, contact the center nearest where you wish to work. These centers are able to give you guidance about local employment trends, conditions in the local job market, names of major employers, and specific occupations that are most needed. Office of Personnel Management, 1900 E Street, NW, Room 1416, Washington, DC 20415, (202) 606-2700.

National Association of Older Worker Employment Services. Referrals to employment services that welcome older workers and offer training in new skills. National Council on Aging, 409 3rd

Street, SW, Washington, DC 20024, (800) 867-2755.

Employment Opportunities

Senior Environmental Employment Program. Part-time or full-time jobs at the Environmental Protection Agency, Washington, DC, and field offices for people over age fifty-five. Mainly technical and support positions, such as laboratory technicians or emissions testers, or clerical jobs. SEEP Program, AARP, Director, 601 E Street, NW, Washington, DC 20049, (800) 424-3410.

Senior Community Service Employment Program (SCSEP). A program for low-income persons age fifty-five or older who are given on-the-job training (with pay) in part-time, nonprofit, or government community service jobs. The goal is to obtain permanent jobs in the private sector after training. Counseling and an annual physical examination included. For a program in your area, contact U.S. Department of Labor, Attention: Division of Older Workers Programs, 200 Constitution Avenue, NW, Room N-4641, Washington, DC 20210, (202) 219-4778.

Publications

Second Careers: New Ways to Work After 50 by Caroline Bird. Encouragement and directions for finding work in a new career. The bulk of the book is devoted to creative suggestions of jobs you can pursue according to your life's interest and experience. For example, people with experience in personal caregiving could get jobs caring for children, hairdressing, home repair, house-sitting. 1992. Little, Brown.

"How to Stay Employable: A Guide for the Mid-Life and Older Worker," American Association of Retired Persons. A discussion of trends in the job market and how to adjust to new developments. FREE. AARP Publications, 601 E Street, NW, Washington, DC 20049.

"Returning to the Job Market: A Woman's Guide to Employment Planning," American Association of Retired Persons. A guide that helps you assess your current skills, compose written documents, prepare for interviews, and develop a job search strategy. FREE. AARP Publications, 601 E Street, NW, Washington, DC 20049.

The Over-40 Job Guide by Kathryn and Ross Petras. Guidance for conducting a job search, writing a résumé, and having an interview. 1993. Poseidon Press.

Employment and Retirement Issues for Women: A Handbook, National Center for Women and Retirement Research. Advice for making job and career decisions, interview strategies, assertiveness, discrimination at work, and other issues. $12. NCWRR, Long Island University, Southampton, NY 11968, (800) 426-7386.

"Working Options: How to Plan Your Job Search, Your Work Life," American Association of Retired Persons. A self-directed job search plan you devise based on your employment goals and your self-assessment. FREE. AARP Publications, 601 E Street, NW, Washington, DC 20049.

"Make More of Your Great American Retirement Dream," National Association of Temporary Services. Explains how temporary help agencies operate and how they can help you find work. FREE with SSE. NATS, 119 South St. Asaph Street, Alexandria, VA 22314, (703) 549-6287.

Retiring to Your Own Business by Gustav Berle. How to start a business, help in deciding if you would like it, and what business might be successful. 1993. Puma Publishing, Santa Maria, CA 93454.

"Information for the Private Sector and State and Local Governments," Equal Employment Opportunity Commission. A description of the laws the EEOC is charged with enforcing, how to file a claim, locations of offices. FREE. EEOC, 1801 L Street, NW, Washington, DC 20507, (800) 669-4000.

"Laws Enforced by the EEOC," Equal Employment Opportunity Commission. Includes the full text of the Age Discrimination in Employment Act. FREE. Office of Communications and Legislative Affairs, EEOC, 1801 L Street, NW, Washington, DC 20507, (800) 669-4000.

Organizations

National Association of Temporary Services. A trade association of temporary help agencies. For a listing of agencies in your state, FREE with SSE, contact NATS, 119 South St. Asaph Street, Alexandria, VA 22314, (703) 549-6287.

National Displaced Homemakers Network. For women making the transition from home to the work force. Assistance and information for continuing education and scholarships. Newsletter, support groups. For a program near you, contact NDHN, 1625 K Street, NW, Suite 300, Washington, DC 20006, (202) 467-NDHN (6346).

Association of Part-Time Professionals. Offers advice and information about alternative work schedules. Publications and networking for job leads. APTP, Crescent Plaza, Suite 216, 77 Leesburg Pike, Falls Church, VA 22043, (703) 734-7975.

VOLUNTEERING YOUR TIME

"Loneliness is not something you choose, being alone is."

When you do something without monetary compensation, your payment is measured against a personal value scheme.

A Volunteer's Pay

- Satisfaction from helping someone else
- Perspective on one's own troubles
- Sense of usefulness
- Improved physical and mental health
- Motivation for keeping healthy, a purpose in living
- *Plus*, most of the benefits of paid employment, such as self-esteem, staying active, involved, stimulated

---

Research finds that people who volunteer are healthier and happier than those who don't, even though there is no certainty that volunteering has made them so. According to the Commonwealth Fund, about 25 percent of all people over age fifty-five, and 45 percent of those sixty to seventy-five, men and women equally, volunteer their time to nonprofit organizations. Nearly fourteen million seniors are doing jobs as tutors, police department aides, advocates for crime victims or abused children, escorts for people who are disabled, mentors for families, mediators in dispute resolution, counselors in shelters, drivers for Meals on Wheels, workers in food banks. If you're considering volunteering, you will be joining about half of

373

all Americans who donate their time each year. The time older Americans volunteer is equivalent to 1.1 million full-time employees, according to calculations by the Commonwealth Fund study. (This doesn't include people who are helping friends or family on an informal basis, outside voluntary organizations.)

How Many Volunteers?

- Salvation Army, which serves 18 million people a year: 1.2 million volunteers
- People taking care of friends and relatives: the equivalent of 7.1 million full-time jobs
- Religious institutions and public service organizations: the equivalent of 1.1 million full-time jobs
- School volunteers: 2.6 million volunteers
- Companions to 30,000 homebound adults: 11,900 senior companions (10 million hours)
- Children with special needs: 23,300 foster grandparents (21 million hours)
- 55,700 community agencies through the Retired Senior Volunteer Program (RSVP): 427,000 retired seniors

---

If you have an idea of the type of work you prefer doing, contact the appropriate institution directly — for example, a nursing home or hospital, the Boy or Girl Scouts, your school district or library, the court system or police department, the Red Cross. For suggestions about where volunteers may be needed check with a senior center, your county offices, or the United Way.

Resources

Services

AARP Volunteer Talent Bank. A clearinghouse for people age fifty and older that connects you with an organization that needs a volunteer with your qualifications. Informational brochure and registration packet. AARP Volunteer Talent Bank, 601 E Street, NW, Washington, DC 20049, (800) 424-3410.

National Association of Partners in Education. Encourages formation of organizations to volunteer in the schools. Contact the association for program nearest you and information and encouragement for starting program in your local schools. NAPE, 209 Madison Street, Suite 401, Alexandria, VA 22314, (703) 836-4880.

Volunteer Opportunities

International Executive Service Corps. Not-for-profit organization that recruits retired, highly skilled executives and technical advisers to share their experiences with businesses in developing nations and countries now entering free market economies. Executives and spouses are sent overseas and given per diem allowances on two- to three-month assignments. IESC, Stamford Harbor Park, 333 Ludlow Street, Stamford, CT 06902, (203) 967-6000.

National Library Service. Volunteers are needed to transcribe books into braille and to proofread materials in braille, also as tape narrators. FREE correspondence courses are available in braille transcription and proofreading. Write for a directory of volunteer groups that produce books for libraries and individuals. NLS, 1291 Taylor Street, NW, Washington, DC 20542, (800) 424-8567.

Service Corps of Retired Executives Association (SCORE). Retired executives counsel small businesses and help organize new businesses. For the local offices nearest you, contact SCORE, 409 3rd Street, SW, 4th Floor, Washington, DC 20024, (800) 634-0245.

National Guardianship Monitoring Program. A project to train volunteers to work with probate courts to monitor guardianships of elderly and incompetent people. Volunteers visit wards of the court and report to the courts regarding the living conditions and needs of individuals who rely on court-appointed guardians, who control their money, assets, and personal affairs with no other supervision. To learn about monitoring in your area, contact the National Guardianship Monitoring Program, c/o American Association of Retired Persons/Legal Council for the Elderly, 601 E Street, NW, Washington, DC 20049, (800) 424-3410.

Court Appointed Special Advocates. Volunteers help attorneys and social workers by representing the best interests of children in family court proceedings. Appointed by the court to investigate, monitor, and serve as a guardian to ensure that a child's interests are heard. National Court Appointed Special Advocates Association,

2722 Eastlake Avenue East, Suite 220, Seattle, WA 98102, (800) 628-3233.

Peace Corps. People with a variety of skills, three to five years' work experience, and/or college degrees for a variety of jobs, in such fields as agriculture, liberal arts, business, nursing, home economy, and teaching. Assignments are for two years plus a training period. FREE informational brochure available: "Senior Volunteers in the Peace Corps." PC, Office of Recruitment, Room P-301, 806 Connecticut Avenue, NW, Washington, DC 20526, (800) 424-8580.

Family Friends. Volunteers fifty-five and over visit ill children to provide emotional support and information. Volunteers are trained and supervised and must make a nine-month commitment. National Council on Aging, 409 3rd Street, SW, 2nd Floor, Washington, DC 20024, (800) 867-2755.

Older American Volunteer Programs. An opportunity to volunteer for those sixty and older who are no longer in the work force. Senior companions and foster grandparents are programs in which low-income seniors serve twenty hours a week and receive small stipends, annual physical examinations, and accident and liability insurance. Senior companions assist homebound adults, especially the frail elderly, helping them maintain independence. Foster grandparents work with children with disabilities, youths needing literacy assistance, teenage parents and their children, and some children in jails. Retired Senior Volunteer Program (RSVP) is the largest such program in the United States. No stipends are available for part-time volunteers, who work four hours per week. For a program office in your area, contact ACTION, 1100 Vermont Avenue, NW, Washington, DC 20525, (202) 606-5108.

Tax-Aide. To be trained by the IRS to assist people who need help filling out their income tax forms. American Association of Retired Persons, 601 E Street, NW, Washington, DC 20049, (800) 424-3410.

Criminal Justice Services. Volunteer jobs in law enforcement. American Association of Retired Persons, 601 E Street, NW, Washington, DC 20049, (800) 424-3410.

Disaster Volunteer. To provide support services after a disaster. Church World Service Disaster Response Program, 475 Riverside Drive, Room 626, New York, NY 10115, (212) 870-3151.

Publications

"Intergenerational Projects: Idea Book," American Association of Retired Persons. Descriptions of seventy-four programs in which seniors can help young people or in which they work together on community service projects. FREE. AARP Publications, 601 E Street, NW, Washington, DC 20049.

"Becoming a School Partner: A Guidebook for Organizing Intergenerational Partnerships in Schools," American Association for Retired Persons and National Association of Partners in Education. Describes a twelve-step process that can help you begin a school volunteer program in your area. FREE. AARP Publications, 601 E Street, NW, Washington, DC 20049.

Organizations

Global Volunteers. Spend one, two, or three weeks working with residents in the United States, a developing country, or an emerging democracy on human and economic development projects, such as teaching English, identifying crop diseases, building schools, painting murals. May be tax-deductible. For example, rural Jamaica, fifteen days, $1,300; language study in Poland, twenty days, $1,825. Airfare *not* included. 375 East Little Canada Road, St. Paul, MN 55117, (800) 487-1074.

Habitat for Humanity. Builds housing in partnership with the families who will be living in the housing. Global Village program or other programs. 121 Habitat Street, Americus, GA 31709, (800) HABITAT (422-4828).

Elderhostel Service Programs. People age sixty or older help people in need of housing or with research projects or other public services in America or abroad. Local accommodations and food not always hotel quality. For example, teaching English in Poland, ten days, about $2,500. Catalog available. Elderhostel Service Programs, 75 Federal Street, Boston, MA 02110, (617) 426-8056.

Health Advocacy Services. A variety of opportunities for volunteers to provide programs and information to older adults on health issues, including diet, Medicare, long-term care. To learn about volunteer opportunities in your area, contact American Association of Retired Persons, 601 E Street, NW, Washington, DC 20049, (800) 424-3410.

"When you need something done, always ask a busy person."

When you're involved in your community, your work, your family, it seems there's never an end of things to be done. Pursuing your interests keeps you challenged, provides opportunities for making friends, and helps you lead a full life. Often leisure-time interests are an extension of lifelong hobbies and activities.

Joining a club is a logical outgrowth that extends your involvement in a pastime as well as a way to find people with whom you're likely to be happy spending time. Leisure-time activities don't have to duplicate what you do for health benefits, like exercise walking; rather these activities are your avocation, what you choose to do in your free time.

Resources

Products

Board Games for People with Low Vision. Backgammon, Monopoly, checkers, and other popular games with larger-print or other easy-to-use features. Lighthouse Consumer Products catalog, (800) 829-0500. Independent Living Aids catalog, (800) 537-2118.

Round Playing Card Holder. Cards are held firmly between two attached disks. Four for $9. AfterTherapy catalog, (800) 235-7054.

Lo Vision Playing Cards. Numerals, suit markings are enlarged on standard-size cards. $6. AfterTherapy catalog, (800) 235-7054.

Playing Cards. 1-inch print of numerals and letters. $4.50. Just for You catalog, (800) 541-7903.

Crossword Puzzle Helper. You enter several letters on a keyboard, and the computer searches the dictionary memory for the whole word, which appears on a digital screen. Pocket size. $50. Signals catalog, (800) 669-9696.

Second Hand Holder. A flexible post clamps to a table and holds knitting, crocheting, embroidering work. Also darning ball. $60. Cleo of New York catalog, (800) 321-0595.

Golf Card. Two FREE eighteen-hole rounds of golf at each of three thousand member courses around the world. Also, discounts and a publication are available. $95 a year. Golf Card, International, 1637 Metropolitan Boulevard, Suite C, Tallahassee, FL 32308, 522-9232.

Services

Presidential Sports Award. Qualify for this award from the President's Council on Physical Fitness and Sports by fulfilling standards specific for each sport. For example, bowling: Bowl a minimum of 150 games with no more than 5 a day and stretching over at least thirty-four days. Award includes personalized presidential certificate of achievement, an emblem, and a congratulatory letter. $6. Presidential Sports Award, P.O. Box 68207, Indianapolis, IN 46268.

Play Tennis America. A program for beginners or players who need to brush up their skills. For a program near you, contact the United States Tennis Association, 70 West Red Oak Lane, White Plains, NY 10604, (914) 696-7000.

Crafts Shops. A list of shops that will take handmade items on consignment. FREE with SSE. The Elder Craftsman, 921 Madison Avenue, New York, NY 10021, (212) 861-5260.

Publications

"Fun and Games Aren't Just for Kids," United States Tennis Association. A brochure explains League Tennis, Senior Division for age fifty and over, including a system for ranking your own ability. FREE. USTA, 70 West Red Oak Lane, White Plains, NY 10604, (914) 696-7000.

World Wide Games. A catalog of quality board games, puzzles, games for developing manual and physical dexterity, familiar and new. FREE. P.O. Box 517, Colchester, CT 06415.

Organizations

National Senior Sports Association. Arranges recreational and competitive events and trips for people age fifty or over in tennis, golf, and bowling. Other membership benefits. NSSA, 1248 Post Road, Fairfield, CT 06430, (800) 282-NSSA (6772).

Senior Softball — USA. Six age divisions from age fifty to age seventy-five and over compete for the annual Senior Softball World Championships. Newsletter available. SS-USA, 9 Fleet Court, Sacramento, CA 95831, (916) 393-8566.

Ski Vacations. Trips to various American and foreign resorts for skiers over fifty. Local chapters sponsor other active outings. Over the Hill Gang International, 3310 Cedar Heights Drive, Colorado Springs, CO 80904, (719) 685-4656. Over the Hill Gang, 13791 East Rice Place, Aurora, CO 80015, (303) 699-6404.

U.S. National Senior Sports Organization. Sponsors biennial National Senior Sports Classic — the Senior Olympics; participants qualify in state competitions for the biennial event. Competitions for people age fifty-five and older in thirty-four sports, including tennis, cycling, badminton, and horseshoes at local, regional, and national levels. Ask for your state's contact. NSSO, 14323 South Outer Forty Road, Suite N300, Chesterfield, MO 63017, (314) 878-4900.

U.S. Senior Athletic Games. No qualifications required for groups from age fifty to compete in shuffleboard, horseshoes, walking, and running events, and others. For information on senior games in your area, or to start one for your sport, contact USSA, 200 Castlewood Drive, North Palm Beach, FL 33408.

United States Masters Swimming. Organized swimming programs, not necessarily competitive, with an opportunity for group practice. For the swim club in your area, contact USMS, National Office, 2 Peters Avenue, Rutland, MA 01543, (508) 886-6631.

A Secure Future

Chapter 20

Managing Your Finances

"I always left it to someone else to think about money. Now it's up to me. While it's a big responsibility, it's also a big challenge. I never make a move without getting a second opinion."

People who have planned their financial futures know how they will pay for the things they need. Despite the old saying that only the very wealthy have to worry about money while the rest of us worry about how to get some money in the first place, the truth is we *all* have to worry — or plan — regardless of the size of our bank accounts. Financial planning in your mature years has three phases: maximizing your income, minimizing expenditures, and directing the distribution of the remainder after your death.

A clear understanding of your finances is essential for genuine independence. Your financial resources will affect your choices of where to live, what clothing to buy, or whether to continue to work. Before you make important decisions about money, it's best to look at your financial status as described by a net worth statement. Your net worth is simply your assets minus your debts. Making such a calculation is often required before you can qualify for a loan, as a way of measuring your financial gains or losses, and as a basis for making decisions about buying or selling assets and how much "disposable" money you have.

To determine your assets, add the following:

- *Cash* in savings accounts, checking accounts, and money market funds
- *Investments* in certificates of deposit, stocks, mutual funds, bonds, and individual retirement accounts
- *Life insurance*
- *Real estate,* such as your home and other properties
- *Possessions,* such as jewelry, a car, and other valuables
- *Pension* and/or *Social Security* benefits

To determine your debts, add up the following:

- Mortgage and personal *loans*
- *Credit card* balances

Your net worth will be the total amount of your debts subtracted from the total amount of your assets.

If you aren't working, your income will be derived from your assets, in particular from retirement investments. A financial planner can help you select investments that maximize your income and can manage your assets so that you can achieve your personal goals. The profession of financial planning, however, does not have uniform defined standards, so you must be alert to avoid unscrupulous individuals who may take advantage of people with money to invest.

Selecting a Financial Planner

- Look for a person with the designation "CFP" (Certified Financial Planner), which is earned on the basis of requirements established by the Certified Financial Planner Board of Standards.
- Find a CFP who works on a *fee-only* basis rather than on commissions from investments you make. This planner will be paid for giving you advice and will not benefit from your following his or her suggestions.

Although credentials are always important for any professional, you will have the best results with a planner with whom you feel comfortable talking, since you must share personal details such as your goals and preferences in order to reach important decisions about your future. You may also consult with an accountant and a lawyer about the effect your eventual plans have on your taxes or estate.

Resources

Products

Easi-Vue Calculator. Large display and large keys with easy-to-read markings. $16. Easy Street catalog, (800) 959-EASY (3279).

Talking Calculator. In addition to a large display, the calculator "speaks" the numerals, functions, and results. $25. Lighthouse Consumer Products catalog, (800) 829-0500.

Big Number Pocket Size Calculator. ⅝-inch-high numerals are displayed on solar or battery-powered calculator, 5 by 3 by ⅜ inches. $15. Lighthouse Consumer Products catalog, (800) 829-0500.

Nitewriter. A ballpoint pen with a light concentrated on the paper beneath the tip, highlighting your work as you write. Enhances the visibility of your writing any time, not only in the dark. $5. LS&S Group catalog, (800) 468-4789.

Retirement Planning Kit. Work sheets and booklets help you devise a financial strategy for retirement. Also describes mutual funds offered by the company. FREE. T. Rowe Price Investment Services, 100 East Pratt Street, Baltimore, MD 21202, (800) 638-5660.

Retirees Financial Guide. Investment guidance specifically for retired persons or for those near retirement. Work sheets to help you determine how much you can spend without depleting your resources. Describes mutual funds offered by the company. FREE. T. Rowe Price Investment Services, 100 East Pratt Street, Baltimore, MD 21202, (800) 638-5660.

"Net Worth Statement: An Important Financial Tool" by Elizabeth Wiegand. A form on which to compute your net worth statement. $1. Cornell Cooperative Extension, Resource Center — GP, 7 Cornell Business and Technology Park, Ithaca, NY 14850, (607) 255-2080.

Services

Institute of Certified Financial Planners. Refers you to a CFP in your area. ICFP, 7600 East Eastman Avenue, Suite 301, Denver, CO 80231, (800) 282-PLAN (7526).

Videotape

Women and Money, National Center for Women and Retirement Research. A step-by-step guide to assessing your current finances, planning for your future, and investing your money. 60 minutes. $30. NCWRR, Long Island University, Southampton, NY 11968, (800) 426-7386.

Computer Programs

Retirement Planning Kit. Work sheets for developing a retirement strategy for those for whom retirement is more than five years in the future. Calculations and "what if" examples are facilitated through use of the computer. $15. T. Rowe Price, P.O. Box 89000, Baltimore, MD 21289, (800) 541-1472.

Retirement Planner. Help in computing investments, taxes, and Social Security benefits. $18. Vanguard, P.O. Box 11004, Des Moines, IA 50336, (800) 876-1840.

Publications

BEST BUY. A Primer on Financial Management for Midlife and Older Women, American Association of Retired Persons. Help for the reader, male or female, who needs guidance in setting financial goals and making investments and other financial decisions. The book offers forms, lists, thought-provoking choices, and options. FREE. AARP Publications, 601 E Street, NW, Washington, DC 20049.

"Financial Planning: A Common Sense Guide for the 1990s," Institute of Certified Financial Planners. Explains various facets of financial planning — tax, retirement, estate, investment — and includes forms to use to calculate your net worth, cash flow, and personal goals. $2. ICFP, 7600 East Eastman Avenue, Suite 301, Denver, CO 80231, (800) 282-PLAN (7526).

"Facts About Financial Planners," American Association of Retired

Persons. Checklists, financial statement form, cash flow form. Also, guidelines for working with a financial planner if you need one. FREE. AARP Publications, 601 E Street, NW, Washington, DC 20049.

Making the Most of Your Money: Smart Ways to Create Wealth and Plan Your Finances in the '90s by Jane Bryant Quinn. A comprehensive resource that can help you understand investments, the rationale behind various financial choices, and other aspects of the financial world. 1991. Simon & Schuster.

Consumer Reports Money Book: How to Get It, Save It, and Spend It Wisely by Janet Bamford and others. A detailed explanation of personal financial issues to use as a reference when you need to make informed decisions. Topics include banking, money management, taxes, insurance, investing, and retirement planning. 1992. Consumer Reports Books.

How to Plan for a Secure Retirement by Barry Dickman and Trudy Lieberman. Explains investment choices for your retirement funds. Discusses the advantages and disadvantages of various investments, insurance policies, and money management methods. Appendix includes work sheets for calculating retirement needs and income. 1992. Consumer Reports Books.

Finances After 50, Financial Planning for the Rest of Your Life, United Seniors Health Cooperative. A self-study guide with twenty work sheets to help you manage your financial life. Helps you assemble the data you need for decisions about insurance, taxes, and investments. 1993. HarperCollins.

Looking Ahead to Your Financial Future, National Center for Women and Retirement Research. A workbook and guide to financial planning. $12. NCWRR, Long Island University, Southampton, NY 11968, (800) 426-7386.

"Focus Your Future: A Woman's Guide to Retirement Planning," American Association of Retired Persons. A comprehensive view of issues to consider in advance of retirement and ways of planning to achieve your goals. FREE. AARP Publications, 601 E Street, NW, Washington, DC 20049.

"Tomorrow's Choices," American Association of Retired Persons. A guide to help you prepare for future legal, financial, and health care decisions. Suggestions, explanations, issues, and ways of preparing for situations that may develop in the future. FREE. AARP

SOURCES OF INCOME

As you contemplate retirement, you may wonder whether you will have enough money to live on, whether Social Security payments will meet your needs, and how to adjust smoothly to your new financial circumstance.

When you retire, income from your assets will replace your salary from work. It's not always a simple matter, however, to switch from generating income to tapping into your nest egg. Most experts estimate that you will need 60 to 80 percent, or even 100 percent, of your preretirement income to maintain your standard of living. One rule of thumb suggests that during your work years you should save 10 percent of your income for retirement. Your retirement income will come from pensions and retirement accounts, Social Security payments, and the return on your investments. Additional income through part-time work may be needed.

Retirement Funds

Part of your retirement income may come from funds you have invested during your working years, such as IRAs, funds invested for you at work, your pension, and Social Security benefits.

IRAs

These special accounts allow you to set aside money and pay income tax at the lower rate in effect when you withdraw the money during your retirement years. The money accrues interest or dividends, compounding with no taxes to pay until it is withdrawn.

IRA Birthdays

- *Age fifty-nine and one-half.* You *may* begin withdrawing from your IRA without penalty.
- *Age seventy and one-half.* You *must* begin withdrawing funds, or there will be a 50 percent tax penalty.

You pay taxes on your IRA withdrawals, which are made according to a formula based on your life expectancy, either fixed at the time of your first withdrawal or recalculated each year. An accountant or the Internal Revenue Service (IRS) can help you decide how to calculate and time your withdrawals for your greatest benefit. If you are still working at age seventy and one-half, you can arrange to withdraw only the minimum required by the IRS so that the tax-deferred compounding continues.

Pensions

Among the decisions you need to make when you retire may be whether to receive your pension benefits for yourself alone (single life) or for yourself and a surviving beneficiary, such as your spouse (joint and survivor). Single life guarantees payments to you for life; joint and survivor extends payments to your surviving spouse when you die. Pensions have different provisions, and you should examine the way your pension works. Payments are usually smaller when you choose joint and survivor and continue at the same rate even if your spouse dies first. Nevertheless, this can be a valuable continuing benefit guaranteed to your spouse.

Social Security

After you have worked for ten years, you are eligible to receive Social Security payments at the minimum eligible age, sixty-two

---

Birthdays for Applying for Social Security

- *Age sixty.* You are eligible for payments if your spouse died and was eligible.
- *Three months before age sixty-two to age sixty-five.* You are eligible to apply for Social Security benefits. Your payments will be at reduced levels permanently if you apply before age sixty-five.
- *Three months before age sixty-five.* Apply for "full" Social Security benefits.
- *Age sixty-five to age sixty-nine.* Your benefits increase if you continue to work (and don't apply for Social Security) each of these years.

---

years. You can apply by telephone or in person at your local Social Security office. Benefits are sent to you, a person you designate, or deposited directly in your bank account.

If you retire between age sixty-two and age sixty-five and therefore no longer are paying into your Social Security base, it may be to your advantage to receive benefits early, even at a reduced rate. Rather than wait for full benefits, you would be receiving three additional years of payments.

When you estimate your retirement income, you can anticipate that Social Security payments will be equivalent to no more than about 30 percent of your income at the time you retire. You must rely on other resources for the bulk of your retirement income. A 1991 survey showed that most people have an unrealistic idea of the contribution Social Security payments make to their retirement income. Almost 60 percent of people age forty-five to sixty-four believed they would be able to rely mainly on Social Security or pensions. Actually, personal savings and investments account for about 40 percent of retirement income. You may also decide to continue to work, perhaps part-time, to augment your income.

Birthdays If You Work and Receive Social Security Benefits

- *Age sixty to age seventy.* You must file an earnings report to Social Security by April 15 (in addition to an income tax return).
- *Age sixty-two to age sixty-nine.* Earned income must be below a certain amount to avoid a reduction in your benefits.
- *Age seventy.* You may earn unlimited income from working, without any reduction in your benefits.

To help you plan your retirement income, you can receive a statement of your Social Security earnings and estimated payments (mailed automatically to those age sixty for whom SS has a current address). Social Security payments are based on past earnings, not on the amount you need, so groups of people who did not pay into the system, such as homemakers, are not eligible on their own for payments.

Services

Personal Earnings and Benefit Estimate Statement. An accounting of your Social Security earnings and how much you have paid in Social Security taxes and an estimate of the benefits you will receive if you retire at age sixty-two, sixty-five, or seventy. If you are sixty or older, you can get an estimate of your retirement benefits by telephone. FREE. For the form (SSA-7004) with which to request your statement, contact Social Security Administration, Office of Public Inquiry, P.O. Box 17743, Baltimore, MD 21235, (800) 772-1213.

National Organization of Social Security Claimants' Representatives. If you are denied benefits you think you deserve, you can get advice from an attorney who specializes in Social Security problems. For referral to an attorney near you, contact NOSSCR, 6 Prospect Street, Midland Park, NJ 07432, (800) 431-2804.

Publications

"Your Pension: Things You Should Know About Your Pension Plan," Pension Benefit Guaranty Corporation. A description of the basic provisions and requirements of pension plans to determine whether you are receiving your full benefits. FREE. PBGC, 1200 K Street, NW, Suite 240, Washington, DC 20006, (202) 326-4000.

"Often-Asked Questions About Employee Retirement Benefits," Pension and Welfare Benefits Administration. Information about the laws governing pension plans presented in a question-and-answer format. FREE. PWBA, U.S. Department of Labor, Room N5619, 200 Constitution Avenue, NW, Washington, DC 20210, (202) 219-8776.

"A Guide to Understanding Your Pension Plan: A Pension Handbook," American Association of Retired Persons. An overview of how certain pension plans function and how to go about learning what your plan offers. FREE. AARP Publications, 601 E Street, NW, Washington, DC 20049.

"What You Should Know About the Pension Law," U.S. Department of Labor. A guide to the Employee Retirement Income Security Act (ERISA), which sets the minimum standards for pension plans. The booklet lets you know what your rights are with respect to your pension plan, what information you are entitled to, and other features as defined by law. FREE. Pension and Welfare Benefits Administration. U.S. Department of Labor, Room N5619, 200 Constitution Avenue, NW, Washington, DC 20210, (202) 219-8776.

"How to File a Claim for Your Benefits," Pension and Welfare Benefits Administration. A guide to the steps you must take to request pension benefits and how to appeal if you are denied. FREE. PWBA, U.S. Department of Labor, Room N5619, 200 Constitution Avenue, NW, Washington, DC 20210, (202) 219-8776.

"Understanding Social Security," Social Security Administration. Describes Social Security programs in general terms, explains how you earn "credits" that add up to eligibility for a benefit when you are older. FREE. SSA, P.O. Box 17743, Baltimore, MD 21235, (800) 772-1213.

"Retirement," Social Security Administration. A brochure to help you understand what to expect when you become eligible for your Social Security benefits so that you can plan your retirement finances. FREE. SSA, P.O. Box 17743, Baltimore, MD 21235, (800) 772-1213.

"The Social Security Book: What Every Woman Absolutely Needs to Know," American Association of Retired Persons. A guide for women on how to apply for benefits, appeal a denial of benefits, and gain understanding of the Social Security system. FREE. AARP Publications, 601 E Street, NW, Washington, DC 20049.

"Survivors," Social Security Administration. Describes who may be eligible to receive benefits as a surviving family member. FREE. SSA, Office of Public Information, P.O. Box 17743, Baltimore, MD 21235, (800) 772-1213.

"SSI: Supplemental Security Income," Social Security Administration. Explains how to apply for SSI and the formula by which your income is evaluated. FREE. SSA, Office of Public Information, P.O. Box 17743, Baltimore, MD 21235, (800) 772-1213.

Organizations

Pension Rights Center. Provides information about pension issues, refers you to a lawyer experienced in pension law, and offers legal assistance to attorneys. PRC, 918 16th Street, NW, Suite 704, Washington, DC 20006, (202) 296-3776.

In 1991, 85 percent of homeowners age sixty-five and older owned their homes free of debt. If you own your home "free and clear," the mortgage paid off, or nearly so, you can consider cashing in its value for additional income. There are several ways of doing this:

- *Trading down.* Sell your current home to purchase a smaller house and invest the difference for income (you may be eligible for a tax benefit too).
- *Family transaction.* Sell your home to your children in exchange for a lifetime annuity, and continue to live in it.
- *Home equity loan.* Actually a second mortgage, this is a loan, backed by the value of your home, that you repay on a monthly basis, with interest. You must qualify for this loan on the basis of your income, not merely the worth of the home. Your home may be foreclosed upon if you fail to meet the monthly payments.
- *Sale/leaseback.* You sell your home but continue to live in it on a rental basis. Mortgage payments may be paid to you, with your rent deducted. Since it is not a debt, you don't pay taxes, insurance, or interest.
- *Reverse mortgage.* This is a refinancing arrangement under which you borrow money against the value of your home. You receive the money, either in regular monthly payments or as you need it, and repay it, with interest, when you move or sell your home. A portable reverse mortgage is backed by a life annuity rather than by the home value, so monthly payments continue even after you leave the home.
- *Special-purpose reverse mortgages.* Some public agencies offer reverse mortgages to use for paying property taxes, making home improvements, or other specific purposes.

The concept of the reverse mortgage is alluring; it is a way of using the value of your home without selling it or moving. You continue living in your home, and you receive payments that augment your income, using the funds for any purpose — and, in the case of a federally insured mortgage, with no concern about the possible decline in your home's value on the real estate market. The maximum amount of equity that can be insured by the Federal Housing Administration is determined by the location of the home, ranging from $67,000 in rural areas to $151,725 in the most expensive housing markets.

The payments from a reverse mortgage are not taxable and, because they are a loan, are not income. They do not affect any Social Security or other government benefits you may be eligible to receive. Insured mortgages are payable when you die, move, or sell your home. Uninsured mortgages must be repaid in full at the end of the term, so they are most practical for people who expect to move at a specific time.

The amount of your payments depends, of course, on how you receive them: as a line of credit to use when you decide, as a regular lifetime monthly amount, as payments for a fixed period, or in a combination of these styles. The older you are, the shorter the amount of time during which you will receive payments, and the larger the payments will be. Usually you can estimate the payments to be about $350 a month for a seventy-five-year-old homeowner (minimum age for applying for a reverse mortgage is usually sixty-two).

For some homeowners the advantages of a reverse mortgage are hard to ignore. Since it is a complicated transaction, counseling is required to be sure you understand how a reverse mortgage will impact on your financial situation and to help you select among the many variables offered. Your lending institution will arrange for you to receive counseling from disinterested professionals who can help you be sure you are making a proper choice for your needs.

Resources

Services

Reverse Mortgage Lenders List. Updated list of all lenders who offer reverse mortgages. FREE. AARP Home Equity Information Center, 601 E Street, NW, Washington, DC 20049, (800) 424-3410.

"Reverse Mortgage Locator," National Center for Home Equity Conversion. State-by-state listing of lenders, with phone numbers, for FHA-insured, privately insured, and uninsured reverse mortgages.

SSE and $1. NCHEC, 7373 147th Street West, Suite 115, Apple Valley, MN 55124, (612) 953-4474.

Publications

"FHA-Insured Reverse Mortgages," Federal National Mortgage Association. A description of reverse mortgages insured by the federal government. Also available: a list of FHA-insured lenders. FREE. Fannie Mae, 3900 Wisconsin Avenue, NW, Washington, DC 20016, (800) 7-FANNIE (732-6643).

Retirement Income on the House: Cashing In on Your Home with a "Reverse" Mortgage by Ken Scholen. A comprehensive guide to all phases of reverse mortgages and help in deciding if you would benefit from using one. $25. National Center for Home Equity Conversion, Suite 115, 7373 147th Street West, Apple Valley, MN 55124, (612) 953-4474.

BEST BUY. "Home-Made Money: Consumers' Guide to Home Equity Conversion" by Ken Scholen. Describes various loans that are based on the value of a home, including reverse mortgages. Explains risks and advantages of each type of loan. FREE. AARP Publications, 601 E Street, NW, Washington, DC 20049.

"Reverse Mortgages," Federal Trade Commission. A brief summary of the features of reverse mortgages. FREE. FTC, Bureau of Consumer Protection, 6th Street and Pennsylvania Avenue, NW, Washington, DC 20580, (202) 326-3650.

"When Your Home Is on the Line: What You Should Know About Home Equity Lines of Credit," Board of Governors of the Federal Reserve System. Explains terminology and options in various plans and provides a checklist to compare features of different plans. FREE. Publications Services, Board of Governors of the Federal Reserve System, Washington, DC 20551.

"Home Equity Credit Lines," Federal Trade Commission. Describes elements of home equity credit plans and includes a checklist with which to compare various offerings. FREE. FTC, Bureau of Consumer Protection, 6th Street and Pennsylvania Avenue, NW, Washington, DC 20580, (202) 326-3650.

Investing

You hope your savings will yield as much as possible at your retirement without jeopardizing the principal. Decisions about where to invest for the best return are highly individual, based on your net worth and your experience with money and investing. Retired people who are careful to conserve their principals may be told they are overly conservative investors, but this may just be a prelude to the suggestion that they invest in something risky. If you have little experience handling investments or little time to devote to the job, don't be tempted by word-of-mouth tips, investment advice from people whom you don't know and who don't know you, or any investment that you don't understand completely. To inform yourself about making investments, you can join an investment club or consult a variety of periodicals that follow financial news and markets. Review the publications in the library — for example, *Changing Times*, *Money Magazine*, *Barron's National Business*, the *Wall Street Journal* — and subscribe to only one a year, but a different one each year to get different perspectives of the financial scene. Complicated transactions may bring you greater returns, but high returns are frequently partners of high risk and may jeopardize your principal. Remember, big profits are often close relatives of big losses.

Your investments can be divided among stocks, bonds, and cash, according to your income needs. Stocks are considered an investment likely to increase in value over the long term. To determine the portion of your portfolio to invest in stocks, one rule of thumb suggests subtracting your age from a hundred. The smaller your portfolio, the less you should have in stocks, since you may need cash for an emergency when the market is down. Similarly, people with a low tolerance for risk should concentrate on insured investments. If you are able to invest for your estate, you can apportion your portfolio according to the age of your heirs; for example, you may invest more heavily into stocks if they are young or in income-producing investments if they are nearer retirement.

Resources

Publications

"What Every Investor Should Know," Securities and Exchange Commission. Explanations of the financial markets, what they are and how they work. FREE. SEC, Washington, DC 20549, (202) 272-5624.

Services

Background Check of Securities Dealers. A hot line that provides information about security brokers who have been the subject of disciplinary action, criminal proceedings, or other professional complaints. National Association of Securities Dealers, (800) 289-9999.

Organizations

National Association of Investment Clubs. You gain experience picking solid growth stocks through the process of learning how to evaluate a company and how to decide when to buy, hold, or sell. Monthly dues (usually $25 to $50) go to purchasing stock, mainly conservative investing. Provides information on starting a club. NAIC, P.O. Box 220, Royal Oak, MI 48067, (313) 543-0612.

Investors Alliance. A nonprofit investment education and research association for individual investors. Various benefits for members, including mutual fund and stock information, a directory of dividend reinvestment plans, discount broker directory. Computer software available. $50. IA, 219 Commercial Boulevard, P.O. Box 11209, Fort Lauderdale, FL 33339, (305) 491-5100.

American Association of Individual Investors. Assists individuals in managing their assets by providing educational materials, information on investing. Tax-planning guide and mutual fund guide; newsletter. $50. AAII, 625 North Michigan Avenue, Chicago, IL 60611, (312) 280-0170.

CONTROLLING EXPENDITURES

More than likely your list of expenses far outnumbers your list of sources of income. After retirement that expense list may seem even longer. While your instinct may be to cut back wherever possible, you should be selective in your economies. Certain essentials, such as food, heat, and health care, are too important to shortchange. Before you can decide how to save money, you should have a clear idea of exactly what your expenses are by creating a cash flow chart.

To create a cash flow chart, try to estimate the amount you spend either monthly or yearly for each category on the following list. One way to do this would be to go through your checkbook stubs over a three-month period.

- Housing: rent, mortgage, property tax, homeowners insurance, housing upkeep, gas, electric, heating, water
- Transportation: public transit, car upkeep, car insurance, car payments, taxis
- Personal: life insurance, health insurance, clothing, vacations, groceries, restaurants, telephone, laundry, medical and dental, prescriptions, hair grooming, entertainment, leisure pursuits, newspapers and periodicals, pet necessities

The largest single category may be housing expenses, which can equal as much as one third of your income. Even if you own your home, taxes and other housing-related expenses may be high, and it is logical to try to economize in this category. The federal government sponsors programs designed to provide housing for people with limited incomes: in publicly supported units; by means of rental subsidies; or by making loans or grants for home repairs, heating costs, or other specific items. If you need to make alterations to continue to live in your home because of a physical limitation, you may be able to deduct the costs from your income tax as medical expenses. Your medical insurance may cover some of the costs, if such improvements mean you don't have to move to a nursing home — a more expensive option. Some costs that could be deducted on your income tax return may include the following:

- Installing entry/exit ramps
- Widening doorways and hallways
- Modifying bathrooms for accessibility
- Adapting kitchen cabinets and equipment
- Relocating electrical outlets and fixtures

Farmers and veterans may be eligible for special housing benefits from the Farmers Home Administration and the Department of Veterans Affairs respectively.

Reducing your housing expenses may reduce other expenses; perhaps your transportation needs will be different or will be provided by the community, or your leisure-time activities less costly. Of course, the range of prices for homes is large and depends on the location, market conditions, and a vast array of other factors, such as taxes, utilities, etc. The rough examples of the costs of various housing options that follow are actual prices noted in recent years.

Housing Costs

- One-bedroom Elder Cottage Housing Opportunity (ECHO) unit: $21,000 to purchase and install.
- College campus retirement community: $50,000 capital investment.
- Studio apartment in an adult community that includes a health care center, two meals a day, housekeeping, transportation, personal health care, and limited health services; nursing care extra: $1,000 a month.
- One-bedroom cooperative apartment in a thirty-five-acre complex next door to a hospital, with housekeeping and one meal a day: $137,000.
- Studio apartment in a continuing care facility with one daily meal, utilities, twenty-four-hour emergency response, transportation, housekeeping; laundry; health services extra: $1,200 a month.
- One-bedroom congregate apartment with two meals a day, housekeeping, transportation, recreation facilities: $2,200 a month.
- Studio apartment with no kitchen in a continuing care community with other facilities available if you need more care: entrance fee $17,500.
- One-bedroom apartment in a life care community with 90 percent refundable purchase price and on-site health care center: $150,000 and $1,500 a month.
- One-bedroom unit in a Hyatt Classic Residence with two meals a day, nursing personnel on duty, housekeeping, transportation: $2,300 a month.
- Group home, including rent, utilities, and food: $800 a month.

Once you have reviewed your housing decisions and possible use of your home's equity, you should determine what community services may be available for you. These may include transportation, meals, chores, socializing, and entertainment opportunities.

Other categories you can consider to reduce expenses include life insurance and automobile insurance. You may not need life insurance if you are single and have no dependents. Some auto policies offer a "good driver discount" if you haven't had an accident or if you have taken a defensive driving course.

Resources

Some changes you may decide to make to keep your home safe for you are included in Chapter 12, "Adapting the Old Homestead."

Refresher driving courses are listed in Chapter 15, "Feeling Safe on the Road."

Services

SelectQuote. Price comparison of insurance policies. FREE. SelectQuote, 595 Market Street, 5th Floor, San Francisco, CA 94105, (800) 253-5577.

Insurance Quote Services. Price comparison of term life insurance policies. FREE. IQ, 3200 North Dobson Road, Building C, Chandler, AZ 85224, (800) 972-1104.

Publications

"Buyer's Guide to Insurance: What the Companies Won't Tell You," National Insurance Consumer Organization. Tips on how to save money when buying personal insurance, auto, homeowner, life, etc. $3 and SSE. CFA, NICO, 414 A Street, SE, Washington, DC 20003, (202) 547-6426.

"Consumer Alert: Coverages Not to Buy," National Insurance Consumers Organization. $1 and SSE. CFA, NICO, 414 A Street, SE, Washington, DC 20003, (202) 547-6426.

Saving on Taxes, Credit, and Banking

Unavoidable expenses, including income and other taxes, and charges for using credit cards and banking services can be kept to a minimum with advice from experts and by comparison shopping.

Volunteer assistance is available to help you file your income tax returns during the months before the April 15 deadline. Some localities may offer an opportunity for you to reduce property or school taxes by volunteering for a certain number of hours of community service.

Many banks offer special services or special fee schedules for their customers over fifty. Although the bank nearest you may seem the most convenient, if a branch that offers better rates is not in your neighborhood, you can bank by mail and use automatic teller machines. Compare the services you use most often at several banks to decide which one will save you money. Look for a checking account with no fees, no minimum balance, and a monthly interest payment.

Using a credit card can save you money by deferring payment on your purchases for up to thirty days. The catch is that you must pay the balance *in full* every month to avoid finance charges. A credit card with no annual fee gives you the most value plus insurance protection for purchases you make with the card.

Charging purchases is an excellent way to establish a credit history. The Equal Credit Opportunity Act protects people age sixty-two and over from being denied credit because of age. If you have no credit history because someone else paid your regular bills or you always paid with cash, you can establish credit by using a credit card or by taking out a small bank loan and making timely payments. A department store charge card and a line of credit from your bank are other good ways of establishing your creditworthiness. A joint account will become part of your credit history if the other person dies. If you have no credit history in your own name, a spouse can change the account name to include you or can help you establish credit on your own with a personal bank loan. Each spouse should have an individual credit record, each with access to credit.

Bank loans are expensive, and unless you pay your credit card balance in full each month, you create a loan transaction. Similarly, a home equity line of credit is a loan using your home as collateral. If you must borrow money, it could be cheaper to arrange a loan with a family member. Naturally you will want to do this formally, with a written legal agreement that details terms and the method of repayment.

If you have had problems with credit in the past, you can get help to reestablish a good credit standing. Credit counseling services can advise you about how to manage your money to repay your debts.

Resources

Products

Large Format Check Register. Twelve entries per 8½- by 11-inch page with fifty spiral-bound pages. $6. Independent Living Aids catalog, (800) 537-2118.

Custom Made Check Stencil. A template that guides you in writing a check with spaces for date, payee, amount, memo, and your signature. Made according to your own check's format. $20. Lighthouse Consumer Products catalog, (800) 829-0500.

Check Writer Rubber Stamp. Adjustable stamp that prints amounts on checks. $10. Harriet Carter catalog, (215) 361-5151.

Credit Card Case. Slim (4¼ by 3 inches) leather case holds twenty cards in swing-out sleeves. Side pockets for driver's license. $5. Harriet Carter catalog, (215) 361-5151.

"Consumer Budget Planner." Compact net worth and budgeting work sheets and advice. FREE with SSE. Consumer Credit Education Foundation, Department CBP, 919 18th Street, NW, Washington, DC 20006, (202) 296-5544.

"Budget Blueprint." A chart for detailing budget expenses and income. FREE with SSE. Credit Union National Association, Public Relations Department, P.O. Box 431, Madison, WI 53701.

"The Consumer's Almanac." A monthly money manager with calendars for recording income and expenses. Includes net worth work sheet and budgeting charts and hints for handling your money. $2. Consumer Credit Education Foundation, Department CA, 919 18th Street, NW, Washington, DC 20006, (202) 296-5544.

Services

"Tax Heaven or Hell: A Guide to the Tax Consequences of Your Retirement Location," Vacation Publications. Cities are rated according to your income, home values, estate taxes. Juneau, Alaska, had the lowest tax burden for retirees of any major U.S. city. Vacation

Publications, 1502 Augusta, Suite 415, Houston, TX 77057, (713) 974-6903.

Tax Preparation Assistance. Two programs sponsored by the Internal Revenue Service — Income Tax Assistance and Tax Counseling for the Elderly — use IRS-trained volunteers to help you with your personal income tax returns. Assistance is available from February 1 to April 15. If you are unable to travel to the site — usually a library, senior center, or community center — a volunteer will visit your home. This service is for basic, uncomplicated returns. You will need to bring your last year's return, all W-2 forms, SSA-1099, 1099s, records of other income, receipts for medical and dental expenses, and receipts for contributions. For the location nearest you, contact the IRS, (800) 424-1040.

Recorded Tax Information. Telephone access to information on about 140 topics relating to federal taxes as recorded by the Internal Revenue Service. A list of topics is available in "Guide to Free Tax Services" (see "Publications") or on the information line when you call. Tele-Tax, (800) 829-4477.

Your Tax Refund Status. An automated status report is available by telephone for a refund you expect from the Internal Revenue Service. Tele-Tax, (800) 829-4477.

Consumer Credit Counseling Service. A nonprofit organization with seven hundred offices nationwide to help you set up a budget, plan future expenses, repay creditors. Also available is a Credit Recovery Program that helps you return to the credit market after repaying your debts. For the office nearest you, contact National Foundation for Consumer Credit, 8611 2nd Avenue, Suite 100, Silver Spring, MD 10910, (800) 388-CCCS (2227).

Publications

Federal Tax Forms and Tax Publications. FREE. IRS Distribution Center, from western states: Rancho Cordova, CA 95743; from central states: P.O. Box 9903, Bloomington, IL 61799; from eastern states: P.O. Box 85074, Richmond, VA 23261; (800) TAX-FORM (829-3676).

"Relocation Tax Guide," American Association of Retired Persons. Describes how the tax laws of different states may affect you. Includes a list of state offices from which to request further information.

FREE. AARP Publications, 601 E Street, NW, Washington, DC 20049.

"Guide to Free Tax Services," Internal Revenue Service. Lists of free publications, telephone services, tax assistance, and tips for filing federal tax returns. Publication 910. FREE. IRS Distribution Center, from western states: Rancho Cordova, CA 95743; from central states: P.O. Box 9903, Bloomington, IL 61799; from eastern states: P.O. Box 85074, Richmond, VA 23261; (800) TAX-FORM (829-3676).

"Tax Information for Older Americans," Internal Revenue Service. Basic tax information that may be of special interest to older Americans, such as how to report pension and annuity income. Includes large-print tax forms to help with preliminary calculations, even though you must use standard forms when you file. Explains how to complete the forms you may need. Publication 554. FREE. IRS Distribution Center, from western states: Rancho Cordova, CA 95743; from central states: P.O. Box 9903, Bloomington, IL 61799; from eastern states: P.O. Box 85074, Richmond, VA 23261; (800) TAX-FORM (829-3676).

Tax Preparation Guides. Four guides are updated each year to reflect changes in the tax law. Each one guides you through each line of the tax forms.

> *Ernst & Young Tax Guide*, Ernst & Young, John Wiley & Sons
> *Guide to Income Tax* by Warren H. Esanu, Barry Dickman, and Elias M. Zuckerman, Consumer Reports Books
> *H & R Block Income Tax Guide*, H & R Block Tax Services, Inc., Collier Books
> *J. K. Lasser's Your Income Tax*, J. K. Lasser Institute, Prentice Hall

"Are You in a Credit Emergency?" National Foundation for Consumer Credit. Ten questions to determine if you should ask for help with budgeting to pay off your debts. FREE. NFCC, 8611 2nd Avenue, Suite 100, Silver Spring, MD 10910, (800) 388-CCCS (2227).

"Using Credit," National Foundation for Consumer Credit. A brief discussion of types of credit, definitions of some terms, explanation of pertinent legislation. FREE. NFCC, 8611 2nd Avenue, Suite 100, Silver Spring, MD 10910, (800) 388-CCCS (2227).

"Equal Credit Opportunity and Age," Federal Deposit Insurance

Corp. A brief review of protections against discrimination for age from creditors. FREE. FDIC, Office of Consumer Affairs, 550 17th Street, NW, Washington, DC 20429, (800) 424-5488.

"What Is Your Credit Report?," National Foundation for Consumer Credit. Explanation of the report creditors will use to decide whether to grant you credit. FREE. NFCC, 8611 2nd Avenue, Suite 100, Silver Spring, MD 20910, (800) 388-CCCS (2227).

"How to Be Credit Smart," Consumer Credit Education Foundation. An overview of issues involved in getting and maintaining credit, including a "credit-ability" questionnaire you can use to evaluate your credit habits. 50 cents. CCEF, Department CS, 919 18th Street, NW, Washington, DC 20006, (202) 296-5544.

"Consumer Handbook to Credit Protection Laws," Federal Reserve. A basic review of various credit situations, such as mortgages and credit cards, with definitions and explanations of your obligations and rights. FREE. Board of Governors of the Federal Reserve System, Washington, DC 20551.

"Building a Better Credit Record: What to Do, What to Avoid," Federal Trade Commission. Explanation of how credit bureaus work and how to check your own credit. Suggestions for improving your credit and dealing with debt. FREE. Federal Trade Commission, Washington, DC 20429.

"How to Manage Your Checking Account," Credit Union National Association. A brochure that explains how to use your checking account, including how to balance your checkbook. FREE. CUNA, Public Relations Department, P.O. Box 431, Madison, WI 53701.

Consumer Problems

When you have a limited income and are taking care to spend it wisely, it's all the more disheartening to encounter unscrupulous people, people who know their products or services are worthless or who want to steal your money with your compliance. Scammers, cheats, thieves, and quacks survive by seeking out people with money, innocence, and credulity.

Beware of these scams that have worked in the past:

- Ketchup drop, also known as mustard drop, egg drop, or ice-cream drop. Something dirties your clothing, and while a passerby is helping you clean up, an associate is cleaning

405

out your pocketbook or jacket pocket.

- Bump and drop. You help someone pick up what he or she dropped on bumping into you, and an accomplice steals your wallet.
- Pigeon drop. Someone approaches you with a wallet or envelope full of phony money asking if it's yours. He or she consults with a "lawyer," who advises him or her to get a show of good faith — money — from you before sharing the proceeds.
- Phony meter reader. A uniformed utility "employee" asks you to pay to avoid having your electric or gas service suspended or urges you to make a down payment for a new meter (with a special discount for seniors!).
- Phony bank guard. As you step outside your bank, a "security guard" tells you that counterfeit money is in circulation and he must check the authenticity of the bills you just withdrew. The "guard" says he'll take it inside the bank to check. He disappears while you wait.
- Ponzi scheme. Someone solicits an investment in a nonexistent enterprise promising a guaranteed high return. The original group of backers is paid off, encouraging others to put up money. A few are paid off, and the number of investors increases until the scamster disappears with the money. (Invest only after obtaining printed information and understanding the risks.)
- Half right all of the time. X calls fifty people telling half that a certain commodity or stock will increase in price; he tells the other half it will decline. The following week X calls the half for whom his prediction was accurate and makes another similar half-and-half prediction. Those who twice missed an opportunity for a profit are often now hooked into sending money. (Inform yourself about investment risks, and be sure to deal with legitimate brokers. Most investment opportunities are available from more than a single source.)
- Phone charges. A telephone "operator" calls to inform you of an investigation into illegal phone use. You are told to accept charges for a call. When it appears on your bill, you may find it was a long-distance, usually international,

call. (Countercheck any unusual requests or solicitations you receive by phone by asking for written descriptions.)

- Gaining entry to steal. Thieves will use a variety of pretexts to enter your home without breaking in. They may say that they need to check the energy efficiency of your furnace or other appliance, check your water quality, or check for radon or that the superintendent sent them to check your windows or plumbing. They may ask to use the bathroom, request a drink of water or other assistance, or ask to use your phone book, for a paper and pencil to leave a message for a neighbor, or for permission to drop off a package for a neighbor. These scammers work in pairs so that while you are talking to one, the other, whom you may never see, is stealing your valuables. Also, when you're doing yard work, one may keep you busy in conversation or asking directions, while the other enters your home. (Although you may dislike feeling suspicious or threatened in your own neighborhood, it is a good policy to lock your doors and close the garage door when you are doing yard work and ask to see identification cards of all unfamiliar servicemen who come without your request.)
- Prizewinner. You are told that you won a prize or are to inherit money and that *for a fee* the caller will help you get it.
- Mortgage change of address. You receive a notice that a new company has taken over your mortgage and that your payments should be sent to a new address. (Contact the previous company and ask for written confirmation before sending money.)
- Scare tactics by fund-raisers. You receive mail from organizations claiming that seniors are about to lose benefits or requests for money from an official-sounding organization, such as Social Security Protection Service, using stationery that resembles official government communications with a disclaimer in small print that states it is not affiliated with any branch of government.
- Mail-order fakery. A $4 coat hanger is a ten-cent nail; a $40 solar clothes dryer is a clothesline and clothespins; "brand-name" perfumes, watches, or other items are shown

with one letter altered, such as Bolova for Bulova.

- Work-at-home schemes. Claims that you can earn thousands of dollars a week from your kitchen table may be a way of selling you the equipment to get started, such as a $500 knitting machine.
- Bogus health cures. These are items that claim to heal conditions for which science has not yet discovered a cure, such as arthritis, overeating, cancer, baldness. While you can't be suspicious of every offer you hear about and many opportunities may be legitimate, it pays to be cautious.

Cautions for Consumers

- Beware of people watching as you withdraw money from the bank or an automatic teller machine. They may follow you as you go shopping or may attempt to enter your house on a pretext.
- When you order by mail, keep receipts, copies of orders, checks sent, and ads that you respond to until you receive and are satisfied with the product.
- Senior citizen seats are often near the entrance to buses, making it easy for a thief to grab your pocketbook, shopping bag, or a package and exit quickly.
- Never give your credit card or account number to solicitors over the phone, unless you call to make a purchase.
- Asking for written material or for time to think something over will generally frighten off a scamster, while legitimate business people and work people are willing to answer questions and show you credentials.
- Making an inquiry to the police, a local newspaper, or the Better Business Bureau can provide information about a company's reliability or reveal prior complaints.

Resources

Products

Safety Wallet. Protect cash and credit cards by attaching this nylon wallet to your belt and tucking it inside your waistband. Can also be worn holster-style and hidden under a shirt. $4. Hanover

House catalog, (717) 633-3366.

Services

Consumer Helpline. Assistance, information, and referrals for consumers with complaints about government agencies or private businesses. U.S. Office of Consumer Affairs, (800) 664-4435.

Consumer Product Safety Hot Line. Information about hazardous consumer products. Consumer Product Safety Commission, 5401 Westbard Avenue, Washington, DC 20207, (800) 638-2772.

Mail Order Action Line. A service to attempt to resolve complaints between consumers and companies that deal directly with the public via catalogs, telephone, or print or TV ads. MOAL, Direct Marketing Association, 1101 17th Street, NW, Suite 705, Washington, DC 20036.

National Fraud Information Center. Provides information, referrals to appropriate agencies, and resources to help you resolve complaints on consumer issues, and advice to consumers about fraud. Publications available. NFIC, 815 15th Street, NW, Suite 928-N, Washington, DC 20005, (800) 876-7060.

National Council Against Health Fraud. Hot line on health fraud and quackery. NCHF, 2800 Main Street, Kansas City, MO 64108, (800) 821-6671.

Publications

BEST BUY. "Consumer's Resource Handbook," U.S. Office of Consumer Affairs. Tips on handling complaints, a sample letter, and contacts for help with consumer problems. Contacts for 750 companies, car manufacturers, Better Business Bureaus, some trade associations, State and local consumer protection offices. FREE. Consumer Information Center, Pueblo, CO 81009.

"Fraud by Phone," Federal Trade Commission. Examples of phony offers made by telemarketers. FREE. FTC, Bureau of Consumer Protection, Washington, DC 20580, (202) 326-3650.

"Quackery and the Elderly," Better Business Bureau. How to identify fraudulent health claims and what you can do if you suspect a product's efficacy. $2. Council of Better Business Bureaus, 4200 Wilson Boulevard, Arlington, VA 22203, (703) 276-0100.

"How to Spot a Con Artist," American Association of Retired Persons. List of schemes and techniques used to fool people into spending money. FREE. AARP Publications, 601 E Street, NW, Washington, DC 20049 (800) 424-3410.

"Investment Swindles: How They Work and How to Avoid Them," National Futures Association. Information to help you recognize and avoid unethical investment advisers, including sixteen questions that can turn off an "investment crook." FREE. NFA, 200 West Madison Street, Suite 1600, Chicago, IL 60606, (800) 621-3570, or in Illinois call (800) 572-9400.

"Swindlers Are Calling," Alliance Against Fraud in Telemarketing. How to recognize a possibly illegitimate call, how to avoid becoming a victim. FREE. National Futures Association, Public Affairs and Education, 200 West Madison Street, Suite 1600, Chicago IL 60606-3447, (800) 621-3570, or in Illinois call (800) 572-9400. Or, also FREE, National Consumers League, 1701 K Street, NW, Suite 1200, Washington, DC 20006, (202) 835-3323.

"Consumer Problems of the Elderly," Better Business Bureau. Situations that attract unethical individuals who take advantage of people's trust or credulity. $2. Council of Better Business Bureaus, 4200 Wilson Boulevard, Arlington, VA 22203, (703) 276-0100.

Organizations

Membership Organizations. These groups focus on senior issues and provide support, information, and other benefits to their members:

Gray Panthers, 1424 16th Street, NW, Suite 602, Washington, DC 20036, (202) 387-3111

National Alliance of Senior Citizens, 1700 18th Street, NW, Suite 401, Washington, DC 20009, (202) 986-0117

Food and Drug Administration. This agency approves the marketing of products and medications according to their safety and efficacy. Provides information about bogus or useless products that claim to alleviate such conditions as obesity, arthritis, wrinkles, and other unproved cures for such problems as sexual dysfunction, cancer, or baldness. FDA, 5600 Fishers Lane, Rockville, MD 20857, (301) 443-3170.

To preserve the assets you spent your life accumulating and to decide how they should be disposed of when you die, you can create certain legal documents yourself or you can consult an expert, a lawyer. Anytime you are presented with papers to sign, you should understand what you are agreeing to and what the other party promises to do. Many complications can be avoided if you consult with a lawyer to be sure the technical language doesn't hide an undesirable limitation or requirement. Advice on legal matters is for your protection and can defend you against being taken advantage of or unwittingly consenting to something not in your best interests. Some situations in which you might benefit from an attorney's advice:

Dealing with documents relating to housing commitments: rental agreements, sale or mortgage transactions, home sharing, nursing home contracts, retirement or continuing care communities
Credit or loan problems
Insurance claims

Legal aid is available FREE for those unable to afford it, and each state's office on the aging is required to have a legal services developer to help you find a lawyer. Your local bar association can recommend a lawyer with specific expertise; information also is available at your library from the *Martindale-Hubbell Law Directory*. For routine matters, such as drawing up a will or certain other documents, you may use standard forms available in most stationery stores and have them reviewed by an attorney.

Resources

Magnifiers to help you read the small print are listed in Chapter 16, "Enhancing Your Memory and Vision."

Services

National Resource Center for Consumers of Legal Services. Consumer Resource Fact Sheets. Information by state on legal service plans that provide legal advice for a monthly fee. Also provides the names of several plans for individuals and an explanation of how they operate. FREE. National Resource Center for Consumers of Legal Services, Tabb House, Main Street, P.O. Box 340, Gloucester, VA 23061, (804) 693-9330 or (202) 842-3503.

National Association of the Deaf Legal Defense Fund. Represents deaf and hard-of-hearing clients before federal courts and those who have been victims of discrimination. Offers advice about legal rights. FREE. NAD, 800 Florida Avenue, NE, P.O. Box 2304, Washington, DC 20002, (202) 651-5343.

National Academy of Elder Law Attorneys. Refers you to members in your area and provides information on how to choose an attorney and how certain issues may affect you. NAELA, 1604 North Country Club Road, Tucson, AZ 85716, (602) 881-4005.

American Bar Association Information Services. Publications and referral to your local bar association that will help you find a lawyer near you. ABA, 750 North Lake Shore Drive, Chicago, IL 60611, (312) 988-5158.

Legal Counsel for the Elderly Hot Line. Legal consultation for callers age sixty and older. You can get advice on simple matters or referral to private, low-cost, or FREE legal services near you. FREE. To find out if your state has this service, contact LCE, P.O. Box 96474, Washington, DC 20090, (800) 424-3410.

Computer Programs

Personal Law Firm. Provides the format for creating a will and other legal documents. $30. Tiger Software, 1 Datran Center, Suite 1500, 9100 Dadeland Boulevard, Miami, FL 33156, (800) 444-3363.

It's Legal. Creates documents, such as wills, durable health care power of attorney, simple power of attorney. $70. Parsons Technology, 1 Parsons Drive, P.O. Box 100, Hiawatha, IA 52233.

Publications

Organizing Your Future: A Guide to Decisionmaking in Your Later Years, Legal Counsel for the Elderly. A manual that describes in question-and-answer format the legal tools you need to control financial and health care decisions. Includes forms and suggestions for finding an attorney who specializes in elder law. Updated annually. $13. LCE, P.O. Box 96474, Washington, DC 20090, (202) 434-2152.

"Question and Answers When Looking for an Elder Law Attorney," National Academy of Elder Law Attorneys. FREE. NAELA, 655 North Alvernon Way, Suite 108, Tucson, AZ 85711, (602) 881-4005.

Important Documents

Your financial and legal status is validated by an assortment of documents that you should keep in a safe place. On the other hand, these documents should be easy to find by you or your family. Your instructions regarding your estate — your will — should be stored *at home,* with a list of all other important papers, where they are located, and a copy of each. The originals of irreplaceable documents, plus those that would be annoying or inconvenient to replace, should be kept in a safe-deposit box.

Important Papers

In a large manila envelope you keep at home, collect the following information and items. Originals of italicized documents should be kept in a safe-deposit box, copies in the envelope.

- Names and addresses of your lawyer, accountant, and financial adviser
- Duplicate keys to your automobile, home, and other property
- List of assets: *stock certificates,* bank account numbers and bank branch names and addresses, *real estate deeds* and *mortgages, life insurance policy*
- *Marriage* and *birth certificates*
- *Military records*
- *Divorce papers*
- *Funeral arrangements*
- *Trust agreements*
- Location of important household and financial files

Also in the envelope should be the location of your safe-deposit box and one key and the location of the second key.

Certain records or copies should be accessible to those who will update and reconcile your accounts. Maintain a file for each stock, recording its purchase price and including any dividend purchase plan statements (place stock certificates in your safe-deposit box);

individual bonds; each mutual fund; checking accounts (keep records for the past three years); savings accounts and certificates of deposit; income tax returns (current and for *all* past years); homeowner records, purchase price, deed, mortgage, homeowner insurance, repairs, and improvements; Social Security records; pension accounts; life insurance policy; credit card accounts; automobile title, repairs, and insurance; funeral plans; receipts for items you own; medical expenses and medical insurance reimbursements.

Resources

Products

File Shuttle. A pine trolley for letter or legal size file folders. $40. Hold Everything catalog, (800) 421-2264.

Net Worth Personal Financial Journal. A passport-style booklet in which you can record financial information and location of important papers. $5. Informative Amenities, P.O. Box 1280, Santa Monica, CA 90406, (800) 553-3886, or in California call (310) 394-6992.

BEST BUY. "Do You Know Your Valuable Papers?" by Elizabeth Wiegand and C. Arthur Bratton. A simple inventory for listing your important papers and other vital information. $1.20. Cornell Cooperative Extension, Resource Center-GP, 7 Cornell Business and Technology Park, Ithaca, NY 14850, (607) 255-2080.

Wall Safe. Mounts flush against the wall so that it can be concealed under a picture frame or in a closet. Mounts between wall studs, steel, combination lock. 13½ by 8½ by 3½-inch interior. $90. Safety Zone catalog, (800) 999-3030.

Can Safes. Fake cleansing, beverage, or cosmetic containers in which to hide valuables under the sink, in the refrigerator, or in the medicine cabinet. Replicas of brand-name products have lids or bottom openings for cash, jewelry, etc. Soda can, $10. Others, $15. Safety Zone catalog, (800) 999-3030.

Book Safe. Hardcover book with hollowed-out felt-lined compartment (4 by 7 inches) for valuables. Compartment is closed so that contents won't spill out if book is removed from shelf. $25. Bruce Medical Supply catalog, (800) 225-8446.

Wall Outlet Safe. Look-alike electric outlet is easily installed in

Sheetrock wall. Locks and unlocks by turning screw. $7. Safety Zone catalog, (800) 999-3030.

Computer Programs

Personal RecordKeeper. A device for organizing and storing your financial, legal, and personal information. Enables you to compute your net worth and keep a property inventory. $50. Ask for a 30 percent discount when you order from the publisher: Nolo Press, 950 Parker Street, Berkeley, CA 94710, (800) 992-6656.

Financial Directives

Certain documents help you retain control over your financial affairs even when you are incapacitated or after your death. You can name a proxy to handle your financial matters, make your own funeral arrangements, and decide on the distribution of your assets.

Durable Power of Attorney

If you are not able to take care of your finances, even temporarily, you can name someone with the legal authority to act for you by executing a durable power of attorney. A simple power of attorney gives someone authority to act in your place, usually for a specified purpose, such as a real estate transaction or to write checks. This document becomes invalid when you are incapacitated. On the other hand, a durable power of attorney continues in effect when you are incapacitated.

By naming a proxy, you avoid having the state appoint a guardian who would make decisions regarding your financial affairs. This would include such transactions as paying your rent, filing your tax returns, selling any possessions, such as a car or house, and making investment decisions. The person named in a durable power of attorney would not be able to make medical decisions for you but would be able to arrange payment, if necessary, for medical treatment authorized by your health care proxy, the medical counterpart (see page 430). Of course, the same person can be named to perform both functions.

Although stationery stores have forms that can be filled out and that would have legal force, a durable power of attorney written by a lawyer will pertain more specifically to your situation. Banks or other financial institutions may require you to use their own forms, so you should verify their procedures before relying on other forms. The key phrase in a durable power of attorney may read: "This power of attorney shall not be affected by the subsequent disability or incompetence of the principal." A springing power of attorney goes into effect only when you are incapacitated and would include a phrase like the following: "This power of attorney will become effective upon my incapacity as certified by my treating physician and one other physician."

Funeral Plans

Making plans regarding what happens to your body after your death may be important to you. This would provide guidance to your relatives, who may not know your wishes, but you must let your family know that you have made such plans. A copy of your organ donor card and any agreements with a medical school or funeral home and cemetery should be attached to your will.

You may want to donate your organs or tissues to others or your body for scientific research or medical study. Hearts to be used for transplantation must be younger than forty years of age, but cornea donors may be up to age seventy.

There is no maximum age to donate your body for anatomical study, but you should register with a medical school near you. In this case your body is prepared according to the needs of the medical school and delivered after the funeral.

You can make funeral and burial arrangements and pay for them in advance. Not only will you be able to indicate your preferences, but you will be saving. The money is placed in a trust fund for the benefit of the funeral home, which guarantees that your payment covers the entire cost of the funeral. The interest that accumulates in the account will compensate the funeral home for inflation or increased costs. The average funeral costs between $3,500 and $8,500, not including the cost of a cemetery plot or gravestone. Veterans and some veterans' dependents can be buried at no charge in national cemeteries, though the estate is responsible for paying the funeral and transportation costs.

A Will

Inexplicably most people die without having wills. Even if your wishes duplicate the laws of inheritance in your state, you might still consider naming an executor to be sure your estate is properly distributed.

Order of Inheritance When There Is No Will

NOTE: Your state's law regarding the distribution of property may be somewhat different from what appears below.

- Half to your spouse, half to be divided among the children
- All to your spouse if there are no children
- All to your children and grandchildren if no spouse survives
- All to your parents if no spouse or children survive
- All to be divided by your siblings or their surviving children if none of the other relatives mentioned above survives

---

Only if you draft a will can *you* designate who is to receive a portion of your estate or alter the division required by law. You also can name alternate beneficiaries and name a person you trust (and an alternate) as executor to be sure your wishes are carried out. If you decide to write your will on your own, it will have legal force if you follow carefully the laws in your state. Will forms are available in stationery stores or from your state or local bar association, and many do-it-yourself books are available. Be sure all witnesses are present when you *and* each of them sign. A lawyer's expertise and knowledge of current state laws may give you added protection, especially if your estate is large or complicated.

You don't have to worry about estate taxes if your estate is valued at less than $600,000 and held jointly. With the advice of a lawyer or a tax professional, you can arrange your assets to reduce your heirs' taxes by making gifts, setting up trusts, and buying stocks. Review your will if you move to a new state, if your beneficiaries die, if your assets change significantly, or if you want to change your executor. When you make your will, evaluate the title in which you hold ownership of property or bank or other accounts to determine the style that is in accord with your wishes or would be most convenient if you become incapacitated.

Resources

Products

"The AICR Will Organizer: Your Personal Planning Worksheet," American Institute for Cancer Research. Not a do-it-yourself will form but a means of organizing your personal information and wishes before visiting an attorney. Helps you assemble financial and legal documents and information, and enumerates other issues you should take into account. FREE. AICR, 1759 R Street, NW, Washington, DC 20009, (800) 843-8114.

Services

National Anatomical Service. Referrals to a medical school near you that needs bodies for its academic programs. NAS, 24 Avon Way, Parlin, NJ 08859, (800) 727-0700.

Computer Programs

WillMaker. Create your legal will by a question-and-answer process. Takes into account your state's requirements (except Louisiana's) and includes a manual containing further information. $70. Ask for a 30 percent discount when you order from the publisher: Nolo Press, 950 Parker Street, Berkeley, CA 94710, (800) 992-6656.

Publications

"Body Donation," University of Medicine and Dentistry of New Jersey — Robert Wood Johnson Medical School Anatomical Association. Information about how to donate your body for anatomical study or medical research. FREE. RWJMSAA, 675 Hoes Lane, Piscataway, NJ 08854, (800) GIFT-211 (443-8211).

"Product Report: Prepaying Your Funeral?," American Association of Retired Persons. Planning and prepaying details and considerations. FREE. AARP Publications, 601 E Street, NW, Washington, DC 20049.

"Funeral Costs," National Funeral Directors Association. A list of services and a range of charges so that you can gauge expenses.

418

FREE. NFDA, Learning Resources Center, 11121 West Oklahoma Avenue, Milwaukee, WI 53227, (414) 541-2500.

"Easing the Burden: Prearranging Your Funeral," National Funeral Directors Association. Questions to consider regarding your funeral, and information about the location of documents indicating your preferences. FREE. NFDA, Learning Resources Center, 11121 West Oklahoma Avenue, Milwaukee, WI 53227, (414) 541-2500.

Simple Will Book: How to Prepare a Legally Valid Will by Denis Clifford, J.D. Sample will forms and work sheets with instructions and explanations for making your own will, including creating a trust. (Not for Louisiana.) 1992. Consumer Reports Books.

Plan Your Estate with a Living Trust by Denis Clifford, J.D. Mainly for people with estates under $600,000 who want to prepare living trusts and wills. Guidance in setting up a legal structure to avoid probate and estate taxes. Includes forms and instructions. (Not for Louisiana.) Request most recent edition. Nolo Press.

Thy Will Be Done: A Guide to Estate Planning for Older Persons by Eugene J. Daly. A practical guide to wills and taxes that encourages you to draw a will and presents issues to think about as you go through the process. Provides suggestions for saving money for yourself and your heirs. 1990. Prometheus Books.

Organizations

The Living Bank. A national registry for people wishing to donate organs and tissue. When the bank is notified that you are near death, a local agency will be informed to comply with your wishes. The Living Bank, P.O. Box 6725, Houston, TX 77005, (800) 528-2971.

Uniform Donor Card. A wallet-size card to note your preferences for donating organs, tissues, or your body. A copy should be kept with your will and other directives. FREE. The National Kidney Foundation, 30 East 33rd Street, New York, NY 10016, (800) 622-9010. Also available from the Organ and Tissue Donor Card Request Line, operated by the United Network for Organ Sharing, (800) 24-DONOR (243-6667).

Chapter 21

Planning Your Health Care

Changes in the nation's health insurance system are not likely to affect us directly in the immediate future. Medicare and any supplemental insurance will still be the primary coverage for medical and hospital expenses for people age sixty-five and over. If you are under age sixty-five and are not covered at work or under your spouse's plan, you must purchase your own health insurance until such time as the government may provide universal coverage.

Health insurance can alleviate worries about catastrophic occurrences that may require expensive long-term solutions. You may express your wishes about the kind of care you would choose if you are very ill.

INSURANCE

Health insurance policies offer a variety of coverages, a choice of how much deductible you pay, and other limitations and options.

Health maintenance organizations (HMOs) are a type of health insurance for which you pay a monthly fee and receive a wide range of health services at little or no additional cost. HMOs generally require you to visit a doctor named by the organization and will not reimburse you, or will do so at a lesser amount, if you see a physician outside their networks. If you don't already have a doctor who knows you well and whom you trust, this would be a low-cost option. An HMO that participates with Medicare would eliminate your having to file claims or to pay a 20 percent copayment or a deductible and may eliminate the need for Medigap coverage. An HMO would not cancel you because of your medical condition, and if you are over a certain age, you may pay less. You would still need to pay for Medicare coverage of physician expenses.

With private traditional health insurance, you may select your own doctors and hospitals and still be reimbursed for some or all of your health care expenses. You must choose a policy that covers major illnesses or accidents, surgeries, hospital care, and physicians' care; these are the most costly eventualities. Many organizations such as AARP offer group health insurance to their members at lower rates than you could obtain on your own.

The federal health insurance program for people age sixty-five and over comes in two parts: Part A for hospital expenses and Part B for medical expenses.

Medicare Birthdays

- *Three months before your sixty-fifth birthday.* Sign up for Part A so that you will be covered at your earliest eligibility. This coverage is automatic if you are receiving Social Security benefits.
- *A seven-month period surrounding your sixty-fifth birthday* — that is, three months prior to the month in which you turn sixty-five and three months after: Sign up for Part B during this period to avoid higher premiums and to be covered at your earliest eligibility (unless you are covered by an employer health plan).

Medicare insurance does not cover all your medical expenses. The hospital is paid directly, financed by payroll taxes, and you receive a bill for the remainder. Part B insurance is financed in part with a monthly premium that you pay, and you will have to pay at least 20 percent of each bill.

Medicaid, a program for people with low incomes and limited resources, has eligibility requirements and coverages that vary by state. People who don't qualify for Medicaid but have limited income and resources may be eligible for the Qualified Medicare Beneficiary program, which will pay their Part B premiums, deductibles, and copayments.

Patients covered by Medicare may not be charged more than a fixed amount above what Medicare approves for a covered service. Doctors participating with Medicare agree to accept assignment — that is, the physician accepts whatever Medicare allows plus your copayment. Of course, Medicare does not cover *all* medical or hospital costs — for example, examinations for eyeglasses or contact lenses, examinations for prescribing and fitting hearing aids or the aids themselves, dental care, long-term nursing home care, or long-term home care. In fact, Medicare pays less than 40 percent of all health care costs. In 1994 the AARP found that out-of-pocket health care costs for people age sixty-five and over averaged $2,800, or 23 percent of their incomes. These expenses were for premiums for insurance, home health care, medical services not covered, and prescription medications.

To cover the costs of health care not covered by Medicare, you can purchase Medigap insurance, which pays the deductibles, copayments, the difference between Medicare's approved amount and the actual charges, and some services not covered at all. Some of the supplemental policies include coverage for prescription medicine.

Medigap Birthday

- *Up to six months after you enroll in Part B insurance* you can purchase a Medigap health insurance policy without being subject to denial because of health problems, though there may be a six-month exclusion of preexisting conditions. No medical exam is necessary.

As noted, Medicare doesn't cover long-term care, either in your home or in a nursing home. This is potentially the biggest drain on your assets since such care can cost a minimum of $40,000 a year. Most long-term care is provided by family members in the family home, but this is a complicated arrangement to maintain, often expensive and often disruptive of the lives of those providing the care.

Long-term care insurance can allow you to receive care in your home and avoid going to a nursing home or pay for a nursing home without dipping into your savings. Individuals with assets of $50,000 or more should consider this insurance if they can afford the premiums, which are higher the older one is. For example, one such policy costs $1,000 a year at age fifty-five and $2,200 at age seventy. If you can't afford it, your children may want to purchase long-term care insurance for you in order to protect their inheritance.

To qualify for Medicaid, you should have reduced assets for a three- to five-year period. For couples to preserve assets for a surviving spouse, arrangements may be made for "spending down" — converting cash assets into protected assets — or for a "Medicaid divorce" — a paper divorce that can transfer assets to one spouse while the other qualifies for Medicaid. This has been labeled "planned impoverishment" and is a means of avoiding spousal impoverishment caused by enormous health care expenses. To be eligible for Medicaid, you must have limited resources, not including your home, household goods, cars, or fine art. This means you could reduce your cash resources by paying off the mortgage, buying a larger home, or making improvements, such as an addition. Your income must be less than the cost of your care.

Of course, Medicaid is intended to provide care for the needy poor, but a legal loophole allows you to qualify by manipulating assets, laws, making gifts, establishing trusts, or other legal maneuvers. Called Medicaid planning, it converts your liquid assets into exempt assets. The three- to five-year waiting period doesn't apply if assets are transferred to a spouse. An irrevocable (or Medicaid) trust shelters your assets from being used to pay for a nursing home but lets you use the income, and at your death the principal goes to your children.

You can reduce your assets by paying relatives or others for home care until your funds are down to levels that would make you eligible for Medicaid. Medicaid pays all nursing home expenses for people with limited assets; nearly 70 percent of nursing home residents receive Medicaid. If you plan to qualify for Medicaid, you can consider purchasing a long-term care policy to cover the period needed to arrange your finances.

What to Look for When Choosing Long-Term Care Insurance

- *Period of nursing home care.* The best is lifetime.
- *Inflation protection.* It should be about 5 percent a year.
- *Home care.* The length of time covered and the level of care vary.
- *Requirement for prior hospitalization or other limitations.* This should not require a hospital stay before coverage begins.
- *Waiting period.* The longer you wait before the policy begins coverage, the smaller the premium you pay.
- *Guaranteed renewable, fixed premium.* Some policies exclude or terminate you for certain illnesses; premiums should be stable.

As more attention is focused on the need for long-term care insurance and as demand for it grows, insurance companies will offer more varied and competitive policies, possibly at more reasonable costs, making it a more attractive option.

To be sure the insurance you buy provides the coverage you need, seek advice from your state's insurance department. All insurance companies are rated for financial stability by A. M. Best, which publishes a guide available in many libraries.

Resources

Products

"Payment Record for Health Insurance Policies," American Association of Retired Persons. A form for recording claims and payments for your various insurance policies. FREE. AARP Publications, 601 E Street, NW, Washington, DC 20049.

Services

List of Federally Qualified HMOs. Office of Health Maintenance Organizations, Division of Qualification, Parklawn Building, 5600 Fishers Lane, Rockville, MD 20857, (301) 443-1976.

List of Health Maintenance Organizations. Group Health Association of America, 624 9th Street, NW, Washington, DC 20001, (202) 737-4311.

National Insurance Consumer Helpline. Response to inquiries regarding all types of insurance. A variety of FREE publications is available about auto and homeowners insurance and how to file an insurance claim. NICH, c/o ACLI, 1001 Pennsylvania Avenue, NW, Washington, DC 20004, (800) 942-4242.

Hot Line for Medicare, Medigap, Second Opinions. For information or to report cases of fraud. Health Care Financing Administration, (800) 638-6833.

Medicare Claims Assistance. Counseling and advocacy services to be sure of receiving your full benefits. Available for people who are unable to afford private assistance. Publications explaining how to look for errors and underpayments, how to apply for refunds, how to qualify for home health benefits, and other topics. Medicare Beneficiaries Defense Fund, 1460 Broadway, 8th Floor, New York, NY 10036, (212) 869-3850.

Partnership for Long-Term Care. An experimental plan to make long-term care insurance more affordable. To find out if your state endorses one of these policies, contact the Partnership's National Program Office, Center on Aging, HHP Building, Room 1240, University of Maryland, College Park, MD 20742, (301) 405-2544.

Publications

"Checkup on Health Insurance Choices," Agency for Health Care Policy and Research. An explanation of various types of health insurance, a work sheet for comparing costs and benefits of several plans, and definitions of insurance terms. FREE. AHCPR Publications Clearinghouse, P.O. Box 8547, Silver Spring, MD 20907, (800) 358-9295.

"Medicare Handbook," Health Care Financing Administration. An explanation of Medicare benefits and how to use the program. Includes a "troubleshooting" chart of whom to contact if you have questions or specific problems. This is an important reference for everyone who has Medicare insurance. Updated annually. FREE. HCFA, 6325 Security Boulevard, Baltimore, MD 21207, or call the Social Security Administration, (800) 772-1213.

"Medicare," Social Security Administration. Explains the outlines of eligibility and coverage of the federal medical and hospital insurance program. FREE. SSA, Office of Information, Room 4-J-10, West

High Rise, 6401 Security Boulevard, Baltimore, MD 21235, (800) 772-1213.

"Guide to Health Insurance for People with Medicare," National Association of Insurance Commissioners and the Health Care Financing Administration. Describes the Medicare program, private health insurance programs and how to evaluate them, and Medigap insurance policies. Lists telephone numbers for Medigap counseling, state insurance departments, state agencies on aging. Updated annually. FREE. HCFA, 7500 Security Boulevard, Baltimore, MD 21244, (410) 786-3000, or Consumer Information Center, Pueblo, CO 81002.

"Medicare: What It Will and Will Not Pay For," American Society of Internal Medicine. A brochure defining the medical and hospital services covered under Medicare and highlighting those services not covered. FREE. ASIM, 2011 Pennsylvania Avenue, NW, Washington, DC 20006, (202) 835-2746.

"Knowing Your Rights," American Association of Retired Persons. How Medicare, your doctor, and the hospital decide what treatment you should receive, how long you should remain in a hospital, and what costs are covered by Medicare. Explains the appeal process. FREE. AARP Publications, 601 E Street, NW, Washington, DC 20049.

Mastering the Medicare Maze by Betsy Abramson, Margie Groom, and Jeffrey Spitzer-Resnick. Explains how Medicare works in practice, highlighting limitations so that you know what to expect. Information on how to file a claim and how to appeal in case you are denied coverage. $11. 1995. May be ordered from the Center for Public Representation, 121 South Pinckney Street, Madison, WI 53703, (800) 369-0388.

"How to Avoid Overpaying Your Doctor Under Medicare Part B," Medicare Beneficiaries Defense Fund. Suggestions for monitoring your doctor bills for correct charges. $2. MBDF, 1460 Broadway, 8th Floor, New York, NY 10036, (212) 869-3850.

"Tips on Medicare and Medigap Insurance," Better Business Bureau. Suggestions for deciding which Medigap insurance policy is most cost-effective and guidance in avoiding unnecessary coverage or expense. SSE and $1. Council of Better Business Bureaus, 4200 Wilson Boulevard, Arlington, VA 22203, (703) 276-0100.

"Medigap: Medicare Supplement Insurance: A Consumer's Guide,"

American Association of Retired Persons. Guidance on comparing policies and understanding the health insurance reimbursement system. FREE. AARP Publications, 601 E Street, NW, Washington, DC 20049.

"Checklist for Purchasing Medicare Supplement Health Insurance" by Andrew Koski, C.S.W. About twenty questions that you should answer to help you decide whether a particular supplemental Medicare policy fills in Medicare's "gaps." FREE. Institute on Law and Rights of Older Adults, Brookdale Center on Aging of Hunter College, 425 East 25th Street, New York, NY 10010, (212) 481-4426.

"Guide to Medicare Supplement Insurance," Health Insurance Association of America. Information to help you make decisions about whether you need Medicare Supplement insurance and which features you should select. FREE. National Insurance Consumer Helpline, c/o ACLI, 1001 Pennsylvania Avenue, NW, Washington, DC 20004, (800) 942-4242.

"Checklist for Purchasing Long-Term Care Insurance Policies" by Andrew Koski, C.S.W. Definitions of terms and answers to pertinent questions to help you understand and evaluate long-term care insurance policies. FREE. Institute on Law and Rights of Older Adults, Brookdale Center on Aging of Hunter College, 425 East 25th Street, New York, NY 10010, (212) 481-4426.

"Guide to Long-Term Care Insurance," Health Insurance Association of America. General information about long-term care insurance. FREE. National Insurance Consumer Helpline, c/o ACLI, 1001 Pennsylvania Avenue, NW, Washington, DC 20004, (800) 942-4242.

"Before You Buy: A Guide to Long-Term Care Insurance," American Association of Retired Persons. Helps you evaluate long-term care insurance and compare different policies. FREE. AARP Publications, 601 E Street, NW, Washington, DC 20049.

"Long-Term Care: A Dollar and Sense Guide" by Susan Polniaszek, M.P.H. Explains sources of financial assistance for long-term health care both at home or in a nursing facility. $9. United Seniors Health Cooperative, 1331 H Street, NW, Suite 500, Washington, DC 20005, (202) 393-6222.

Beat the Nursing Home Trap: A Consumer's Guide to Choosing and Financing Long-Term Care by Joseph Matthews. Discusses options for how to provide for the time when you need long-term care, including housing choices, insurance, community programs. Request most recent edition. Nolo Press.

"Directory of Medicare Providers and Suppliers of Services." A list of all Medicare-approved hospitals, physicians, skilled nursing facilities, home health agencies, visiting nurses, outpatient physical therapy facilities, independent laboratories, portable X-ray units, renal disease treatment centers. Medicare-approved services are charged according to Medicare's fee schedule. $2.70. Available from your local Medicare office. For the office nearest you, contact the Health Care Financing Administration, (800) 638-6833.

HEALTH CARE CONSUMERS

Your health care expenses will be reduced if you can take advantage of free or low-cost services. Pharmacies may offer special discounts to seniors, and in some states special prescription payment programs are available to provide medications at lower cost.

Keep careful records of all your expenses and reimbursements so that you are sure to receive what you are due. It's a good idea to discuss your doctor's fee structure and payment policy when you call to make an appointment to avoid future misunderstandings. If you are frank about your need to economize, a sympathetic doctor may let you pay monthly amounts, adjust his or her fee, or decide to accept Medicare assignment.

It's a good idea to get copies of all reports — blood tests, X rays, prescriptions, and so on — for your records. After all, these test results and reports belong to you. A primary care physician can coordinate your care, recommend doctors for consultations or second opinions, and help you make decisions about your care.

Make inquiries about medications you are given or procedures that are recommended for your treatment. It's always best to know as much as possible about your health and how to take good care of yourself.

Resources

Some mail-order pharmacies that may offer discounts are listed in Chapter 14, "Preparing for Emergencies."

Services

Veterans Hospitals. To find out if you are eligible for care in a veterans hospital, contact the Department of Veterans Affairs, 810 Vermont Avenue, NW, Washington, DC 20420, (800) 827-1000.

FREE Hospital Care. To find out if you are eligible for FREE hospital care, contact Hill-Burton Hospital Free Care Program, BHMORD-JRSA, 5600 Fishers Lane, Rockville, MD 20857, (800) 638-0742.

National Health Information Center. Source of information and referral for health questions, the latest treatment options, medications, etc. NHIC, P.O. Box 1133, Washington, DC 20013, (800) 336-4797.

"Directory of Pharmaceutical Manufacturers Programs," Special Committee on Aging, U.S. Senate. Describes programs of drug manufacturers that make medications available FREE to patients who cannot pay for them. If a drug you are taking is listed, your doctor should contact the company. FREE. Special Committee on Aging, Dirksen Senate Office Building, Room G-31, Washington, DC 20510, (202) 224-5364. To learn if a specific medication is included in the program, call Pharmaceutical Research and Manufacturers Association, (800) 762-4636.

Publications

"Health Care Shopper's Guide: 59 Ways to Save Money," Office of the Maryland Attorney General. Suggestions for avoiding extra expenses, how to select health care services, and ways of getting good medical care for the least cost. FREE. Superintendent of Documents, Washington, DC 20402, (202) 512-1800.

"Healthy Questions," American Association of Retired Persons. Suggestions about how to talk to and select physicians, pharmacists, dentists, and vision care specialists. FREE. AARP Publications, 601 E Street, NW, Washington, DC 20049.

Health Care Choices for Today's Consumer, Families USA. A practical guide to choosing a health plan, a doctor, a hospital. Also, advice for keeping your medical costs low. 1994. Families USA, 1334 G Street, NW, 3rd Floor, Washington, DC 20005, (800) 699-6960.

Organizations

National Organization for Rare Disorders. A central source for information about unusual diseases and for networking to exchange information. Newsletter for members. Maintains computerized data on more than one thousand conditions. Provides names of experts, treatment, and self-help groups. NORD, 100 Route 37, P.O. Box 8923, New Fairfield, CT 06812, (203) 746-6518.

National Easter Seal Society. Information, referrals, and support to those with disabilities; not limited to people with polio. NESS, 230 West Monroe, Suite 1800, Chicago, IL 60606, (800) 221-6827.

People's Medical Society. Membership consumer health organization. Newsletter and publications with information geared to helping you get the best health care at the best price. PMS, 462 Walnut Street, Allentown, PA 18102, (800) 624-8773.

United Seniors Health Cooperative. Guidance to members regarding Medicare supplemental insurance or long-term care insurance. Information available on a wide range of health subjects. USHC, 1331 H Street, NW, Suite 500, Washington, DC 20005, (202) 393-6222.

MEDICAL DIRECTIVES

If you are in the hospital, you must sign a consent form to authorize treatment, or you can refuse to submit to treatment, surgery, or any medical procedure. To prepare for a situation in which you are unable to make such decisions yourself, you can execute an advance directive that names someone to assume this responsibility for you. A health care proxy named in a durable power of attorney for health care will make medical decisions for you and carry out your wishes about health care when you can't. This is similar to the durable power of attorney for financial matters (see page 415) since it continues in effect when you are no longer able to direct your own medical care.

According to a 1991 survey, most people would refuse life-sustaining treatment if they were terminally ill. Of those queried, 90 percent favored advance directives, although only 15 percent had made them. Most people say they would refuse treatment, but medical personnel are not authorized to withhold life-support measures when patients cannot communicate this desire themselves and have not named proxies.

Ideally the person you designate as your health care proxy will know your personal preferences regarding the treatment you want under specified circumstances. You and your proxy should discuss your beliefs about death and dying, dependency and disability, and your concept of what constitutes being "alive." These thoughts may also be conveyed in a living will, which applies to circumstances in which you are near death or have an incurable or irreversible condition that leaves you with diminished cognition or in which life-sustaining measures will simply prolong dying. A living will can give you control over the way you live and how you want to die. The Supreme Court requires that a person's wishes be followed when there is evidence that they are clearly and definitely stated.

To enable your proxy and your physicians to carry out your wishes, each individual should know the names of the others and have a copy of your health care proxy with an indication of where the original can be found. Only your proxy need have a copy of the living will.

Resources

Products

BEST BUY. **Living Will and Health Care Proxy Forms.** Your own state's forms for these advance directives with instructions for completing them. FREE. Choice in Dying, 200 Varick Street, 10th Floor, New York, NY 10014, (800) 989-WILL (9455).

Values History Form. A means for listing the locations of advance directives and recording your beliefs and preferences regarding what life means to you. Offers a way of raising these issues and a structure for thinking about them. $3. Values History, Institute of Public Law, 1117 Stanford, NE, Albuquerque, NM 87131.

"Planning for Incapacity: A Self-Help Guide," Legal Counsel for the Elderly. A step-by-step guide to advance directives, health care powers of attorney, and living wills. Each guide is for a specific state and contains forms for that state. Includes living will, health care power of attorney forms, instructions. $5. LCE, P.O. Box 96474, Washington, DC 20090, (202) 434-2152.

Publications

"A Matter of Choice: Planning Ahead for Health Care Decisions," American Association of Retired Persons. A discussion of the options you have as you plan your future. Includes legal issues, living wills, forms, and resources. FREE. AARP Publications, 601 E Street, NW, Washington, DC 20049.

Living Wills and More: Everything You Need to Ensure That All Your Medical Wishes Are Followed by Terry J. Barnett. Legal issues and personal and medical considerations are explained to help you control your medical future. Model documents for every state. 1992. John Wiley.

The Complete Guide to Living Wills: How to Safeguard Your Treatment Choices by Evan R. Collins, Jr., with Doron Weber. A guide to formulating your thoughts and wishes about treatment at the end of life. Includes forms and legal guidelines for living wills in every state. 1991. Bantam Books.

Organizations

Choice in Dying. Counseling, advice, and up-to-date information on your state's legal requirements for advance directives. Choice in Dying, 200 Varick Street, 10th Floor, New York, NY 10014, (800) 989-WILL (9455).

AARP Pharmacy Service, (800) 456-2277.

Accent on Living, P.O. Box 700, Bloomington, IL 61702, (800) 787-8444.

Accessolutions, Harc Mercantile, P.O. Box 3055, Kalamazoo, MI 49003, (800) 445-9968.

Active Living, 7 Green Tree Drive, South Burlington, VT 05403, (800) 522-3393.

AdaptAbility, P.O. Box 515, Colchester, CT 06415, (800) 243-9232.

Adaptations, 1758 Empire Central, Dallas, TX 75235, (800) 688-1758.

AfterTherapy, NCM Consumer Products Division, P.O. Box 6070, San Jose, CA 95150, (800) 235-7054.

American Printing House for the Blind, 1839 Frankfort Avenue, P.O. Box 6085, Louisville, KY 40206, (800) 223-1839.

Ann Morris Enterprises, 890 Fams Court, East Meadow, NY 11554, (516) 292-9232.

Atlanta Thread and Supply Company, 695 Red Oak Road, Stockbridge, GA 30281, (800) 847-1001.

Avenues, 1199 Avenida Acaso, Camarillo, CA 93012, (800) 848-2837.

B.A. Mason, 1251 First Avenue, Chippewa Falls, WI 54729, (800) 422-1000.

Back to Basics Soft-Wear, 1107 West Main Street, Suite 201, Durham, NC 27701, (919) 477-5669.

Beautiful Times, 4700 Westside Avenue, North Bergen, NJ 07047, (800) 223-1216.

Blair Mail Order Clothing, 220 Hickory Street, Warren, PA 16366, (800) 458-6057.

Bossert Specialties, P.O. Box 15441, Phoenix, AZ 85060, (800) 776-5885.

Brookstone Hard-To-Find Tools, 1655 Bassford Drive, Mexico, MO 65265, (800) 926-7000.

Bruce Medical Supply, 411 Waverly Oaks Road, P.O. Box 9166, Waltham, MA 02254, (800) 225-8446.

Buckeye Beans & Herbs, Inc., P.O. Box 28220, Spokane, WA 99228, (800) 449-2121.

Cabot Creamery, P.O. Box 128, Cabot, VT 05647, (802) 563-2650.

Campmor, P.O. Box 700-B, Saddle River, NJ 07458, (800) CAMPMOR (226-7667).

Carol Wright Gifts, 340 Applecreek Road, P.O. Box 8503, Lincoln, NE 68544, (402) 474-4465.

Chef's Catalog, 3215 Commercial Avenue, Northbook, IL 60062, (800) 338-3232.

Cleo of New York, Trent Building, South Buckhout Street, Irvington, NY 10533, (800) 321-0595.

Collage Video Specialties, 5390 Main Street, NE, Minneapolis, MN 55421, (800) 433-6769.

Comfort House, 189-203 Frelinghuysen Avenue, Newark, NJ 07114, (800) 359-7701.

Community Kitchens, 2 North Maple Avenue, Ridgely, MD 21660, (800) 535-9901.

A Cook's Wares, 211 37th Street, Beaver Falls, PA 15010, (412) 846-9490.

Critics' Choice Video, P.O. Box 749, Itasca, IL 60143, (800) 367-7765.

Delty Sugar Free Chocolate, 412 North Coast Highway, No. 356, Laguna Beach, CA 92651, (800) 962-3355.

Dr. Leonard's Health Care Products, 42 Mayfield Avenue, Edison, NJ 08837, (800) 785-0880.

Easier Ways, 1101 North Calvert Street, Suite 405, Baltimore, MD 21202, (410) 659-0232.

Easy Street, 8 Equality Park West, Newport, RI 02840, (800) 959-EASY (3279).

Enrichments, 145 Tower Drive, P.O. Box 579, Hinsdale, IL 60521, (800) 323-5547.

Equipment Shop, P.O. Box 33, Bedford, MA 01730, (617) 275-7681.

Fashion Ease, 1541 60th Street, Brooklyn, NY 11219, (800) 221-8929.

Fatwise, P.O. Box 25, Colonia, NJ 07067, (800) 773-8822.

Fitness Wholesale, 895-A Hampshire Road, Stow, OH 44224, (800) 537-5512.

Fuller Brush, 1 Fuller Way, Great Bend, KS 67530, (800) 522-0499.

Gaylord Inc., Box 4901, Syracuse, NY 13221, (800) 448-6160.

Great Valley Mills, 1774 County Line Road, Barto, PA 19504, (800) 688-6455.

Hale Indian River Groves, Indian River Plaza, P.O. Box 217, Wabasso, FL 32970.

Hanover House, P.O. Box 2, Hanover, PA 17333, (717) 633-3366.

Harriet Carter, North Wales, PA 19455, (215) 361-5151.

Harris Communications, 6541 City West Parkway, Eden Prairie, MN 55344, (800) 825-6758.

Harvest Direct, P.O. Box 4514, Decatur, IL 62525, (800) 835-2867.

Hear-More, P.O. Box 3413, Farmingdale, NY 11735, (800) 881-HEAR (4327).

HeartyMix, 1231 Madison Hill Road, Rahway, NJ 07065, (908) 382-3010.

Hear You Are, 4 Musconetcong Avenue, Stanhope, NJ 07874, (800) 278-EARS (3277).

Hello Direct, 5884 Eden Park Place, San Jose, CA 95138, (800) 444-3556.

Hitec Group International, 8160 Madison, Burr Ridge, IL 60521, (800) 288-8303.

Hold Everything, P.O. Box 7807, San Francisco, CA 94120, (800) 421-2264.

Home Delivery Incontinent Supplies Company, 1215 Dielman Industrial Court, Olivette, MO 63132, (800) 2MY-HOME (269-4663).

Home Health Products, 949 Seahawk Circle, Virginia Beach, VA 23452, (800) 284-9123.

Home Trends, 1450 Lyell Avenue, Rochester, NY 14606, (716) 254-6520.

Improvements, 4944 Commerce Parkway, Cleveland, OH 44128, (800) 642-2112.

Independent Living Aids, 27 East Mall, Plainview, NY 11803, (800) 537-2118.

JC Penney's Easy Dressing Fashions, P.O. Box 2021, Milwaukee, WI 53201, (800) 222-6161.

Just for You, P.O. Box 941621, Atlanta, GA 30341, (800) 541-7903.

Kimbo Educational, Box 477, Long Branch, NJ 07740, (800) 631-2187.

King Arthur Flour, P.O. Box 876, Norwich, VT 05055, (800) 827-6836.

Kingsmill Foods, Med Diet, Plymouth, MN 55447, (800) 633-3438.

Lighthouse Consumer Products, 36-20 Northern Boulevard, Long Island City, NY 11101, (800) 829-0500.

LS&S Group, P.O. Box 673, Northbrook, IL 60065, (800) 468-4789.

Magellan's, P.O. Box 5485, Santa Barbara, CA 93150, (800) 962-4943.

Mail Order Medical Supply, P.O. Box 922, Santa Clarita, CA 91380, (800) 232-7443.

Maxi-Aids, P.O. Box 3209, Farmingdale, NY 11735, (800) 522-6294.

Miles Kimball, 41 West 8th Avenue, Oshkosh, WI 54906, (414) 231-4886.

National Incontinent Supplies, Inc., Home Delivery Service, P.O. Box 1277, St. Charles, MO 63302, (800) 228-2718.

National Wholesale Company, 400 National Boulevard, Lexington, NC 27294, (704) 249-0211.

Northern, P.O. Box 1499, Burnsville, MN 55337, (800) 533-5545.

Pillows for Ease, Inc., 4225 Royal Palm Avenue, Miami, FL 33140, (800) 347-1486.

Potomac Technology, 1 Church Street, Suite 101, Rockville, MD 20850, (800) 433-2838.

Real Goods, 966 Mazzoni Street, Ukiah, CA 95482, (800) 762-7325.

Safety Zone, Hanover, PA 17333, (800) 999-3030.

Science Products Magnilog, Box 888, Southeastern, PA 19399, (800) 888-7400.

Sears Home HealthCare, 20 Presidential Drive, Roselle, IL 60172, (800) 326-1750.

Self Care, 5850 Shellmound Street, Emeryville, CA 94607, (800) 345-3371.

Sense-Sations, 919 Walnut Street, Philadelphia, PA 19107, (800) 876-5456.

Seventh Generation, 49 Hercules Drive, Colchester, VT 05446, (800) 456-1177.

Sharper Image, 650 Davis Street, San Francisco, CA 94111, (800) 344-4444.

Signals, WGBH Education Foundations, P.O. Box 64428, St. Paul, MN 55164, (800) 669-9696.

Signatures, 19465 Brennan Avenue, Perris, CA 92599, (909) 943-2021.

Smith & Nephew Rolyan, 1 Quality Drive, P.O. Box 578, Germantown, WI 53022, (800) 558-8633.

Solutions, P.O. Box 6878, Portland, OR 97228, (800) 342-9988.

Sonoma Cheese Factory, (800) 535-2855.

Sun Precautions, 2815 Wetmore Avenue, Everett, WA 98201, (800) 882-7860.

Support Plus, 99 West Street, Box 500, Medfield, MA 02052, (800) 229-2910.

TASH ADL, Unit 1, 91 Station Street, Ajax, Ontario, Canada L1S 3H2, (416) 686-4129.

TechnoLog, c/o Maxi-Aids, 42 Executive Boulevard, Farmingdale, NY 11735, (800) 522-6294.

Technology for Independence, 529 Main Street, Boston, MA 02129, (800) 331-8255.

TravelSmith, 3140 Kerner Boulevard, San Rafael, CA 94901, (800) 950-1600.

Vermont Country Store, P.O. Box 3000, Manchester Center, VT 05255, (802) 362-2400.

Very Special Clothing, Inc., P.O. Box 603, Maplewood, NJ 07040, (800) 283-3094.

Visual Aids, National Association for Visually Handicapped. Western United States: 3201 Balboa Street, San Francisco, CA 94121, (415) 221-3201. Eastern United States: 22 West 21st Street, 6th Floor, New York, NY 10010, (212) 889-3141.

Walnut Acres, Penns Creek, PA 17862, (800) 433-3998.

Wax Orchards, 22744 Wax Orchards Road, Vashon, WA 98070, (800) 634-6132.

Williams-Sonoma, P.O. Box 7456, San Francisco, CA 94120, (800) 541-2233.

Woodbury Products, Inc., 4410 Austin Boulevard, Department 250, Island Park, NY 11558, (800) 879-3427.

The Wooden Spoon, P.O. Box 931, Clinton, CT 06413, (800) 431-2207.

Xenejenex, 300 Brickstone Square, Andover, MA 01810, (800) 228-2495.

Zabar's, 2245 Broadway, New York, NY 10024, (212) 496-1234.

Index